Advances in Experimental Medicine and Biology

Volume 994

More information about this series at http://www.springer.com/series/5584

Mark Jesus M. Magbanua • John W. Park
Editors

Isolation and Molecular Characterization of Circulating Tumor Cells

Springer

Editors
Mark Jesus M. Magbanua
Division of Hematology & Oncology
University of California San Francisco
San Francisco, CA, USA

John W. Park
Division of Hematology & Oncology
University of California San Francisco
San Francisco, CA, USA

ISSN 0065-2598 ISSN 2214-8019 (electronic)
Advances in Experimental Medicine and Biology
ISBN 978-3-319-55946-9 ISBN 978-3-319-55947-6 (eBook)
DOI 10.1007/978-3-319-55947-6

Library of Congress Control Number: 2017939867

Printed on acid-free paper

This Springer imprint is published by Springer Nature
The registered company is Springer International Publishing AG
The registered company address is: Gewerbestrasse 11, 6330 Cham, Switzerland

In memory of Teresita Mendoza Magbanua and all the women and men we have lost to cancer.

Foreword

The advent of targeted tumor therapies in the clinic during the last 20 years coincided with increasing activities to develop companion diagnostics that allow stratification of patient populations for such therapies. The aim of these continuing efforts is to increase the likelihood of detecting early signs of efficacy during clinical drug development and, after approval, to target patient populations with the best efficacy and safety profiles.

The concept of liquid biopsy, i.e., methods for retrieving molecular and/or cellular information from blood draws, holds the potential to obtain information from primary or metastatic lesions that are inoperable or difficult to access by needle biopsy. It allows clinicians to longitudinally follow the course of cancer evolution in an individual patient through sequential blood analyses. This approach provides great opportunities to closely monitor the response of cancer patients to therapy, which, in turn, can facilitate treatment decisions that can lead to early changes in treatment.

Over the last decade, circulating tumor cells (CTCs) have received growing attention in the field of diagnostics, due to the regulatory approval of the Veridex (now Janssen Diagnostics) CellSearch® platform by the US Food and Drug Administration in 2004, as the first liquid biopsy-based in vitro diagnostic (IVD) product. With this technology, epithelial tumor cells are isolated using magnetic beads coated with EpCAM antibodies. Since then, an increasing amount of data has shown the prognostic value of CTCs in breast, colorectal, and prostate cancers. While the number of EpCAM-positive CTCs detected in a standard blood draw is clearly associated with poor survival, presumably due to their capacity to form distant metastases, it became evident that EpCAM-negative tumor cells also do exist within the bloodstream. The latter are, however, missed by the CellSearch® system, and their numbers are not reflected in the analysis. These EpCAM-negative cells are presumed to be the result of epithelial-mesenchymal transition (EMT), and their phenotype might be related to the dissemination of cells from the primary tumor and possibly resistance to therapy. However, the true nature of the EMT-status of CTCs and the clinical relevance of EpCAM-negative CTCs are still under investigation.

Next-generation technologies for CTC isolation, like filtration and microfluidic devices, have been designed to capture higher numbers of CTCs by using additional markers (e.g., EMT or stem cell-like markers) or by exploiting the biophysical differences (e.g., size and rigidity) between CTCs and normal blood cells. Increasing the yield of CTCs from a blood draw may, in the future, help expand the use of CTC technologies to indications like lung or pancreatic cancer, where CTC counts are low. In addition, CTCs detected in early disease stages or during minimal residual disease may become accessible to molecular analyses (e.g., detection of potentially resistance-conferring mutations). An important upside along these lines is the possibility of performing single-cell analyses, which can ultimately provide a better reflection of the tumor heterogeneity and enable the detection of rare disease-relevant mutations that are not found in tissue biopsies. Showing concordance of molecular features detected in CTCs with those derived from established conventional biopsies is also an important task. Needle tissue biopsy, which is currently the "gold standard," may be inadequate since it may not reflect the extent of tumor heterogeneity and, therefore, miss clinically relevant tumor subclones. Moreover, metastases at different sites in individual patients can also harbor distinct genomic characteristics.

Fundamental biological questions in the field such as the viability of CTCs in the bloodstream await further elucidation. To this end, the option to isolate viable CTCs from microfluidic devices offers new opportunities for research and may provide essential insights regarding the use of CTCs as pharmacodynamic biomarkers. Cultivation protocols and in vivo propagation in patient-derived xenograft models are already being explored for testing drugs with the goal of applying these technologies in the framework of personalized medicine. In addition, CTC-based pharmacodynamic markers could be of particular interest for immuno-oncology therapies. Here, novel markers for prediction of treatment response to new therapy standards, like PD-1-/PD-L1-targeted approaches, are needed. Single CTC analysis can potentially address this unmet need, as individual cells can be isolated based on relevant protein marker expression, tested in short-term in vitro assays, and emerging markers for immuno-oncology like expression of PD-L1, as well as mutational load and neo-antigen expression, can be analyzed. This may result in a more complete picture of activated pathways for tumor immune evasion and help stratify patients to the best treatment available.

The use of CTC enrichment, isolation, and analysis in the clinical setting critically depends on stability, reproducibility, and "plug-and-play" properties of the technologies. In order to avoid technical day-by-day variation and observer bias, a human component should be avoided or minimized. Obviously, automation is key to achieve this and to ensure sufficient throughput and fast data turnaround times. Optimization and evaluation of cell-based technologies to demonstrate that they are fit for purpose in the intended context of use are crucially dependent on standardization. Interdisciplinary multi-stakeholder consortia like the Innovative Medicines Initiative (IMI) CANCER-ID have been initiated to address these challenges and hoped to support further developments in the field (www.cancer-id.eu).

The authors of this volume highlight new developments in the analysis of CTCs. Their contributions range from the description of new markers for CTC subpopulations to the relevance of these subpopulations for disease progression. Issues of clinical implementation of CTC technologies and guidance of clinical decisions based on CTC expression of pharmacologically relevant targets are discussed. We hope that this book may stimulate further progress in research on CTC-based companion diagnostics, which can ultimately lead to improved cancer therapies.

Biomarker Research, Bayer AG, Leverkusen, Germany Thomas Schlange
Department of Tumor Biology Klaus Pantel
University Medical Center Hamburg-Eppendorf
Hamburg, Germany

Preface

Circulating tumor cells (CTCs) shed by the primary tumor into circulation provide unique opportunities for elucidating mechanisms involved in cancer progression, metastasis, and development of resistance to therapy. Numerous clinical studies, including meta-analyses, have now unequivocally demonstrated the strong association between the levels of CTCs in the blood of cancer patients and poor prognosis.

While the question regarding the clinical relevance of CTCs has been largely settled, the molecular nature and the biology of CTCs are just beginning to be unraveled. The slower progress in efforts towards molecular profiling of CTCs has been attributed mainly to the technical difficulties in isolating these rare cells from blood, as well as the complexities involved in molecular characterization of single or small numbers of cells.

In this book, key leaders in the field of CTC research present state-of-the-art approaches for the detection and isolation of CTCs, along with innovative strategies for molecular profiling of these cells. In addition, the book provides excellent discussions regarding the current understanding of the molecular biology of CTCs. This book will serve as an important source of information for bench scientists as well as clinical researchers who are interested in pursuing research to elucidate the biology of CTCs and their potential utility as biomarkers in the clinic.

University of California San Francisco
San Francisco, CA, USA

Mark Jesus M. Magbanua
John W. Park

Acknowledgments

The editors thank Tulasi Solanki and Feng Hsiao for their assistance in reviewing manuscripts and for preparing this book for publication. We also thank all the authors for their highly informative chapter contributions, without which this book project would have not been possible.

Contents

Chapter 1
Circulating Tumor Cells as Cancer Biomarkers in the Clinic

Ludmilla Thomé Domingos Chinen, Emne Ali Abdallah, Alexcia Camila Braun, Bianca de Cássia Troncarelli de Campos Parra Flores, Marcelo Corassa, Solange Moraes Sanches, and Marcello Ferretti Fanelli

Abstract It is believed that the development of metastatic cancer requires the presence of circulating tumor cells (CTCs), which are found in a patient's circulation as rare abnormal cells comingled with billions of the normal red and white blood cells. The systems developed for detection of CTCs have brought progress to cancer treatment. The molecular characterization of CTCs can aid in the development of new drugs, and their presence during treatment can help clinicians determine the prognosis of the patient. Studies have been carried out in patients early in the disease course, with only primary tumors, and the role of CTCs in prognosis seems to be as important as it is in patients with metastatic disease. The published studies on CTCs have focused on their prognostic significance, their utility in real-time monitoring of therapies, the identification of therapeutic and resistance targets, and understanding the process of metastasis. The analysis of CTCs during the early stages, as a "liquid biopsy," helps to monitor patients at different points in the disease course, including minimal residual disease, providing valuable information about the very early assessment of treatment effectiveness. Finally, CTCs can be used to screen patients with family histories of cancer or with diseases that can lead to the development of cancer. With standard protocols, this easily obtained and practical tool can be used to prevent the growth and spread of cancer. In this chapter, we review some important aspects of CTCs, surveying the disease aspects where these cells have been investigated.

Keywords Circulating tumor cells • Prognosis • Biomarker • Clinical utility

---

L.T.D. Chinen (✉) • E.A. Abdallah • A.C. Braun • B.d.C.T.d.C.P. Flores
International Research Center, A. C. Camargo Cancer Center, Rua Taguá 440, São Paulo, SP 01508-010, Brazil
e-mail: ltdchinen@gmail.com

M. Corassa • S.M. Sanches • M.F. Fanelli
Department of Medical Oncology, A. C. Camargo Cancer Center, Rua Professor Antônio Prudente, São Paulo, SP 01509-010, Brazil

M.J.M. Magbanua, J.W. Park (eds.), *Isolation and Molecular Characterization of Circulating Tumor Cells*, Advances in Experimental Medicine and Biology 994,
DOI 10.1007/978-3-319-55947-6_1

1.1 Circulating Tumor Cells (CTCs) as Prognostic Factors in the Metastatic Setting

It is believed that the dissemination of cancer requires the presence of CTCs, which are defined as isolated single or clusters of cancerous cells in the blood or lymphatic fluids co-mingled with billions of normal hematopoietic cells (Mego et al. 2010). The presence of CTCs in the peripheral blood was first reported by Thomas Ashworth (1869), an Australian doctor at Melbourne Hospital. He studied material obtained from the autopsy of a patient with metastatic subcutaneous tumors located in the anterior wall of the chest and abdomen. He noted circulating cells (obtained from the saphenous vein of the right leg) identical to those from tumors and postulated that these cells were derived from an existing tumor structure, they must have traversed a large part of the circulatory system to reach the inside of the saphenous vein the right leg.

The development of enrichment systems and immunohistochemical detection of CTCs represents significant progress for the scientific community. The best known is the CellSearch® System, which separates the cells with magnetic beads coated with anti-epithelial cell adhesion molecule (EpCAM) antibody followed by flow cytometry of cells captured with anti-cytokeratin fluorescence. Reading is done in semi-automated microscope (revised by Riethdorf and Pantel 2008). In 2007, the U.S. Food and Drug Administration (FDA) approved the system for monitoring patients with metastatic breast, prostate, and colorectal tumors (www.accessdata.fda.gov/cdrh_docs/reviews/K071729).

The overall majority of metastases are localized in internal organs, such as lung, bone, or liver. Because of this, conventional biopsies of metastatic lesions are invasive, painful and expensive. Accordingly, both the isolation and characterization of CTCs might serve as a real time "liquid biopsy" (Hayes and Paoletti 2013).

Using the CellSearch® System, Cristofanilli et al. (2004) reported a study of 177 patients with metastatic breast cancer, performing the CTC counts before and after the start of treatment for metastatic disease. Patients with ≥5 CTCs/7.5 ml of blood when compared to those with less <5 CTCs/7.5 ml, had lower progression-free survival (2.7 versus 7 months, $p < 0.001$) and reduced overall survival (10.1 versus 18 months, $p < 0.001$). After the first segment following the beginning of treatment, this difference between the groups persisted (in relation to the survival and the number of CTCs). Multivariate analysis of CTCs levels before and after the start of treatment proved the significance of these predictors of overall survival (OS) and progression-free survival (PFS). Furthermore, it was observed that about 70% of patients with metastatic disease had CTC counts above 1/7.5 ml of peripheral blood. This study provided key evidence for the use of CTCs and was used to clear CellSearch® by the FDA.

Using the same CTC detection system, Nolé et al. (2008) studied 80 patients with metastatic breast cancer and evaluated them at the beginning of treatment, at 4 and 8 weeks after the first clinical assessment, and then every 2 months thereafter. Before the start of the treatment, 49 patients had ≥5 CTCs. In multivariate analysis, the CTC levels before treatment were significantly associated with PFS (relative risk [RR] 2.5, 95% CI). Patients with persistent levels of CTCs ≥5 had increased risk of progression compared to those with CTCs <5 (RR 6.4, 95% CI). These studies indicate the likely utility of CTCs in assessing the responses of patients with metastatic breast tumors.

For colorectal cancers (CRC), the primary strategy for treatment is complete resection of the primary lesion (Katsumata et al. 2006). However, despite this, some patients experience recurrences that are believed to reflect residual micrometastases. Conventional diagnostic methods are not capable of detecting CTCs present in these sites that are eventually released into the circulation. Katsumata et al. (2006) used the reverse transcription polymerase chain reaction (RT-PCR) to detect CTCs, through the identification of cytokeratin genes and carcinoembryonic antigen (CEA). They analyzed 57 patients with CRC who underwent surgery. The presence of cytokeratin 20 (CK20) in peripheral blood was evaluated. The CK20 mRNA was found in 42.1% of patients and was correlated with lymph node metastasis ($p = 0.037$). The 5-year overall survival (5y–OS) for CK20 positive patients was 62.5% whereas for CK20 negative it was 87.5% ($p = 0.048$). Therefore, the authors advocate the idea of looking at CTCs as being one of the best predictors of disease recurrence. However, it is known that hematopoietic cells may express "not legitimate" antigens associated with tumor or epithelial cells, and pseudogenes can lead to PCR products identical to imprinted genes, which can lead to false positive results by RT-PCR (Gunn et al. 1996).

Sastre et al. (2008) observed a positive correlation between the number of CTCs and clinical stage in 97 patients with the following characteristics: non-metastatic CRC newly diagnosed or rectal cancer without neoadjuvant chemo-radiotherapy; metastatic CRC newly diagnosed; and CRC recurrence. They used a control group of 30 healthy patients. A cut-off of 2 CTCs/7.5 ml was chosen for this study. There was an observed relationship between CTCs and location of the primary tumor, increased levels of CEA, lactate dehydrogenase and degree of differentiation.

De Giorgi et al. (2010) evaluated the relation between the detection and prognostic significance of CTCs and sites of metastases detected by 2 [fluorine-18]-fluoro-2-deoxy-D-glucose-positron emission tomography/computed tomography (FDG-PET/CT) in patients with metastatic breast cancer. The study included 195 patients. Higher numbers of CTCs were observed in patients with bone metastases (detected by PET/CT) than in patients without these metastases (mean 65.7 versus 3.3; $p = 0.012$) as well as in patients with multiple metastases in relation to one or two bone lesions (mean 77.7 versus 2.6; $p < 0.001$). CTCs were OS predictors in 108 patients with multiple metastases, including bone ($p \leq 0.0001$) but not in 58 without bone metastasis ($p = 0.411$) and in 29 involving bone alone ($p = 0.3552$). In multivariate analysis, the CTCs, but not bone metastasis, remained as significant predictors of SG.

A meta-analysis of 36 CTC studies with 3094 CRC patients was published by Rahbari et al. (2010). The authors concluded that CTC detection in peripheral blood was an indicator of poor prognosis in patients with primary CRC (Rahbari et al. 2010).

Hofman et al. (2011) evaluated CTC detection, by CellSearch®, in lung cancer patients after surgical resection and correlated it with pathologic findings and clinical outcomes. They analyzed the blood of 208 patients with non-small cell lung cancer (NSCLC) with diverse histology before surgery and also blood of 39 healthy volunteers. Of these, 44% were in stage I, 25% in stage II, 28% in stage III, and 6% in stage IV. CTCs were detected in 37% of the NSCLC patients but there were no CTCs detected in the healthy individuals. There was no correlation between the presence of CTCs and the different stages, but equal counts or those above 50 CTCs were related to worse OS ($p = 0.002$) and PFS ($p = 0.001$) compared to counts less than 50 CTCs.

Krebs et al. (2011) studied 101 patients with NSCLC in stages III and IV without prior treatment, to determine the ability of CTCs to indicate the response to therapy to a standard cycle of chemotherapy. CTCs were evaluated by CellSearch® and their numbers were higher in patients with stage IV (n = 60) than in patients with stage IIIB (n = 27) and IIIA (n = 14), where no CTC was detected (n = 14). PFS was 6.8 vs. 2.4 months ($p < 0.001$) and OS was 8.1 vs. 4.3 months ($p < 0.001$) in patients with less than 5 CTCs compared with patients with 5 or more CTCs before chemotherapy. In multivariate analysis, the number of CTCs was the strongest predictor of OS (hazard ratio [HR] = 7.92; 95% CI: 2.85 to 22.01; $p < 0.001$) and the estimated HR increased with the second sample of CTC harvested after the first cycle of chemotherapy (HR = 15.65; 95% CI: 3.63 to 67.53; $p < 0.001$).

In concordance with this study, Punnoose et al. (2012) performed CTC collections before treatment of NSCLC and on days 14, 28 and 56 after the start of this study. The response ratings were evaluated by PET-CT on days 14, 28, and 56 after start of treatment. Patients who had partial or complete response by PET-CT showed greater reduction of CTCs from baseline ($p = 0.014$) as did patients with partial response in CT at day 56 ($p = 0.019$). Recently, Muinelo-Romay et al. (2014), used CellSearch® and found a statistically significant difference in PFS (8.5 versus 4.2 months; $p = 0.016$) before the second cycle of chemotherapy among patients who had CTCs drop to less than 2 CTCs/mL compared to those who maintained levels above that. Patients whose CTCs counts remained at or above the top after the first chemotherapy cycle showed greater radiographic progression rates compared to patients whose scores decreased after the first cycle.

Our group (Chinen et al. 2013) reported the case of a patient with NSCLC where two methods were used to detect CTCs: one method was antibody-based and similar to CellSearch®, while the other method was size based (ISET®, or the Isolation by Size of Tumor cells method, Rarecells, France). The levels of CTCs detected by ISET® had correlation with image exams and showed circulating tumor microemboli (CTM), which is known as a poor prognostic factor. In fact, the patient had disease progression just 1 month after the detection of CTM.

Some studies indicated that CTCs have the ability to form clusters of CTCs, named CTM, in the circulation. CTM were demonstrated in a variety of tumor types, providing pro-metastatic capabilities compared to solitary CTCs in circulation (Brandt et al. 1996; Hou et al. 2012). Hou et al. (2012) hypothesized that because CTM appear to lack apoptotic features, they may be more resistant to anoikis and hence have a survival advantage in circulation as compared to singular CTCs. Some authors believe that CTM, at least in some cases, result in clinically detectable metastases (Brandt et al. 1996; Hou et al. 2012; Caixeiro et al. 2014).

Recently, we observed the presence of CTM by ISET® in 43 patients with locally advanced head and neck squamous cell carcinoma (LAHNSCC), who had been treated with curative intention and evaluated as to their drug resistance and to their protein expression (excision repair cross-complementation 1 [ERCC1] and multidrug resistance protein 7 [MRP-7] related to cisplatin and taxane resistance, respectively) with PFS (De Oliveira et al. 2016). The median number of CTCs at baseline (before any treatment) was 2.0 CTCs/ml (0–8), and 27 of 43 patients had CTCs analyzed after treatment, with a median count of 3.0 CTCs/ml (0–12). Patients with CTC counts under the median had better PFS after treatment (11.66 versus 9.5 months; $p = 0.132$). The presence of CTM was strongly correlated with worse PFS after treatment; about 2 months after the beginning of treatment (first follow-up; $p = 0{,}012$), especially if ERCC1 (7.2 versus 17.9 months; $p < 0.001$) or MRP-7 staining (10.4 versus 17.4 months; p = 0.025) were positive in these CTM (Fig. 1.1). These results show that not only the presence of CTM but also their molecular features can help physicians to understand the biology of these diseases and their evolution, and to provide better treatment for their patients.

There a few studies about the role of CTCs in epithelial ovarian carcinoma (EOC), probably because the primary route of metastasis in this type of cancer is peritoneal spread in the abdominal cavity, with distant metastases occur in only about one-third of the patients (reviewed by Van Berckelaer et al. 2016). The few studies that exist, made with diverse methods, have shown the role of hematogenous spread in EOC and that CTC levels $\geq$2 CTC/7.5 mL (CellSearch®) or $\geq$1 tumor-associated transcript above threshold (Adnatest) is associated with poor PFS and OS (Poveda et al. 2011; Aktas et al. 2011; Kuhlmann et al. 2014). However, as for all solid tumors, the prognostic role of CTCs in EOC is dependent on the isolation and detection methods. Recently, we (Corassa et al. 2016, submitted) reported a case of a 19-year-old woman with advanced low-grade serous papillary adenocarcinoma that relapsed disease with no corresponding cancer antigen 125 (CA 125). CTCs were evaluated by ISET® method and compared with CA 125 levels and image exams. Although relapses were not correspondent to elevations of CA 125, they were related to CTC counts, which were proportional to disease relapse. After exposure to two different chemotherapy regimens, CA 125 could not detect uncontrolled disease, remaining low despite the ongoing symptoms and novel imaging findings. CTCs, on the other hand, if used in clinical practice, would be helpful in determining the quality of treatment decision-making, as their levels were related to clinical outcome. In a disease where the unique biomarkers have had controversial roles CTC monitoring seems promising (Fig. 1.2).

As for EOC, there are few studies with pancreatic cancer (PC), with a large variety of CTC platforms, limiting the balance among the studies. Kurihara et al. (2008) analyzed the CTC count in 26 patients with metastatic pancreatic cancer by CellSearch® System and correlated it with various clinical findings. They could not

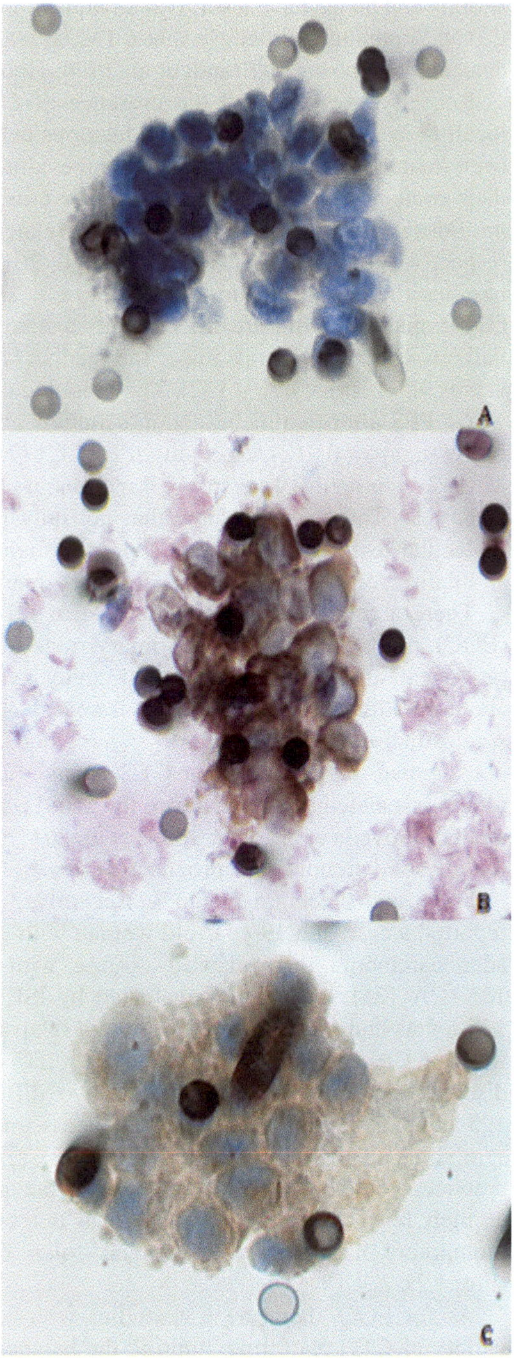

Fig. 1.1 Immunostaining of CTMs (**a**) CTM from rectum cancer patient visualized with haematoxilin-eosin (HE) (×40) (**b**) CTM from LAHNSCC stained for ERCC1, visualized with DAB (3,3′-diaminobenzidine) and counterstained with HE (×20) (**c**) CTM from LAHNSCC stained for MRP-7, visualized with DAB (diaminobenzidine) and counterstained with HE (×40). Photomicrograps were taken using a light microscope (Research System Microscope BX61—Olympus, Tokyo, Japan) coupled to a digital camera (SC100—Olympus, Tokyo, Japan)

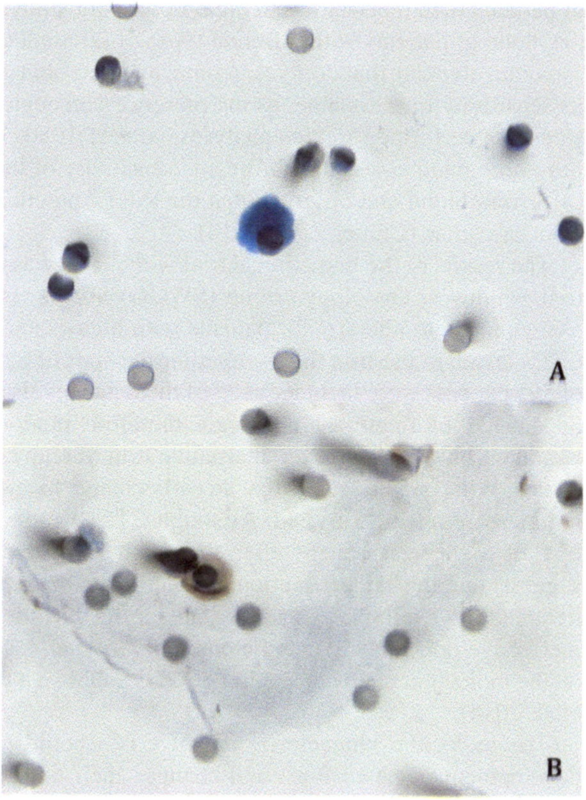

Fig. 1.2 (**a**) CTC from a patient with epithelial ovarian cancer. CTC was visualized with haematoxilin-eosin (HE) (×40) (**b**) Leucocyte stained for CD45, visualized with DAB (3,3′-diaminobenzidine) and counterstained with HE (x40). Photomicrographs were taken using a light microscope (Research System Microscope BX61—Olympus, Tokyo, Japan) coupled to a digital camera (SC100—Olympus, Tokyo)

observe statistically significant differences in tumor size; blood invasion; or splenic vein, portal vein, superior mesenteric artery, or vascular invasion. However, patients with CTC ≧1/7.5 ml serum showed higher CA 19.9 levels compared to the negative CTC (15,496 ± 22,572 U/ml versus 1452 ± 3800 U/ml; $p < 0.05$), demonstrating positive correlation between the number of CTCs and serum CA 19.9. They also found a correlation between CTC levels and OS ($p < 0.001$). Bidard et al. (2013) found the same results with another cohort. A meta-analysis recently published by Han et al. (2014) showed that patients who had any CTC in their blood had a lower PFS ($p = 0.001$) and OS ($p < 0.001$) compared to patients who did not present these cells. The results held for PFS, whether dividing the sample by the detection method of CTC by CellSearch® ($p < .001$) or by RT-PCR ($p = 0.032$). According to the author, these results indicate that the prognosis of patients with PC is associated with the presence of CTCs. Despite these results, limitations such as the small number of studies and patients, different methods of detection, and various treatments can lead to controversial results.

Although CTCs have been exhaustively explored in solid tumors, these cells can be recognized in the blood of patients with mesenchymal tumors. Our group was successful in demonstrating the possibility of ISET® in isolating CTCs from blood of patients with metastatic sarcoma. Before our study, others had detected CTCs in the blood of patients with different types of sarcoma (rhabdomyosarcoma, Ewing's sarcoma, alveolar rhabdomyosarcoma, and neuroblastoma) by RT-PCR, which has its sensitivity questionable, as the presence leucocytes can mask the result. In our study, we performed spiking analyses with HT 1080 cell line derived from a human fibrosarcoma to assess the ability and sensitivity of the ISET® in isolating sarcoma cells from blood and observed that the ISET® practically does not lose tumor cells from sarcomas (Chinen et al. 2014).

The results of the first clinical trial with CTCs was reported in 2013. The clinical trial Southwest Oncology Group (SWOG) S0500 assessed the benefit of an early change in chemotherapy for patients with breast cancer with persistent increase of CTCs levels in the first follow-up after the start of first-line chemotherapy. A total of 595 patients were included: 123 of them had levels of CTCs persistently elevated on day 21 of treatment and were therefore randomized to continue the same treatment or switched to an alternative drug therapy, by their treating physician's choice. What can be seen is that an early change to an alternative chemotherapy did not increase overall survival. Although CTCs were a potent prognostic factor, the lack of a survival benefit after switching from treatment based on high scores suggests that the early detection of relapse can be important when a more effective treatment is available. Changing an ineffective therapy to another that also is ineffective does not change the outcome. Instead, a change of the treatment based on the molecular characterization of CTC could be a promising approach (Smerage et al. 2014).

The molecular characterization of CTCs could potentially play a role in the development of new drugs, and changes their counts during treatment may help oncologists to evaluate the patient's status. The COU-AA-301 (A Phase 3, Randomized, Double-Blind, Placebo-Controlled Study of Abiraterone Acetate (CB7630) Plus Prednisone in Patients with Metastatic Castration-Resistant Prostate Cancer Who Have Failed Docetaxel-Based Chemotherapy) study was the first phase III trial aimed to evaluate CTC counts as an outcome measure for new therapies for castration-resistant, metastatic prostate cancer in patients previously treated with docetaxel. This study demonstrated that abiraterone inhibition of the cytochrome P450 17 (CYP17) enzyme required for androgen synthesis significantly prolonged the OS of the patients. The conversion of CTC from unfavorable to favorable (using the cut-off $\geq$5 CTCs/7.5 mL) demonstrated a significant effect on OS, suggesting a key role of access to serially CTCs as a predictor of survival (Scher et al. 2015).

Bidard et al. (2014) published the first pooled analysis on clinical validity of CTC in 1944 patients with metastatic breast cancer diagnosed between 2003 and 2012 in 17 centers in Europe. This was the largest pooled analysis of the clinical utility of CTC count by CellSearch® system. As Cristofanilli et al. (2004), these authors showed that more than 5 CTCs/7.5 ml at baseline were associated with shorter PFS and OS. They also showed that the analysis of patients was improved by adding CTC counts at baseline to the clinicopathologic features, whereas CEA and cancer antigen 15–3 (CA15–3) levels at this point and during therapy did not add significant benefit.

Although he acknowledged methodology limitations, Cristofanilli (2014) states that a critical review of the data suggests that enumeration of CTCs provides a baseline therapeutic benefit ratio, independent of the treatment selected. Patients with indolent disease (≤ 5 CTCs) might derive benefit, such as better OS, from sequential standard treatments. Bidard et al. (2014) showed that longitudinal monitoring enabled early identification of patients with a refractory disease (no decrease <5 CTCs/7.5 mL or unchanged ≥ 5 CTCs/7.5 mL).

In prostate cancer, CTC levels have been measured in about 2000 patients. The collective data show that CTC measurements have potential to identify patients with primary resistance 4–8 weeks after treatment initiation, making it possible to monitor treatment efficacy, study drug target interactions, and identify mechanisms of resistance at an individual level (Mehra et al. 2015).

After conducting this review of the history of research on CTCs, we observed that the discovery of their existence mainly involved metastatic cancer. In recent years research addressing non-metastatic tumors suggests that CTCs may have promise for early diagnosis of primary lesions.

1.2 CTCs as Prognostic Factors in Advanced Stages of Disease

Studies have been done with non-metastatic cancer and the role of CTCs in prognosis also seems to be as important as it is in metastatic disease. In the study of Magni et al. (2014), 16 of 90 patients (19%) had CTCs ≥ 1 at the outset (t0) and a reduction in CTC number in cases of objective remissions. The proportion of patients with CTCs ≥ 1 decreased over time as the therapeutic course proceeded. Increasing CTC detection rate by enhancing the available laboratory tests and achieving better patient characterization would be productive (Magni et al. 2014).

Nesteruk et al. (2014) analyzed the CTC prevalence in 162 patients with rectal cancer after preoperative short-term radiotherapy. CTCs were evaluated by RT-PCR, based on expression of CEA, CK20, and/or cancer stem cells marker CD133 (CEA/CK20/CD133). CTC detection 7 days after surgery was a prognostic factor for local recurrence ($p = 0.006$). However, CTC detected preoperatively and after 24 hours of resection was not. There was a significant relationship between the presence of lymph node metastasis (positive node 1–2 [pN1–2]) and CTC prevalence after 24 hours of the surgery. These results indicate that in these patients with advanced rectal disease, preoperative sampling was not significant for prognosis.

In the study of Murray et al. (2015), primary CTC counts are said to have a role in colorectal cancer screening. But analyzing primary CTCs - detected before surgical removal – did not predict clinicopathologic features of the primary tumor. However, the same group described the secondary CTC levels as associated with these features after surgical removal, and suggested that this secondary count may be important in identifying patients at high risk of relapse.

Hinz et al. (2015) analyzed the response after chemoradiation (RCTX) in patients with rectal cancer with locally advanced disease and found that responders had a lower incidence of CTCs compared to non-responders, which might be a reflection of effective systemic and local treatment prior to surgery. They also found no correlation between CTCs and tumor stage, which is in agreement with Tsai et al. (2016).

Using immunofluorescence and immunohistochemistry techniques, Hong et al. (2016) isolated and identified CTCs in 100% of (29) patients with early (non-metastatic) breast cancer, indicating that this procedure allowed detection of these cells with greater accuracy, sensitivity, and specificity. In addition, they demonstrated *in situ* "naked eye" identification of the captured cancer cells via a simple colorimetric immunoassay.

The use of CTC in non-metastatic colorectal cancer requires very sensitive and specific detection methods. An international consensus on the assessment of detection method and markers needs to be finalized before incorporating CTC detection into risk stratification in the clinical setting (Thorsteinsson and Jess 2011).

1.3 CTCs as a Predictor of Drug Resistance

It is well described that cancer is a heterogeneous disease composed of various differing cell clones in different patients, with each clone having different characteristics, including metabolism, mutations, gene regulation, gene expression, and protein translation as well as signaling pathway alterations (Fearon and Vogelstein 1990; Gerlinger et al. 2012). These different characteristics reflect the natural history of the disease, resulting in different tumor behavior, and therefore, tumor prognosis, depending on how the neoplastic cells respond to treatment. This theory can explain why patients with the same tumor localization, histopathological classification, and stage have different outcomes and treatment responses (Marusyk and Polyak 2010).

Advanced and metastatic solid tumors are commonly treated with chemotherapy, one of the most aggressive types of treatment. Because its lack of specificity ensures that it will affect many different kinds of cancer cells. Although chemotherapy has high potential activity against tumor cells, the toxicity of these drugs on normal growing cells is a significant problem (Phillips et al. 2001; Roden and George 2002). Even with targeted therapies, resistance mechanisms as well as toxic side effects occur frequently (Holohan et al. 2013). The pharmacokinetics and tolerability of the chemotherapy agents can also differ in cancer patients, and many patient characteristics have to be taken into account before a specific chemotherapy treatment is selected.

Resistance to chemotherapy is a very common issue in cancer (Haber et al. 2011). It can be an early or late event, which is attributed to intrinsic and acquired resistance, respectively (Holohan et al. 2013). When chemotherapy agents affect their target cancer cells, the sensitive cells undergo cell cycle arrest and as consequence the tumors eventually show shrinkage. But resistant clones in the tumor can persist and grow again, increasing the tumor mass, with cancer cells with characteristics completely different from the previous ones. The process of mutation and deregulation in gene expression is continuous. Chemotherapy can also lead to such modulations, making it difficult for clinicians to choose the best sequence of treatment to control tumor growth (Holohan et al. 2013; Kuczynski et al. 2013).

There are some genes and proteins that have been described as factors that contribute to resistance or to the responses to chemotherapy treatment, by transporting drugs inside or outside of cells, repairing DNA damage, and/or evading cell death (Holohan et al. 2013).

Acquired chemo-resistance is one of the recurrent issues in almost all tumors after the exposition to chemotherapy. Many types of cancer cells have plasma membrane proteins that transport chemicals and toxins out of the cytoplasm. These proteins are mainly from the multi-drug resistance (MDR) family and have been widely studied (Flens et al. 1996; Cui et al. 1999; Doyle and Ross 2003). Their functions are ATP dependent, and they act as efflux pumps, with different membrane proteins functioning to transport specific classes of drugs.

CTCs shed by the both primary and metastatic cancers during tumor formation and progression are now considered to be a real-time "liquid biopsy" reflecting the disease complexity (Salvianti et al. 2016). Thus far, studies on CTCs have been focused on their prognostic significance, their utility for real-time monitoring of therapies, the identification of therapeutic and resistance targets, and understanding the process of metastasis (Salvianti et al. 2016).

CTCs can be considered pharmacological markers, and their analysis may allow researchers to (a) provide proof of the mechanisms of action of a drug; (b) select optimal doses and scheduling of antineoplastic drug administration; (c) gain an understanding of both the therapeutic and resistance mechanisms of anti-cancer drugs; (d) design rational combination therapies; and (e) predict treatment outcomes, as postulated for pharmacodynamic biomarkers by Sarker and Workman (2007) (reviewed by Devriese et al. 2011). Recently, it has been postulated that molecular characterization of CTCs is key for increasing the diagnostic specificity of CTC assays and investigate therapeutic targets and their downstream pathways (Gasch et al. 2013).

CTCs have been demonstrated to be efficient markers for providing tumor information, presenting predictive markers, optimizing choices of therapeutic strategies, and thus opening new perspectives to achieve personalized medicine (Gazzaniga et al. 2010; Gradilone et al. 2011a, b; Abdallah et al. 2015, 2016). Some MDR-related markers were successfully derived from CTCs, correlating with drug resistance (MRP1, MRP2, MRP4, MRP5, and MRP7). Gazzaniga and colleagues (2010) performed a drug-resistance profile of CTCs from 105 patients with epithelial tumors (bladder, colorectal, breast, gastric, urothelial, ovarian, esophageal, head and neck cancers, and NSCLC), who received adjuvant or palliative chemotherapy by analyzing messenger RNA expression. They analyzed mRNA from CTCs looking for drug transporters (MRP1, MRP2, MRP4, MRP5, MRP7, human equilibrative nucleoside transporter [hENT] and deoxycytidine kinase [dCK]) as markers of resistance. They found presence of CTCs by the CELLection™ Dynabead® method in 51% of samples and the drug resistance profiles were correlated with DFS ($p = 0.001$) and time to progression (TTP; $p = 0.001$) (for adjuvant and metastatic settings, respectively), and predicted the treatment resistance in 98% of the cases. The same group (Gradilone et al. 2011a), using the same principle, was able to evaluate MRP1 and MRP2 messenger RNA expression in CTCs from metastatic breast cancer (mBC) patients treated with conventional anthracyclines or nonpegylated liposomal doxorubicin. They observed that patients treated with conventional anthracyclines showing CTCs expressing MRP1 and MRP2 had a significant shorter progression-free survival (PFS; $p < 0.005$).

In our study (Abdallah et al. 2016), the same results were observed working with MRP1 in metastatic colorectal cancer (mCRC). MRP1 expression was linked to short PFS in mCRC patients when it was found expressed in CTCs in relation to negative ones ($p = 0.003$). This relation of MRP-1 to poor PFS was not observed in primary or metastatic tissues.

Another interesting result from Gradilone et al. (2011b) involved MRPs, human epidermal growth factor receptor 2 (HER-2/neu), estrogen receptor α (ERα), and aldehyde dehydrogenase 1 (ALDH1) expression in CTCs from mBC patients. Patients who had CTCs expressing two or more MRPs had shorter PFS. Moreover, the expression of ALDH1 (a stemness marker) was statistically correlated with the number of MRPs. This suggests potential retention of stem cell properties within the MRPs-expressing CTCs group, therefore resisting chemotherapeutic treatment, and becoming more invasive and with high migratory capabilities.

The expression of stemness and epithelial-mesenchymal transition (EMT)-related genes detected in CTCs seem to have a crucial role in chemo-resistance in several tumors, such as castration-resistant prostatic cancers compared to castration-sensitive ones (Chen et al. 2013), and breast cancer (Mego et al. 2012; Nadal et al. 2013). These two cellular conditions are correlated. Studies have shown that stem cell properties can be acquired during the EMT process (Mani et al. 2008; Morel et al. 2008).

Continuing with well-known markers of drug resistance, our group (Abdallah et al. 2015) compared the expression of thymidylate synthase (TYMS), an enzyme involved in the process of metabolism of 5-fluorouracil (5-FU) in primary tumors (mCRC), CTCs, and metastatic tissue. TYMS is constitutively expressed in leucocytes and is found with augmented expression in some tumors, and confers resistance to the effects of 5-FU (Popat et al. 2004). Surprisingly, the expression of TYMS in CTCs (analyzed by immunocytochemistry) but not in primary tumors or in metastatic tissue, was associated with rapid disease progression. We observed that the expression of TYMS was statistically associated with high CTC's levels in the blood of mCRC patients.

Studies performing analysis of molecular profiles and molecular markers like CEA, epidermal growth factor receptor (EGFR), Kirsten rat sarcoma viral oncogene homolog (KRAS), v-rapidly accelerated fibrosarcoma (RAF) murine sarcoma viral oncogene homolog B (BRAF), vascular endothelial growth factor (VEGF), adenomatous polyposis coli (APC), and tumor protein p53 (TP-53) in the CTCs have raised hope that personalized treatments can be more effective and less aggressive (Fina et al. 2015; Buim et al. 2015; Sawada et al. 2016; Bredemeier et al. 2016; Huang et al. 2016).

Increasing attention has been given in recent years to CTCs from castration-resistant prostate cancer (CRPC) patients. CTC counts were reported to predict poor overall survival (OS) in patients with progressive CRPC starting a new line of therapy (de Bono et al. 2008). Both CTC count and CTC characterization were reported in patients with androgen-receptor splice variant 7 messenger RNA (AR-V7) in CTCs, mainly because it was correlated with resistance to enzalutamide or abiraterone. Mutations in androgen receptor genes were reported in CTCs (Jiang et al. 2010). Antonarakis and colleagues (2014) were able to detect AR-V7 positivity in CTCs from metastatic CRPC patients and to significantly associate these results with low prostate-specific antigen (PSA) response rates, PSA PFS, clinical or radiographic PFS, and OS in both arms, whose received enzalutamide and abiraterone.

ERCC1 is a protein involved in nucleotide excision repair pathway, mainly repairing helix-distorting DNA damage induced by ultraviolet light or electrophilic compounds, such as cisplatin (Houtsmuller et al. 1999). ERCC1 was already evaluated in CTCs from breast (Somlo et al. 2011), NSCLC (Das et al. 2012) and ovarian cancer (Kuhlmann et al. 2014). Somlo and colleagues (2011) found weak correlation of expression of ERCC1 among CTCs, primary tumors and metastases. Das et al. (2012) correlated lack of ERCC1 expression in CTCs with better PFS ($p < 0.02$, HR: 4.2). Ovarian cancer patients whose CTCs had ERCC1 expression had worse PFS and OS ($p = 0.02$ and $p = 0.009$, respectively) (Kuhlmann et al. 2014).

Hoshimoto and colleagues (2012a) performed CTC (blood) analysis by multimarker RT-quantitative PCR assay (melanoma-specific proteins: melanoma antigen recognized by T cells 1 [MART-1], melanoma-associated antigen 3 [MAGE-A3], and GalNac-T) in 331 patients with melanoma with sentinel lymph node (SLN) metastases after complete metastasis resection. They found that patients with two or more positive biomarkers had worse distant metastasis DFS (HR = 2.13, $p = 0.009$) and reduced recurrence-free survival (HR = 1.70, $p = 0.046$) and melanoma-specific survival (HR = 1.88, $p = 0.043$) by multivariable analysis, suggesting they are good biomarkers to stratify patients with respect to additional aggressive adjuvant therapy.

Regarding prognosis, CTC measurements have demonstrated to be useful in paired analysis to primary tumors. Ilie and colleagues (2012) were able to detect in CTCs isolated from 87 lung cancer patients by ISET® technology, anaplastic lymphoma kinase (ALK)-rearrangement by fluorescence in situ hybridization (FISH), and immunocytochemistry, demonstrating consistent results when compared with matched primary tumors. Similarly, Pailler and colleagues (2013) found 18 of 18 NSCLC ALK-positive patients also positive in CTCs. However, among the

14 NSCLC ALK-negative patients, they found 10 patients with at least 1 - ALK-positive CTC. This is an important result, because lung biopsies are difficult and obtaining enough cellular content to provide for a definitive tissue diagnosis coveys significant risk.

BRAF mutations (V600E) in circulating melanoma cells (CMCs) can be identified by immunocytochemistry using anti-VE1 antibodies. This can reach a high specificity and sensitivity compared with mutation status for corresponding primary tumors (by pyrosequencing and immunohistochemistry), making it possible to monitor patients focusing on a targeted therapy (Hofman et al. 2013). We (Buim et al. 2015) also observed an interesting level of correlation between the primary tumor and CTCs from mCRC patients in relation to levels of KRAS mutations (71%), similar to results found in other studies (Mostert et al. 2013; Fabbri et al. 2013; Gasch et al. 2013; Raimondi et al. 2014). Kalikaki et al. (2014) evaluated CTCs from 31 mCRC patients (14 primary tumors with mutant KRAS and 17 primary tumors wild-type KRAS). CTCs were isolated, counted, and captured for further DNA analysis for KRAS status evaluation. The blood collections ranged from one to four, and CTC ranged from 0 to 865/7.5 mL of blood. It was observed that: (a) some patients had the same variations of mutations between CTC and tumor: (b) some patients with mutations in the primary tumor lost the mutation in CTCs over the course of treatment as well as returning to the prior mutation status, and (c) patients with wild-type tumors and mutations in CTC. They were able to find similar tumor mutation variants in only 3 CTCs from patients and by contrast, they did not find mutations in 865 CTCs from patients with mutations in the primary tumor. This shows the importance of follow-up of such patients by CTC analysis as well as for genotypic changes, in order to change treatments as needed in a timely fashion.

HER-2 overexpression and amplification in breast cancer is an important prognostic and predictive marker. It predicts a good response to HER-2 inhibitors (trastuzumab and lapatinib) in both adjuvant and metastatic lesions (Paik et al. 2008). HER-2 was observed in CTCs from breast cancer patients by laser microdissection (Pinzani et al. 2006). They could compare the DNA of matched CTCs and primary tumors from 7 CTC+ cases and found a good correlation of HER-2 amplification in these two sites ($R = 0.918$; $p < 0.01$). This result could represent an advance in the follow-up of these patients in order to evaluate the status of HER-2 by CTC counts, reflecting the primary tumor as well as the response to trastuzumab over time. Interestingly, Gasch and colleagues (2016) demonstrated the feasibility in detecting CTCs with strong HER-2 positivity from mBC HER-2-negative patients. Furthermore, they found mutations in phosphatidylinositol 4,5-bisphosphate 3-kinase catalytic subunit alpha (PIK3CA) in 12 of 33 patients by micromanipulation, whole genome amplification, and Sanger sequencing of their CTCs. These results move us toward use of personalized mBC treatment, giving a better understanding of some mechanisms to HER-2 blockade resistance by single cell analysis.

Recently, much effort has been expended to assess proteins with potential predictive and therapeutic interest in CTCs. Some examples follow: B-cell lymphoma 2 (Bcl-2) (Smerage et al. 2013): Kiel-67 (Ki-67) (Paoletti et al. 2015): γ-H2A histone family, member X (γ-H2AX) (Garcia-Villa et al. 2012): programmed death-ligand 1 (PDL1) (Mazel et al. 2015; Satelli et al. 2016): and folate receptors, mainly in NSCLC (Yu et al. 2013; Lou et al. 2013; Chen et al. 2015).

Finally, CTCs can be also expanded and cultivated *in vitro*, allowing molecular characterization, and may even provide drug sensitivity data, to select patients who will benefit from specific drug combinations (Yu et al. 2014; Cayrefourcq et al. 2015).

In this brief summary, we have addressed role and feasibility of CTCs as a mirror of tumor signatures and identified them as a potentially valuable tool to monitor the response to treatment. Further study should yield increased benefits over time. The contents of Table 1.1 show an overview of studies with drug resistance gene detection in CTCs and their relation with clinical outcome. Beyond the quantification of CTCs, their molecular analysis can provide clinicians insights into the pattern of a patient's disease and provide tools for better management and treatment.

With the advance of techniques for detection and purification of CTCs, it should be possible to develop better individualized patient care, at different time-points, thus continually re-evaluating a cancer throughout the course of treatment. Furthermore, studies with larger numbers of patients should be performed in order to evaluate the accuracy and the substantial clinical gains that molecular analysis of CTCs can provide for clinical cancer therapy.

1.4 CTCs as Prognostic Factors in Early Stages of Cancer

It has been demonstrated in several clinical studies that the presence of malignant cells in the blood is associated with a poor prognosis, even in the context of early-stage disease. Lucci et al. (2012) carried out a prospective study involving 302 women with early-stage breast cancer. They observed, using the CellSearch® system to isolate CTCs, that 73 of 302 (24%) patients had ≥1 CTCs/7.5 mL of blood before surgery. These patients had poor PFS (log-rank $p = 0.005$; HR = 4.62, 95% CI 1.79–11.9) and OS (log-rank $p = 0.01$; HR = 4.04, CI 1.28–12.8). Although this study showed the prognostic value of initial CTCs in malignant disease, the CTCs were not monitored during the follow-up period nor was minimal residual disease analyzed. Prospective studies with standard procedures to detect CTCs, with well-established inclusion criteria, are currently needed (Hayes and Paoletti 2013).

CTC detection in non-metastatic breast cancer is more difficult because the cells occur at a lower frequency. Pierga et al. (2008) found CTC ≥1/7.5 ml in 23% of 97 patients before administering neoadjuvant chemotherapy and in 17% of 86 patients after neoadjuvant chemotherapy. The detection of CTC ≥1/7.5 ml prior to neoadjuvant chemotherapy, after neoadjuvant chemotherapy, or at both

Table 1.1 Overview of drug resistance gene detection in CTCs and their relation with clinical outcome

Authors	Year	Tumor	Stage	Method	Markers	No. patients	Main results
Pinzani et al.	2006	Breast cancer	I, II, and III	ISET®/ICC/LM/Quantitative real-time RT-PCR	HER2/neu amplification	44	There was found a good correspondence ($R = 0.918$; $P < 0.01$) between microdissected CTCs and primary tumor, for HER2 amplification.
Maheswaran et al.	2008	NSCLC	IV	CTC-chip/Scorpion Amplification Refractory Mutation	EGFR: deletions within exon 19, insertions within exon 20, and mutations	27	EGFR activating mutations in CTCs were found in 11/12 patients (92%) and in matched free plasma DNA from 4 of 12 patients (33%) ($P = 0.009$).
Gazzaniga et al.	2010	Bladder, colorectal, breast, NSCLC, gastric, urothelial, ovarian, esophageal, and head and neck cancers.	I, II, III and IV	CELLsection™Dynabeads coated with EpCAM/RT-PCR	MRP1, MRP2, MRP4, MRP5, MRP7, dCK, and hENT1	105	CTCs were found in 51% of the samples. Drug resistance profile was correlated with DFS ($P = 0.001$) and TTP ($P = 0.001$),for adjuvant and metastatic settings, respectively, and predicted the treatment resistance in 98% of the cases.
Gradilone et al.	2010	Breast cancer	IV	CELLection™Dynabeads coated with EpCAM/PCR	MRPs, ALDH1, Erα, and HER2/neu expression	42	PFS was shorter in patients with a 'drug resistance' CTCs profile and in patients whose

							CTCs expressed two or more MRPs.
Jiang et al.	2010	Prostate cancer	IV	Cellsearch® system/RNA extraction from CTCs/ Amplification of AR gene/ SURVEYOR Digestion and dsDNA Sizing/Fractionation and Sequencing	AR mutations	40	RNA from CTCs could be amplified in 35/40 samples and mutations were found in 20/35 samples.
Riethdorf et al.	2010b	Breast cancer	I, II, and III	CellSearch® system	HER2/neu amplification	213	HER2-overexpressing CTC were observed in 14/58 CTC-positive patients (24.1%), including 8 patients with HER2-negative primary tumors and 3 patients after trastuzumab treatment. CTC scored HER2-negative or weakly HER2-positive before or after NT were present in 11/21 patients with HER2-positive primary tumors. HER2 overexpression on CTC was restricted to ductal carcinomas and associated with high tumor stage (P = 0.002).
Somlo et al.	2011	Breast cancer	II, III and IV	WBC magnetic depletion/ Immunofluorescence	HER2, ER, and ERCC1	36	There was fund poor correlation between scores of ERCC1 expression on CTCs and

(continued)

Table 1.1 (continued)

Authors	Year	Tumor	Stage	Method	Markers	No. patients	Main results
							the primary tumor ($r = -0.16$). There was also poor correlation ($r = 0.15$) of ERCC1 between the primary and biopsied metastatic sites ($N = 8$).
Das et al.	2012	NSCLC	IV	WBC magnetic depletion/ Immunofluorescence	ERCC1	17	Lack of ERCC1 expression in CTCs was correlated with better PFS (HR: 4.2; $P < 0.02$).
Hoshimoto et al.	2012a	Melanoma With Sentinel Lymph Node Metastasis	III	Multimarker reverse-transcriptase quantitative polymerase chain reaction (RT-qPCR)	MART-1, MAGE-A3, and GalNAc-T expression	331	Two or more positive biomarkers was significantly associated with worse distant metastasis DFS (HR: 2.13, $P = 0.009$) and reduced RFS (HR: 1.7, $P = 0.046$) and melanoma-specific survival (HR: 1.88, $P = 0.043$).
Ilie et al.	2012	Lung cancer	I, II, III and IV	ISET®/FISH/ Immunoreactivity.	ALK-rearrangement	87	5 patients showed ALK-gene rearrangement and strong ALK protein expression in CTCs and in the corresponding

							tumour samples. Both ALK-FISH and ALK immunoreactivity analyses showed negative results in CTCs and corresponding tumour samples.
Mego et al.	2012	Breast cancer	I, II, and III	AdnaTest™ Breast Cancer Select/Detect test/Depletion of CD45+ leukocytes/ Quantitative RT-PCR assay	TWIST, SNAIL1, SLUG, ZEB1, FOXC2 and EpCAM	52	15.4% of patients overexpressed at least one of the EMT-inducing TF transcripts. Patients who received NT had overexpression of any EMT-inducing TF transcripts when compared to patients who did not receive ($P = 0.003$).
Miyamoto et al.	2012	Prostate cancer	IV	CTC-chip/ Immunofluorescence	AR signaling	25	Presence of "AR-on" CTC signatures was frequently found in untreated patients, compared to heterogeneous ("ARon, AR-off, and AR-mixed") CTC populations in patients with CRPC. Presence of "AR-mixed" CTCs and increasing "AR-on" cells were associated with an adverse treatment outcome.

(continued)

Table 1.1 (continued)

Authors	Year	Tumor	Stage	Method	Markers	No. patients	Main results
Chen et al.	2013	Prostate cancer	IV	ScreenCell®CC filtration kit/CellsDirect™ one-step qRT-PCR	84 EMT-related and reference genes	8	Genes that promote mesenchymal transitioning into a more malignant state, were commonly observed in CTCs. An additional subset of EMT-related genes were expressed in CTCs of CRPC, but less frequently in castration-sensitive cancer.
Hofman et al.	2013	Melanoma	IV	ISET®/ICC	BRAFV600E mutation	98	There was statistical correlation between the mutational status of the BRAFV600E detected by pyrosequencing on tumor specimens and expression of the protein detected by ICC on circulating melanoma cells ($P < 0.001$).
Nadal et al.	2013	Breast cancer	I, II, and III	Immunomagnetic techniques/ICC	CD133	98	CTCs positive for CD133 were more found in luminal tumor subtypes before the treament ($P = 0.006$). There was a relative enrichment of CTC positive for CD133 after the systemic treatment in non-luminal tumor subtypes.

Pailler et al.	2013	NSCLC	NS	ISET®/Filter-adapted-FISH	ALK-rearrangement	32	18 ALK-rearranged patients and 14 - ALK-negative patients were included. All ALK-positive patients had 4 or more ALK-rearranged CTCs/1 mL of blood. Only one ALK-rearranged CTC was detected in ALK-negative patients.
Smerage et al.	2013	Breast cancer	IV	CellSearch® system	M30 and Bcl2 expression		Patients with elevated CTC count, and higher levels of CTC-M30 were associated with worse prognosis, while higher CTC-Bcl-2 levels correlated with better outcomes.
Antonarakis et al.	2014	Prostate cancer	IV	Quantitative reverse-transcriptase–PCR	AR-V7 splice variant	62	Patients treated with enzalutamide ($n = 31$) and abiraterone ($n = 31$), respectively 39% and 19% had detectable AR-V7 in CTCs. In both groups there was observed better survival in AR-V7 negative patients.

(continued)

Table 1.1 (continued)

Authors	Year	Tumor	Stage	Method	Markers	No. patients	Main results
Kalikaki et al.	2014	Colorectal cancer	IV	CellSearch® system/Peptide Nucleic Acid (PNA)-based qPCR	KRAS mutations: G12D, G13D, G12R, G12C, G12S, G12 V, and G12A	31	KRAS mutation analysis in CTC-enriched specimens showed that 45% and 16.7% of patients with mutant and wild type primary tumors, respectively, had detectable mutations in their CTCs. Serial blood samples revealed different mutational status of KRAS during treatment.
Kuhlmann et al.	2014	Ovarian cancer	I, II, III, and IV	Immunomagnetic enrichment/Multiplex RT-PCR	ERCC1 and CA125	143	ERCC1 expression in CTCs was significantly associated with poor PFS ($P = 0.026$) and OS ($P = 0.009$) and correlated with platinum resistance ($P = 0.01$).
Abdallah et al.	2015	Colorectal cancer	IV	ISET®/ICC	TYMS expression	54	TYMS expression in CTCs was associated with quick disease progression ($P = 0.07$) and with ≥2 CTCs/ml ($P = 0.02$).
Pailler et al.	2015	NSCLC	Advanced	Isolation by Size of Epithelial Tumor Cells (ISET®)/Filter-adapted-	ROS1-rearrangements	8	4 ROS1-rearranged patients and 4 ROS1-negative patients were included. ROS1 copy

				fluorescence in situ hybridization (FA-FISH)			number was significantly higher in baseline CTCs compared with paired tumor biopsies in the three patients experiencing partial response or stable disease ($P < 0.0001$). ROS1-rearranged CTCs increased significantly in two patients who progressed ($P < 0.02$).
Punnoose et al.	2015	Prostate cancer	IV	Epic CTC platform/FISH	PTEN gene status	76	PTEN gene status detected in CTCs was concordant with PTEN status in matched fresh tissues and archival tissue in 32/38 patients (84%) and 24/39 patients (62%), respectively. PTEN loss in CTCs associated with worse survival in univariate analysis (HR 2.05; $P = 0.01$).
Steinestel et al.	2015	Prostate cancer	Advanced	AdnaTest ProstateCancerSelect Kit/AdnaGen ProstateCancerDetect Kit/ Real-Time PCR system/ DNA pyrosequencing	AR-V7 splice variant: AR-V567 AR-V7/AR point mutations (8 point mutations were evaluated)	47	51% patients with detectable CTCs carried AR-modifications. 17 patients carried the AR-V7 splice variant. Positive predictive value for response/non-response to therapy by AR status in CTCs was ~94%.

(continued)

Table 1.1 (continued)

Authors	Year	Tumor	Stage	Method	Markers	No. patients	Main results
Miyamoto et al.	2015	Prostate cancer	Localized and advanced	CTC-chip/Single-cell RNA-sequencing (RNA-Seq)	RNA sequencing	22	RNA sequencing was made in 77 CTCs from 13 patients. Single CTCs from each individual display considerable heterogeneity, including expression of AR gene mutations and splicing variants. Retrospective analysis of CTCs from patients progressing under treatment with an AR inhibitor, compared with untreated cases, indicates activation of noncanonical Wnt signaling ($P = 0.0064$).
Abdallah et al.	2016	Colorectal cancer	IV	ISET®/ICC	MRP1, MRP4, and ERCC1 expression	34	MRP1 expression CTCs was significantly associated with shorter PFS ($P = 0.003$).
Satelli et al.	2016	Colorectal cancer and prostate cancer	IV and IV	Magnetic separation with the cell-surface vimentin (CSV)-specific 84–1 monoclonal antibody/confocal microscopy	PD-L1 expression	62 and 30	Nuclear PD-L1 (nPD-L1) expression in these patients was significantly associated with short survival. Colorectal cancer (OS: $P = 0.0264$); Prostate

							cancer (PFS: P = 0.0215).
Scher et al.	2016	Prostate cancer	IV	Immunofluorescence	AR-V7 splice variant	161	AR-V7–positive CTCs were found in 34 samples (18%). Patients whose samples had AR-V7–positive CTCs before ARS inhibition had shorter PFS, shorter time on therapy, and shorter OS than those without AR-V7–positive CTCs. The presence of AR-V7-positive CTCs before the treatment predicted better OS in patients treated with taxanes than with ARS inhibitors (P = 0.035).

Abbreviations: *AR* androgen receptor, *ARS* androgen receptor signaling, *ISET*® Isolation by Size of Epithelial Tumor Cells ICC immunocytochemistry, *LM* laser microdissection, *DFS* disease free survival, *TTP* time to progression, *NT* neoadjuvant treatment, *NSCLC* non-small-cell lung cancer, *WBC* white blood cells, *PCR* polymerase chain reaction, *RFS* recurrence free survival, *FISH* Fluorescence in situ hybridization, *OS* overall survival, *CRPC* castrate resistant prostate cancer time points in the above study was associated with worse distant metastasis-free and OS at a median follow-up period of 36 months (Bidard et al. 2010). Moreover, it was associated to poor clinical outcome, especially in patients with estrogen receptor (ER)-negative, triple negative, and HER2-positive cancer (Ignatiadis et al. 2007). When the CTC detection occurs before and after neoadjuvant chemotherapy, it appears that the detection of ≥1 CTCs/7.5 ml of blood can accurately predict the poor overall survival of patients (Pierga et al. 2008).

Studies demonstrating CTC detection in non-metastatic CRC require specific and sensitive methods, because of the low incidence of these cells in the initial stage of the tumor, as in breast cancer. The presence of CTCs in the peripheral blood of CRC patients is a potential marker of poor DFS (Thorsteinsson and Jess 2011).

Wong et al. (2009) examined 101 patients with tumor, node, metastasis (TNM) stage I e III CRC, detecting CTC with a gastrointestinal-specific CK20. Sixty-two of 101 patients were followed for a period of 24 months and the association between preoperative elevated CK20 and recurrence was found to be highly significant ($p < 0.001$). The CTCs were an independent prognostic factor of survival ($p < 0.005$) in a multivariate regression analysis including TNM-stage, lymph node status, age, sex, tumor stage and degree of differentiation. In accordance, Iinuma et al. (2006) was also able to demonstrate poor DFS for CRC patients with preoperatively elevated CTC using a RT-PCR based method.

Allen-Mersh et al. (2007) demonstrated that poor DFS was associated with the occurrence of CEA or CK20 24 hours postoperatively ($p < 0.001$). Uen et al. (2008) used a multi-marker membrane array method to detect CTC in 438 patients with TNM stage I e III colorectal cancer. Presence of all four markers (human telomerase reverse transcriptase [hTERT], CK19, CK20, and CEA) was considered as a positive result for CTC. The authors demonstrated that patients with persistent presence of CTC after surgery had a significantly poorer relapse-free survival compared with patients without CTC ($p < 0.001$).

The CTCs analysis may also be useful for patients with melanoma. The detection of CTCs in these patients may help for determining prognosis. Hoshimoto et al. (2012a) reviewed the clinical usefulness of an RT-qPCR MultiMarker (MART-1, MAGE-A3, and GalNAc-T) for detection of CTCs in 331 melanoma patients who were clinically free of disease after lymphadenectomy. The individual detection of CTCs ranged from 13.4 to 17.5% and there was no stated association of CTC with known clinical or pathological prognostic variables. However, the presence of two or more positive biomarkers was significantly associated with distant metastasis and recurrence-free survival.

Lowes et al. (2012) were able to detect CTCs in patients with early stage prostate cancer and suggested the possibility that the reduction after treatment of CTC levels may be indicative of response to radiotherapy.

The main advantage of CTC analysis in early stages is based on the ease of obtaining a "liquid biopsy" and thus being able to monitor patients over the course of the disease, providing valuable information about the very early assessment of treatment effectiveness and helping towards establishing individualized therapies that will improve the efficiency with less cost and fewer side effects for cancer patients.

More studies on the molecular characterization of CTCs in early stage may provide important information for the identification of therapeutic targets and understand resistance to therapies (Lianidou et al. 2013). According to Lianidou et al. (2014) CTCs characterization is promising in combination with sequencing technologies that will allow the elucidation of molecular pathways in these cells, generating new molecular therapies. The real-time monitoring of therapy in early stages will have a major impact on personalized medicine in many types of cancers, allowing the choice of more effective and less toxic therapies.

1.5 Role of CTCs in Minimal Residual Disease

Minimal residual disease (MRD) has usually been studied after surgery and treatment with targeted therapies (Maheswaran et al. 2008). Defined as micrometastatic cells undetectable by laboratory tests and conventional imaging, some MRD "substitutes" are detected in the peripheral blood (CTCs) and bone marrow (disseminated tumor cells [DTCs]). The detection of CTCs and DTCs leads to new strategies for personalized treatment and therapeutic agents for breast cancer, and brings new knowledge of tumor biology (Riethdorf and Pantel 2010).

DTC and CTC detection is a challenge, and different enrichment techniques are applied for each. The techniques are based on physical properties or immunological characteristics of these cells. Braun et al. (2005) detected micrometastases in 30.6% of the patients with stage I, II, or III breast cancer. The presence of micrometastases was a significant prognostic factor with respect to poor OS, breast-cancer-specific survival, poor DFS, and distant-DFS during a 10-year observation period. Micrometastasis was an independent predictor of a poor outcome. In the univariate subgroup analysis, breast-cancer-specific survival among patients with micrometastasis was significantly shortened ($p < 0.001$ for all comparisons) among those receiving adjuvant endocrine treatment (mortality ratio, 3.22) or cytotoxic therapy (mortality ratio, 2.32) and among patients who had tumors no larger than 2 cm in diameter without lymph-node metastasis and did not receive systemic adjuvant therapy (mortality ratio, 3.65).

Several authors performed studies comparing CTCs and DTCs and demonstrated correlation between them (Bidard et al. 2014; Goldkorn et al. 2014). Furthermore, given that blood is more easily obtained than bone marrow, CTCs are now being widely used as surrogate markers for DTCs.

Kasimir-Bauer et al. (2012), detected CTCs in 97 of 502 (19%) patients and DTCs in 107 of 502 (21%) patients, showing the value of CTCs and DTCs, despite the detection method for CTCs not being as efficient for identifying circulating tumor cells undergoing EMT.

At the time of initial diagnosis, patients often have DTCs (at bone marrow) or even undetected micrometastasis. The long dormancy period of MRD offers an opportunity to develop agents that can eradicate clinically relevant metastatic sites (Wan et al. 2013). *In vivo* experiments suggest that DTCs from bone marrow (BM) can be turned into CTCs and return to the primary tumor, a process called "tumor self-seeding," leading to aggressive metastatic variants (Kim et al. 2009).

Gao et al. (2016) adopted an integrated cellular and molecular approach of subtraction enrichment and immunostaining-fluorescence in situ hybridization (SE-iFISH (SE-iFISH, to investigate the chromosome 8 polyploidy, found in many solid tumors) to detect CTCs in the peripheral blood of patients with glioma, a disease considered restricted to brain, as very few cases with extracranial metastases has been observed (Fonkem et al. 2011; Kalokhe et al. 2012). However, the idea that brain glioma cells never enter the bloodstream has been put in doubt recently. Müller et al. (2014) were the first to find CTCs in the peripheral blood of patients with glioblastoma multiform (GBM) and declared that CTC is the "intrinsic property" of GBM biology. However, it is important to consider the methodological deficiencies in previous studies, the low incidence of CTCs and the fact that results were exclusively limited to high-grade gliomas (Gao et al. 2016). So, these authors investigated 31 patients with 7 different pathologic features (grade II-IV) of primary gliomas. They identified CTCs in 24 of 31 (77%) patients with no statistical difference of CTC incidence/count in different pathological subtypes or World Health Organization (WHO) grades of glioma. Clinical data demonstrate that CTCs, to some extent, was superior to magnetic resonance imaging (MRI) in monitoring the treatment response and differentiating radionecrosis from recurrence of glioma. The authors propose the use of CTCs to monitor the microenvironment of gliomas dynamically, as a complement to radiographic imaging.

The role of CTCs in micrometastatic disease is not completely understood, as CTCs compose a very heterogeneous population of cells, Meng et al. (2004) showed that the presence of documented micrometastases by CTCs detection does not imply absolute risk of subsequent recurrence. These authors reported that 13 of 36 (36%) women who had no evidence of clinical disease 7–22 years after mastectomy had detectable aneusomic CTCs. In other study (Wiedswang et al. 2004) it was reported that 53 of 356 (15%) patients who were disease-free after 3 years of follow-up had bone marrow micrometastases. After a follow-up of about 3 years, only 21% of these patients with documented persistent bone marrow metastases relapsed.

Studies suggest that simply finding cells using high sensitivity assays may not have clinical implications and that future studies using next-generation capture devices need to be planned carefully, taking into consideration clinical outcomes and not just diagnostic comparisons with the current gold standard. Molecular characterization of captured CTCs might provide insight into the future clinical behavior of the cancer, especially in relation to targeted therapy. However, it is not clear that CTCs actually reflect the biology of the tissue-based cancer. It is possible that the detected cells identified by currently available techniques are merely those that were shed and are only the "tip of the iceberg", as stained by Hayes and Paoletti (2013). Or, these are terminally differentiated cells that reflect the presence of more malignant cancer stem cells that are not captured by CellSearch®, (Hayes and Paoletti 2013), which can be captured by other antibody independent methods.

1.6 Role of CTCs in Screening and Diagnosis

Kohn and Liotta (1995) published a study showing that *in situ* breast cancer is a clonal precursor of breast carcinoma and that tumor invasion starts 5–10 years before cancer diagnosis. According to Paterlini-Bréchot (2014), this raises the hypothesis that it should be possible to detect cancer at a pre-diagnostic stage through the very sensitive detection techniques for "sentinel" cancer cells in blood.

More recently, Ilie et al. (2014) collected blood samples from 168 individuals with chronic obstructive pulmonary disease (COPD), a disease that typically results from long-term cigarette smoking, causing breakdown of lung tissues, and an increased risk of lung cancer. They also studied 77 control subjects. They looked for CTCs by ISET® in the blood of all 245 subjects, to investigate CTCs as a possible new marker for early lung cancer. They also obtained annual CT-scans in the COPD (68.6%) and control subjects (31.4%), none of whom were known to have lung cancer. CTCs were identified by cytomorphological analysis and characterized by expression of epithelial and mesenchymal markers. CTCs were detected during the study in 5 of the COPD patients (3%). The annual evaluation of the CTC-positive COPD patients by CT-scan screening then detected lung nodules 1–4 years later and led to surgical resection of early-stage lung cancers. Follow-up of these 5 cancer patients (by CT-scan and ISET®) 12 months after surgery showed no tumor recurrence. CTCs detected in COPD patients had a heterogeneous expression of epithelial and mesenchymal markers. No CTCs were detected in the 77 control subjects.

So, maybe, the utility of CTCs will not be only for follow-up of patients with well-known disease but also prove to be useful for screening of patients with family history of cancer, or with underlying diseases that can predispose to the development of cancers. With standardized protocols, we may be able to develop a practical tool for the early detection and prevention of untoward outcomes in this difficult, harmful, and deadly disease.

1.7 Conclusions

Raimondi et al. (2014) started his paper with a statement: "If one could translate the "Divina Commedia" into a scientific language and try to imagine where Dante Alighieri would have placed circulating tumor cells (CTCs), the answer would be, without a doubt, "in limbo". These authors affirm that despite the increasing scientific evidence collected in the last decade, "which is enough to avert the danger of Hell," the use of CTC in clinical practice is still "far from the light that suits to Heaven." They support their idea based on disappointing results obtained in the Phase III SWOG S0500 trial, concluding that CTCs are not a good marker to help to decide when to choose chemotherapy in women with metastatic breast cancer. They wrote a very interesting paper arguing that CTCs are "not in heaven yet."

These authors also discuss the CellSearch® system, which is the most used method to isolate CTCs in clinical trials. It was cleared by the FDA in 2004, but its clinical utility is still to be fully demonstrated. To date, no large prospective studies using CellSearch® have shown any predictive value for CTCs, and their clinical utility is therefore limited. The effect of the type of treatment on the prognostic and predictive value of CTCs has not been directly evaluated, and the ability of targeted therapies to modify the predictive value of CTC count has not yet been demonstrated. CellSearch® is based on the capture of cells expressing an epithelial antigen, without morphological verification of the neoplastic nature of the captured cells. This is a weakness of the test, because it therefore can misidentify nonmalignant circulating epithelial cells as CTCs. In addition, CellSearch® is unable to detect cells that have undergone epithelial mesenchymal transition, which explains the absence of CTCs in the subset of patients with metastatic cancer with documented progression of the disease in many clinical trials (Paterlini-Bréchot and Benali 2007; Pantel et al. 2012; Hofman et al. 2014, 2016).

Alternatively, there are investigators, who argue that the prognostic significance of CTC counts should not be ignored, even when the system used to evaluate CTCs—the CellSearch® System-has well known limitations (Kang and Pantel 2013; Paterlini-Bréchot 2014; Hofman and Popper 2016). Thus, CTC evaluations are included as a biomarker in more than 400 clinical trials using various assays (see Table 1.2).

We believe that CTCs studies have potential to help physicians use a more rational approach for management of both metastatic and non-metastatic tumors, reflecting solid tissue or mesenchymal cancers. However, we will need to develop a standard system and protocol in order to be able to use CTCs in routine clinical settings. There are systems that provide for CTC isolation in a marker independent manner, by cytopathological analysis, which seems promising in capturing all malignant cells.

Even considering their weak points, CTCs are one of the most promising and versatile biomarkers in translational oncology (Mehra et al. 2015). As highlighted by Kang and Pantel (2013), viewing CTCs as a "liquid biopsy" opens new opportunities for genotyping and phenotyping micrometastatic cells derived from various distant sites, which, if adequately developed, may provide clinical oncology with more complete pictures of the evolution of cancers compared to those provided by biopsies of single metastatic sites.

Table 1.2 Clinical trials that considered CTCs as a secondary endpoint on final analysis

Study	Year	Population	Intervention	Commentary
GEPARQuattro (Riethdorf et al.)	2010b	BC neoadjuvant therapy, multiple subtypes, focus on HER2 positive BC	Trastuzumab addition to anthracycline based chemotherapy and CTC related response	Decrease in CTC detection rate after neoadjuvan therapy (22% → 11%). Absent correlation between CTC decrease and pathological complete response. Evaluation of survival variables not performed. CTC evaluation performed in the HER2 positive subgroup
GEPARQuinto (Riethdorf et al.)	2010a	BC neoadjuvant therapy, multiple subtypes	Addition of targeted therapy to anthracycline based chemotherapy	Decrease in CTC detection rate after neoadjuvant therapy (23% → 11%). Absent correlation between CTC decrease and pathological complete response. Evaluation of survival variables not performed. CTC evaluation performed in the multiple subgroups (bevacizumab in triple negative BC and trastuzumab in HER2 positive BC)
Behbakht et al.	2011	Relapsed/recurrent ovarian cancer after 1–3 lines of treatment.	CTC analysis in phase II trial of Temsirolimus monotherapy.	Positivity for CTC on baseline was associated with shorter PFS (5.4 months for CTC negative and 2.3 for CTC positive patients). Statistical significance was lost after 12 months. Decreasing counts of CTC after therapy demonstrated improved numeric PFS
COU-AA-31 (de Bono et al.)	2011	CRPC, 2nd line post docetaxel	Abiraterone versus placebo: CTC prognostic evaluation	Elevated baseline CTC counts and decrease in 30% in 4 weeks were an independent predictor of OS with abiraterone

(continued)

Table 1.2 (continued)

Study	Year	Population	Intervention	Commentary
Poveda et al.	2011	Relapsed/recurrent ovarian cancer after platinum therapy	CTC analysis for association of trabectedin to PLD.	CTC counts ≥2 at baseline had higher risk of progressive disease (1.89) and death 2.06, both with statistical significance. Multivariate analysis including CA-125, platinum sensitivity status, performance and tumor grade sustained isolated numeric differences
AFFIRM (Scher et al.)	2012	CRPC, 2nd line post-docetaxel	Enzalutamide versus placebo: CTC prognostic evaluation	CTC counts ≥5 at baseline were an independent predictor of poor OS in both arms. Decline in CTC below defined threshold (<5) after treatment with enzalutamide was predictor of greater benefit and survival
MMAIT (Hoshimoto et al.)	2012b	Melanoma, stage IV, adjuvant.	CTC analysis related to peptide vaccine administration	CTC biomarker detection demonstrated worst prognosis related to RFS, distant metastasis and melanoma specific survival. Worst prognosis was seen with expression of more biomarkers. CTC levels were not associated with prognosis
SUCCESS (Franken et al.; Rack et al.)	2012; 2014	BC adjuvance, multiple subtypes	Evaluation of CTC impact on survival. Evaluation of different chemotherapy schemes	Survival analysis for primary endpoints still pending. For CTC analysis there was no morphologic or histologic difference between groups. CTC detection was associated with poor DFS (93.7% × 88.1%), including local and distant DFS, and also

(continued)

Table 1.2 (continued)

Study	Year	Population	Intervention	Commentary
				poor OS (97.3% × 93.2%), with statistical significance. Prognostic impact was sustained before and after chemotherapy
LAP 07 – CirCe 07 (Bidard et al.)	2013	LAPC: erlotinib addition to gemcitabine and RT evaluation.	CTC as a prognostic marker to LAPC treatment	CTC ≥ 1 at baseline is directly correlated with worst prognosis for OS, with statistical significance. No impact of CTC status on PFS. Study is underpowered due to complications in accrual and low acceptance for CTC analysis
MACRO (Sastre et al.)	2013	mCRC: XELOX + Bevacizumab in 1st line → bevacizumab maintenance therapy	Evaluation of prognostic CTC impact despite of KRAS analysis	Patients with CTC counts <3 and KRAS wild type tumors had a greater statistical significant survival (PFS 14.2 and OS 28.9 months) compared to patients with CTC counts ≥3 and KRAS mutated tumors (PFS 6.2 and OS 13.7 months). Both high CTC counts and KRAS mutated status were independent prognostic factors for mCRC
NeoALTTO (Azim et al.)	2013	HER2 positive BC, neoadjuvant therapy	Addition of lapatinib and trastuzumab to chemotherapy	Lower pathologic complete response rate observed in patients with detectable CTCs (27.3% versus 42.5%) without statistical significance. Study was underpowered (only 51 patients accepted participation on CTC analysis)

(continued)

Table 1.2 (continued)

Study	Year	Population	Intervention	Commentary
BEVERLY-1 (Bertucci et al.)	2016	HER2 negative	Addition of bevacizumab to neoadjuvant therapy	Significant decrease in CTC In both BEVERLY-1 (40 → 11%) and BEVERLY-2 (37–7%), without correlation to pathologic complete response, but with demonstrating CTC as a strong predictor for survival variables
BEVERLY-2 (Pierga et al.)	2012	HER2 positive		
		Inflammatory BC		

Only phase II or III prospective clinical trials were considered for the selection. In all studies, CTC analysis was performed by CellSearch® System (Veridex, Raritan, NJ). This table shows a sample of current studies, already with published results. Many more papers are to come with CTC considered as an endpoint for analysis

Abbreviations: *OS* overall survival, *PFS* progression-free survival, *DFS* disease free survival, *RT* radiotherapy, *CRPC* castration resistant prostate cancer, *BC* breast cancer, *mCRC* metastatic colorectal cancer, *LAPC* locally advanced pancreatic cancer, *PLD* pegylated liposomal doxorubicin

References

Abdallah EA, Fanelli MF, Buim ME et al (2015) Thymidylate synthase expression in circulating tumor cells: a new tool to predict 5-fluorouracil resistance in metastatic colorectal cancer patients. Int J Cancer 137(6):1397–1405

Abdallah EA, Fanelli MF, Souza E, Silva V et al (2016) MRP1 expression in CTCs confers resistance to irinotecan-based chemotherapy in metastatic colorectal cancer. Int J Cancer 139 (4):890–898

Aktas B, Kasimir-Bauer S, Heubner M et al (2011) Molecular profiling and prognostic relevance of circulating tumor cells in the blood of ovarian cancer patients at primary diagnosis and after platinum-based chemotherapy. Int J Gynecol Cancer 21(5):822–830

Allen-Mersh TG, McCullough TK, Patel H et al (2007) Role of circulating tumour cells in predicting recurrence after excision of primary colorectal carcinoma. Br J Surg 94(1):96–105

Antonarakis ES, Lu C, Wang H, Luber B et al (2014) AR-V7 and resistance to enzalutamide and abiraterone in prostate cancer. N Engl J Med 371(11):1028–1038

Ashworth TR (1869) A case of cancer in which cells similar to those in the tumours were seen in the blood after death. Med J Aust 14:146–147

Azim HA Jr, Rothé F, Aura CM et al (2013) Circulating tumor cells and response to neoadjuvant paclitaxel and HER2-targeted therapy: a sub-study from the NeoALTTO phase III trial. Breast 22(6):1060–1065

Behbakht K, Sill MW, Darcy KM et al (2011) Phase II trial of the mTOR inhibitor, temsirolimus and evaluation of circulating tumor cells and tumor biomarkers in persistent and recurrent epithelial ovarian and primary peritoneal malignancies: a Gynecologic Oncology Group study. Gynecol Oncol 123(1):19–26

Bertucci F, Fekih M, Autret A et al (2016) Bevacizumab plus neoadjuvant chemotherapy in patients with HER2-negative inflammatory breast cancer (BEVERLY-1): a multicentre, single-arm, phase 2 study. Lancet Oncol 17(5):600–611

Bidard FC, Mathiot C, Delaloge S et al (2010) Single circulating tumor cell detection and overall survival in nonmetastatic breast cancer. Ann Oncol 21(4):729–733

Bidard FC, Huguet F, Louvet C et al (2013) Circulating tumor cells in locally advanced pancreatic adenocarcinoma: the ancillary CirCe 07 study to the LAP 07 trial. Ann Oncol 24(8):2057–2061

Bidard FC, Peeters DJ, Fehm T et al (2014) Clinical validity of circulating tumour cells in patients with metastatic breast cancer: a pooled analysis of individual patient data. Lancet Oncol 15 (4):406–414

Brandt B, Junker R, Griwatz C et al (1996) Isolation of prostate-derived single cells and cell clusters from human peripheral blood. Cancer Res 56(20):4556–4561

Braun S, Vogl FD, Naume B et al (2005) A pooled analysis of bone marrow micrometastasis in breast cancer. N Engl J Med 353:793–802

Bredemeier M, Edimiris P, Tewes M et al (2016) Establishmernt of a multimarker qPCR panel for the molecular characterization of circulating tumor cells in blood samples of metastatic breast cancer patients during the course of palliative treatment. Oncotarget 7:41677–41690

Buim ME, Fanelli MF, Souza VS et al (2015) Detection of KRAS mutations in circulating tumor cells from patients with metastatic colorectal cancer. Cancer Biol Ther 16(9):1289–1295

Caixeiro NJ, Kienzle N, Lim SH et al (2014) Circulating tumour cells—a bona fide cause of metastatic cancer. Cancer Metastasis Rev 33(2–3):747–756

Cayrefourcq L, Mazard T, Joosse S et al (2015) Establishment and characterization of a cell line from human circulating colon cancer cells. Cancer Res 75(5):892–901

Chen CL, Mahalingam D, Osmulski P et al (2013) Single-cell analysis of circulating tumor cells identifies cumulative expression patterns of EMT-related genes in metastatic prostate cancer. Prostate 73(8):813–826

Chen X, Zhou F, Li X et al (2015) Folate receptor-positive circulating tumor cell detected by LT-PCR-based method as a diagnostic biomarker for non-small-cell lung cancer. J Thorac Oncol 10(8):1163–1171

Chinen LT, de Carvalho FM, Rocha BM et al (2013) Cytokeratin-based CTC counting unrelated to clinical follow-up. J Thorac Dis 5(5):593–599

Chinen LT, Mello CA, Abdallah EA et al (2014) Isolation, detection, and immunomorphological characterization of circulating tumor cells (CTCs) from patients with different types of sarcoma using isolation by size of tumor cells: a window on sarcoma-cell invasion. Onco Targets Ther 7:1609–1617

Corassa M, Fanelli M, Guimarães APG et al (2016) Circulating Tumor Cells (CTCs) as a new and additional approach to follow-up patients with serous papillary low-grade ovarian adenocarcinoma – a case report and review of the literature (submitted)

Cristofanilli M (2014) Circulating tumour cells: telling the truth about metastasis. Lancet Oncol 15 (4):365–366

Cristofanilli M, Budd GT, Mathew JE et al (2004) Circulating tumor cells, disease progression, and survival in metastatic breast cancer. N Engl J Med 351(8):781–791

Cui Y, König J, Buchholz JK et al (1999) Drug resistance and ATP-dependent conjugate transport mediated by the apical multidrug resistance protein, MRP2, permanently expressed in human and canine cells. Mol Pharmacol 55(5):929–937

Das M, Riess JW, Frankel P et al (2012) ERCC1 expression in circulating tumor cells (CTCs) using a novel detection platform correlates with progression-free survival (PFS) in patients with metastatic non-small-cell lung cancer (NSCLC) receiving platinum chemotherapy. Lung Cancer 77(2):421–426

de Bono JS, Scher HI, Montgomery RB et al (2008) Circulating tumor cells predict survival benefit from treatment in metastatic castration-resistant prostate cancer. Clin Cancer Res 14 (19):6302–6309

de Bono JS, Logothetis CJ, Molina A et al (2011) Abiraterone and Increased Survival in Metastatic Prostate Cancer. N Engl J Med 364(21):1995–2005

De Giorgi U, Valeo V, Rohren E et al (2010) Circulating tumor cells and bone metastases as detected by FDG-PET/CT in patients with metastatic breast cancer. Ann Oncol 21(1):33–39

De Oliveira TB, Nicolau UR, Braun AC et al (2016) Detection of drug resistance proteins in CTC from patients with locally advanced head and neck squamous cell carcinoma and their relation with survival. 7th ECHNO (European Congress on Head and Neck Oncol) abstract OP011

Devriese LA, Voest EE, Beijnen JH et al (2011) Circulating tumor cells as pharmacodynamic biomarker in early clinical oncological trials. Cancer Treat Rev 37(8):579–589

Doyle L, Ross DD (2003) Multidrug resistance mediated by the breast cancer resistance protein BCRP (ABCG2). Oncogene 22(47):7340–7358

Fabbri F, Carloni S, Zoli W et al (2013) Detection and recovery of circulating colon cancer cells using a dielectrophoresis-based device: KRAS mutation status in pure CTCs. Cancer Lett 335 (1):225–231

Fearon ER, Vogelstein B (1990) A genetic model for colorectal tumorigenesis. Cell 61 (5):759–767

Fina E, Reduzzi C, Motta R et al (2015) Did circulating tumor cells tell us all they could? The missed circulating tumor cell message in breast cancer. Int J Biol Markers 30(4):e429–e433

Flens MJ, Zaman GJ, van der Valk P et al (1996) Tissue distribution of the multidrug resistance protein. Am J Pathol 148(4):1237–1247

Fonkem E, Lun M, Wong ET (2011) Rare phenomenon of extracranial metastasis of glioblastoma. J Clin Oncol 29(34):4594–4595

Franken B, de Groot MR, Mastboom WJ et al (2012) Circulating tumor cells, disease recurrence and survival in newly diagnosed breast cancer. Breast Cancer Res 14(5):R133

Gao F, Cui Y, Jiang H et al (2016) Circulating tumor cell is a common property of brain glioma and promotes the monitoring system. Oncotarget 7:71330–71340

Garcia-Villa A, Balasubramanian P, Miller BL et al (2012) Assessment of γ-H2AX levels in circulating tumor cells from patients receiving chemotherapy. Front Oncol 2:128

Gasch C, Bauernhofer T, Pichler M et al (2013) Heterogeneity of epidermal growth factor receptor status and mutations of KRAS/PIK3CA in circulating tumor cells of patients with colorectal cancer. Clin Chem 59(1):252–260

Gasch C, Oldopp T, Mauermann O et al (2016) Frequent detection of PIK3CA mutations in single circulating tumor cells of patients suffering from HER2-negative metastatic breast cancer. Mol Oncol pii: S1574-7891(16)30065-5

Gazzaniga P, Naso G, Gradilone A et al (2010) Chemosensitivity profile assay of circulating cancer cells: prognostic and predictive value in epithelial tumors. Int J Cancer 126 (10):2437–2447

Gerlinger M, Rowan AJ, Horswell S et al (2012) Intratumor heterogeneity and branched evolution revealed by multiregion sequencing. N Engl J Med 366(10):883–892

Goldkorn A, Ely B, Quinn DI et al (2014) Circulating tumor cell counts are prognostic of overall survival in SWOG S0421: a phase III trial of docetaxel with or without atrasentan for metastatic castration-resistant prostate cancer. J Clin Oncol 32(11):1136–1142

Gradilone A, Naso G, Raimondi C et al (2010) Circulating tumor cells (CTCs) in metastatic breast cancer (MBC): prognosis, drug resistance and phenotypic characterization. Ann Oncol 22 (1):86–92

Gradilone A, Raimondi C, Naso G et al (2011a) How circulating tumor cells escape from multidrug resistance: translating molecular mechanisms in metastatic breast cancer treatment. Am J Clin Oncol 34(6):625–627

Gradilone A, Naso G, Raimondi C et al (2011b) Circulating tumor cells (CTCs) in metastatic breast cancer (MBC): prognosis, drug resistance and phenotypic characterization. Ann Oncol 22(1):86–92

Gunn J, McCall JL, Yun K et al (1996) Detection of micrometastases in colorectal cancer patients by K19 and K20 reverse-transcription polymerase chain reaction. Lab Investig 75(4):611–616

Haber DA, Gray NS, Baselga J (2011) The evolving war on cancer. Cell 145(1):19–24

Han L, Chen W, Zhao Q (2014) Prognostic value of circulating tumor cells in patients with pancreatic cancer: a meta-analysis. Tumour Biol 35(3):2473–2480

Hayes DF, Paoletti C (2013) Circulating tumour cells: insights into tumour heterogeneity. J Intern Med 274(2):137–143
Hinz S, Röder C, Tepel J et al (2015) Cytokeratin 20 positive circulating tumor cells are a marker for response after neoadjuvant chemoradiation but not for prognosis in patients with rectal cancer. BMC Cancer 15:953
Hofman P, Popper HH (2016) Pathologists and liquid biopsies: to be or not to be? Virchows Arch 469:601–609
Hofman V, Ilie MI, Long E et al (2011) Detection of circulating tumor cells as a prognostic factor in patients undergoing radical surgery for non-small-cell lung carcinoma: comparison of the efficacy of the CellSearch Assay™ and the isolation by size of epithelial tumor cell method. Int J Cancer 129(7):1651–1660
Hofman V, Ilie M, Long-Mira E et al (2013) Usefulness of immunocytochemistry for the detection of the BRAF(V600E) mutation in circulating tumor cells from metastatic melanoma patients. J Invest Dermatol 133(5):1378–1381
Hofman V, Ilie M, Long E et al (2014) Detection of circulating tumor cells from lung cancer patients in the era of targeted therapy: promises, drawbacks and pitfalls. Curr Mol Med 14 (4):440–456
Hofman VJ, Ilie M, Hofman PM (2016) Detection and characterization of circulating tumor cells in lung cancer: why and how? Cancer Cytopathol 124(6):380–387
Holohan C, Van Schaeybroeck S, Longley DB et al (2013) Cancer drug resistance: an evolving paradigm. Nat Rev Cancer 13(10):714–726
Hong W, Lee S, Chang HJ et al (2016) Multifunctional magnetic nanowires: a novel breakthrough for ultrasensitive detection and isolation of rare cancer cells from non-metastatic early breast cancer patients using small volumes of blood. Biomaterials 106:78–86
Hoshimoto S, Shingai T, Morton DL et al (2012a) Association between circulating tumor cells and prognosis in patients with stage III melanoma with sentinel lymph node metastasis in a phase III international multicenter trial. J Clin Oncol 30(31):3819–3826
Hoshimoto S, Faries MB, Morton DL et al (2012b) Assessment of prognostic circulating tumor cells in a phase III trial of adjuvant immunotherapy after complete resection of stage IV melanoma. Ann Surg 255(2):357–362
Hou JM, Krebs MG, Lancashire L et al (2012) Clinical significance and molecular characteristics of circulating tumor cells and circulating tumor microemboli in patients with small-cell lung cancer. J Clin Oncol 30(5):525–532
Houtsmuller AB, Rademakers S, Nigg AL et al (1999) Action of DNA repair endonuclease ERCC1/XPF in living cells. Science 284(5416):958–961
Huang MY, Tsai HL, Huang JJ et al (2016) Clinical implications and future perspectives of circulating tumor cells and biomarkers in clinical outcomes of colorectal cancer. Transl Oncol 9(4):340–347
Ignatiadis M, Perraki M, Apostolaki S et al (2007) Molecular detection and prognostic value of circulating cytokeratin-19 messenger RNA-positive and HER2 messenger RNA-positive cells in the peripheral blood of women with early-stage breast cancer. Clin Breast Cancer 7 (11):883–889
Iinuma H, Okinaga K, Egami H et al (2006) Usefulness and clinical significance of quantitative real-time RTPCR to detect isolated tumor cells in the peripheral blood and tumor drainage blood of patients with colorectal cancer. Int J Oncol 28(2):297–306
Ilie M, Long E, Butori C et al (2012) ALK-gene rearrangement: a comparative analysis on circulating tumour cells and tumour tissue from patients with lung adenocarcinoma. Ann Oncol 23(11):2907–2913
Ilie M, Hofman V, Long-Mira E et al (2014) "Sentinel" circulating tumor cells allow early diagnosis of lung cancer in patients with chronic obstructive pulmonary disease. PLoS One 9 (10):e111597
Jiang Y, Palma JF, Agus DB et al (2010) Detection of androgen receptor mutations in circulating tumor cells in castration-resistant prostate cancer. Clin Chem 56(9):1492–1495

Kalikaki A, Politaki H, Souglakos J et al (2014) KRAS genotypic changes of circulating tumor cells during treatment of patients with metastatic colorectal cancer. PLoS One 9(8):e104902
Kalokhe G, Grimm SA, Chandler JP et al (2012) Metastatic glioblastoma: case presentations and a review of the literature. J Neuro-Oncol 107(1):21–27
Kang Y, Pantel K (2013) Tumor cell dissemination: emerging biological insights from animal models and cancer patients. Cancer Cell 23(5):573–581
Kasimir-Bauer S, Hoffmann O, Wallwiener D et al (2012) Expression of stem cell and epithelial-mesenchymal transition markers in primary breast cancer patients with circulating tumor cells. Breast Cancer Res 14(1):R15
Katsumata K, Sumi T, Mori Y et al (2006) Detection and evaluation of epithelial cells in the blood of colon cancer patients using RT-PCR. Int J Clin Oncol 11(5):385–389
Kim MY, Oskarsson T, Acharyya S et al (2009) Tumor self-seeding by circulating cancer cells. Cell 139(7):1315–1326
Kohn EC, Liotta LA (1995) Molecular insights into cancer invasion: strategies for prevention and intervention. Cancer Res 55(9):1856–1862
Krebs MG, Sloane R, Priest L et al (2011) Evaluation and prognostic significance of circulating tumor cells in patients with non–small-cell lung cancer. J Clin Oncol 29(12):1556–1563
Kuczynski EA, Sargent DJ, Grothey A et al (2013) Drug rechallenge and treatment beyond progression—implications for drug resistance. Nat Rev Clin Oncol 10(10):571–587
Kuhlmann JD, Wimberger P, Bankfalvi A et al (2014) ERCC1-positive circulating tumor cells in the blood of ovarian cancer patients as a predictive biomarker for platinum resistance. Clin Chem 60(10):1282–1289
Kurihara T, Itoi T, Sofuni A et al (2008) Detection of circulating tumor cells in patients with pancreatic cancer: a preliminary result. J Hepato-Biliary-Pancreat Surg 15(2):189–195
Lianidou ES, Mavroudis D, Georgoulias V (2013) Clinical challenges in the molecular characterization of circulating tumour cells in breast cancer. Br J Cancer 108(12):2426–2432
Lianidou ES, Strati A, Markou A (2014) Circulating tumor cells as promising novel biomarkers in solid cancers. Crit Rev Clin Lab Sci 51(3):160–171
Lou J, Ben S, Yang G et al (2013) Quantification of rare circulating tumor cells in non-small cell lung cancer by ligand-targeted PCR. PLoS One 8(12):e80458
Lowes LE, Lock M, Rodrigues G et al (2012) Circulating tumour cells in prostate cancer patients receiving salvage radiotherapy. Clin Transl Oncol 14(2):150–156
Lucci A, Hall CS, Lodhi AK et al (2012) Circulating tumour cells in non-metastatic breast cancer: a prospective study. Lancet Oncol 13(7):688–695
Magni E, Botteri E, Ravenda PS et al (2014) Detection of circulating tumor cells in patients with locally advanced rectal cancer undergoing neoadjuvant therapy followed by curative surgery. Int J Color Dis 29(9):1053–1059
Maheswaran S, Sequist LV, Nagrath S et al (2008) Detection of mutations in EGFR in circulating lung-cancer cells. N Engl J Med 359(4):366–377
Mani SA, Guo W, Liao MJ et al (2008) The epithelial mesenchymal transition generates cells with properties of stem cells. Cell 133(4):704–715
Marusyk A, Polyak K (2010) Tumor heterogeneity: causes and consequences. Biochim Biophys Acta 1805(1):105–117
Mazel M, Jacot W, Pantel K (2015) Frequent expression of PD-L1 on circulating breast cancer cells. Mol Oncol 9(9):1773–1782
Mego M, Mani SA, Cristofanilli M (2010) Molecular mechanisms of metastasis in breast cancer-clinical applications. Nat Rev Clin Oncol 7(12):693–701
Mego M, Mani SA, Lee B et al (2012) Expression of epithelial-mesenchymal transition-inducing transcription factors in primary breast cancer: the effect of neoadjuvant therapy. Int J Cancer 130(4):808–816
Mehra N, Zafeiriou Z, Lorente D et al (2015) CCR 20th anniversary commentary: circulating tumor cells in prostate cancer. Clin Cancer Res 21(22):4992–4995

Meng S, Tripathy D, Frenkel EP et al (2004) Circulating tumor cells in patients with breast cancer dormancy. Clin Cancer Res 10(24):8152–8162

Miyamoto DT, Lee RJ, Stott SL et al (2012) Androgen receptor signaling in circulating tumor cells as a marker of hormonally responsive prostate cancer. Cancer Discov 2(11):995–1003

Miyamoto DT, Zheng Y, Wittner BS et al (2015) RNA-Seq of single prostate CTCs implicates noncanonical Wnt signaling in antiandrogen resistance. Science 349(6254):1351–1356

Morel AP, Lievre M, Thomas C et al (2008) Generation of breast cancer stem cells through epithelial mesenchymal transition. PLoS One 3(8):e2888

Mostert B, Jiang Y, Sieuwerts AM et al (2013) KRAS and BRAF mutation status in circulating colorectal tumor cells and their correlation with primary and metastatic tumor tissue. Int J Cancer 133(1):130–141

Muinelo-Romay L, Vieito M, Abalo A et al (2014) Evaluation of circulating tumor cells and related events as prognostic factors and surrogate biomarkers in advanced NSCLC patients receiving first-line systemic treatment. Cancers (Basel) 6(1):153–165

Müller C, Holtschmidt J, Auer M et al (2014) Hematogenous dissemination of glioblastoma multiforme. Sci Transl Med 6(247):247ra101

Murray NP, Albarran V, Perez G et al (2015) Secondary Circulating Tumor Cells (CTCs) but not primary CTCs are associated with the clinico-pathological parameters in Chilean patients with Colo-rectal cancer. Asian Pac J Cancer Prev 16(11):4745–4749

Nadal R, Ortega FG, Salido M et al (2013) CD133 expression in circulating tumor cells from breast cancer patients: potential role in resistance to chemotherapy. Int J Cancer 133 (10):2398–2407

Nesteruk D, Rutkowski A, Fabisiewicz S et al (2014) Evaluation of prognostic significance of circulating tumor cells detection in rectal cancer patients treated with preoperative radiotherapy: prospectively collected material data. Biomed Res Int 2014:712827

Nolé F, Munzone E, Zorzino L et al (2008) Variation of circulating tumor cell levels during treatment of metastatic breast cancer: prognostic and therapeutic implications. Ann Oncol 19 (5):891–897

Paik S, Kim C, Wolmark N (2008) HER2 status and benefit from adjuvant trastuzumab in breast cancer. N Engl J Med 358(13):1409–1411

Pailler E, Adam J, Barthélémy A et al (2013) Detection of circulating tumor cells harboring a unique ALK rearrangement in ALK-positive non-small-cell lung cancer. J Clin Oncol 31 (18):2273–2281

Pailler E, Auger N, Lindsay CR et al (2015) High level of chromosomal instability in circulating tumor cells of ROS1-rearranged non-small-cell lung cancer. Ann Oncol 26(7):1408–1415

Pantel K, Denève E, Nocca D et al (2012) Circulating epithelial cells in patients with benign colon diseases. Clin Chem 58(5):936–940

Paoletti C, Muñiz MC, Thomas DG et al (2015) Development of circulating tumor cell-endocrine therapy index in patients with hormone receptor-positive breast cancer. Clin Cancer Res 21 (11):2487–2498

Paterlini-Bréchot P (2014) Circulating tumor cells: who is the killer? Cancer Microenviron 7 (3):161–176

Paterlini-Brechot P, Benali NL (2007) Circulating tumor cells (CTC) detection: clinical impact and future directions. Cancer Lett 253(2):180–204

Phillips KA, Veenstra DL, Oren E (2001) Potential role of pharmacogenomics in reducing adverse drug reactions: a systematic review. JAMA 286(18):2270–2279

Pierga JY, Bidard FC, Mathiot C et al (2008) Circulating tumor cell detection predicts early metastatic relapse after neoadjuvant chemotherapy in large operable and locally advanced breast cancer in a phase II randomized trial. Clin Cancer Res 14(21):7004–7010

Pierga JY, Petit T, Delozier T et al (2012) Neoadjuvant bevacizumab, trastuzumab, and chemotherapy for primary inflammatory HER2-positive breast cancer (BEVERLY-2): an open-label, single-arm phase 2 study. Lancet Oncol 13(4):375–384

Pinzani P, Salvadori B, Simi L et al (2006) Isolation by size of epithelial tumor cells in peripheral blood of patients with breast cancer: correlation with real-time reverse transcriptase-polymerase chain reaction results and feasibility of molecular analysis by laser microdissection. Hum Pathol 37(6):711–718

Popat S, Matakidou A, Houlston RS (2004) Thymidylate synthase expression and prognosis in colorectal cancer: a systematic review and meta-analysis. J Clin Oncol 22(3):529–536

Poveda A, Kaye SB, McCormack R et al (2011) Circulating tumor cells predict PFS and overall survival in patients with relapsed/recurrent advanced ovarian cancer. Gynecol Oncol 122 (3):567–572

Punnoose EA, Atwal S, Liu W et al (2012) Evaluation of circulating tumor cells and circulating tumor DNA in non-small cell lung cancer: association with clinical endpoints in a phase II clinical trial of pertuzumab and erlotinib. Clin Cancer Res 18(8):2391–2401

Punnoose EA, Ferraldeschi R, Szafer-Glusman E et al (2015) PTEN loss in circulating tumour cells correlates with PTEN loss in fresh tumour tissue from castration-resistant prostate cancer patients. Br J Cancer 113(8):1225–1233

Rack B, Schindlbeck C, Jückstock J et al (2014) Circulating tumor cells predict survival in early average-to-high risk breast cancer patients. J Natl Cancer Inst 106(5):dju066

Rahbari NN, Aigner M, Thorlund K et al (2010) Meta-analysis shows that detection of circulating tumor cells indicates poor prognosis in patients with colorectal cancer. Gastroenterol 138 (5):1714–1726

Raimondi C, Nicolazzo C, Gradilone A et al (2014) Circulating tumor cells: exploring intratumor heterogeneity of colorectal cancer. Cancer Biol Ther 15(5):496–503

Riethdorf S, Pantel K (2008) Disseminated tumor cells in bone marrow and circulating tumor cells in blood of breast cancer patients: current state of detection and characterization. Pathobiology 75(2):140–148

Riethdorf S, Pantel K (2010) Advancing personalized cancer therapy by detection and characterization of circulating carcinoma cells. Ann N Y Acad Sci 1210:66–77

Riethdorf S, Müller V, Zhang L et al (2010a) Detection and HER2 expression of circulating tumor cells: prospective monitoring in breast cancer patients treated in the neoadjuvant GeparQuattro trial. Clin Cancer Res 16(9):2634–2645

Riethdorf S, Mueller V, Mauermann O et al (2010b) Abstract PD04-06: changes in circulating tumor and endothelial cells in peripheral blood of patients treated in the neoadjuvant chemotherapy plus targeted treatment breast cancer study "GeparQuinto". Cancer Res 70(24 Suppl): PD04-6-PD-6

Roden DM, George AL Jr (2002) The genetic basis of variability in drug responses. Nat Rev Drug Discov 1(1):37–44

Salvianti F, Pazzagli M, Pinzani P (2016) Single circulating tumor cell sequencing as an advanced tool in cancer management. Expert Rev Mol Diagn 16(1):51–63

Sarker D, Workman P (2007) Pharmacodynamic biomarkers for molecular cancer therapeutics. Adv Cancer Res 96:213–268

Sastre J, Maestro ML, Puente J et al (2008) Circulating tumor cells in colorectal cancer: correlation with clinical and pathological variables. Ann Oncol 19(5):935–938

Sastre J, Vidaurreta M, Gómez A et al (2013) Prognostic value of the combination of circulating tumor cells plus KRAS in patients with metastatic colorectal cancer treated with chemotherapy plus bevacizumab. Clin Colorectal Cancer 12(4):280–286

Satelli A, Batth IS, Brownlee Z et al (2016) Potential role of nuclear PD-L1 expression in cell-surface vimentin positive circulating tumor cells as a prognostic marker in cancer patients. Sci Rep 6:28910

Sawada T, Watanabe M, Fujimura Y et al (2016) Sensitive cytometry based system for enumeration, capture and analysis of gene mutations of circulating tumor cells. Cancer Sci 107 (3):307–314

Scher HI, Fizazi K, Saad F et al (2012) Increased survival with enzalutamide in prostate cancer after chemotherapy. N Engl J Med 367(13):1187–1197

Scher HI, Heller G, Molina A et al (2015) Circulating tumor cell biomarker panel as an individual-level surrogate for survival in metastatic castration-resistant prostate cancer. J Clin Oncol 33 (12):1348–1355
Scher HI, Lu D, Schreiber NA et al (2016) Association of AR-V7 on circulating tumor cells as a treatment-specific biomarker with outcomes and survival in castration-resistant prostate cancer. JAMA Oncol 2:1441–1449
Smerage JB, Budd GT, Doyle GV et al (2013) Monitoring apoptosis and Bcl-2 on circulating tumor cells in patients with metastatic breast cancer. Mol Oncol 7(3):680–692
Smerage JB, Barlow WE, Hortobagyi GN et al (2014) Circulating tumor cells and response to chemotherapy in metastatic breast cancer: SWOG S0500. J Clin Oncol 32(31):3483–3489
Somlo G, Lau SK, Frankel P et al (2011) Multiple biomarker expression on circulating tumor cells in comparison to tumor tissues from primary and metastatic sites in patients with locally advanced/inflammatory, and stage IV breast cancer, using a novel detection technology. Breast Cancer Res Treat 128(1):155–163
Steinestel J, Luedeke M, Arndt A et al (2015) Detecting predictive androgen receptor modifications in circulating prostate cancer cells. Oncotarget. doi:10.18632/oncotarget.3925
Thorsteinsson M, Jess P (2011) The clinical significance of circulating tumor cells in non-metastatic colorectal cancer—a review. Eur J Surg Oncol 37(6):459–465
Tsai WS, Chen JS, Shao HJ et al (2016) Circulating tumor cell count correlates with colorectal neoplasm progression and is a prognostic marker for distant metastasis in non-metastatic patients. Sci Rep 6:24517
Uen YH, Lu CY, Tsai HL et al (2008) Persistent presence of postoperative circulating tumor cells is a poor prognostic factor for patients with stage I-III colorectal cancer after curative resection. Ann Surg Oncol 15(8):2120–2128
Van Berckelaer C, Brouwers AJ, Peeters DJ et al (2016) Current and future role of circulating tumor cells in patients with epithelial ovarian cancer. Eur J Surg Oncol 42:1772–1779
Wan L, Pantel K, Kang Y (2013) Tumor metastasis: moving new biological insights into the clinic. Nat Med 19(11):1450–1464
Wiedswang G, Borgen E, Karesen R et al (2004) Isolated tumor cells in bone marrow three years after diagnosis in disease-free breast cancer patients predict unfavorable clinical outcome. Clin Cancer Res 10(16):5342–5348
Wong SC, Chan CM, Ma BB et al (2009) Clinical significance of cytokeratin 20-positive circulating tumor cells detected by a refined immunomagnetic enrichment assay in colorectal cancer patients. Clin Cancer Res 15(3):1005–1012
Yu Y, Chen Z, Dong J et al (2013) Folate receptor-positive circulating tumor cells as a novel diagnostic biomarker in non-small cell lung cancer. Transl Oncol 6(6):697–702
Yu M, Bardia A, Aceto N et al (2014) Cancer therapy. Ex vivo culture of circulating breast tumor cells for individualized testing of drug susceptibility. Science 345(6193):216–220

Chapter 2
Strategies for Isolation and Molecular Profiling of Circulating Tumor Cells

Jia-Yang Chen and Ying-Chih Chang

Abstract Cancer is the leading cause of death by disease worldwide, and metastasis is responsible for more than 90% of the mortality of cancer patients. Metastasis occurs when tumor cells leave the primary tumor, travel through the blood stream as circulating tumor cells (CTCs), and then colonize secondary tumors at sites distant from the primary tumor. The capture, identification, and analysis of CTCs offer both scientific and clinical benefits. On the scientific side, the analysis of CTCs could help elucidate possible genetic alterations and signaling pathway aberrations during cancer progression, which could then be used to find new methods to stop cancer progression. On the clinical side, non-invasive testing of a patient's blood for CTCs can be used for patient diagnosis and prognosis, as well as subsequent monitoring of treatment efficacy in routine clinical practice. Additionally, investigation of CTCs early in the progression of cancer may reveal targets for initial cancer detection and for anti-cancer treatment. This chapter will evaluate strategies and devices used for the isolation and identification of CTCs directly from clinical samples of blood. Recent progress in the understanding of the significance of both single CTCs and circulating tumor microemboli will be discussed. Also, advancements in the use of CTC-based liquid biopsy in clinical diagnosis and the potential of CTC-based molecular characterization for use in clinical applications will be summarized.

Keywords Circulating tumor cells • CTC isolation • Molecular characterization • CTC Clinical relevance and utility • Liquid biopsy

J.-Y. Chen • Y.-C. Chang (✉)
Genomics Research Center, Academia Sinica, 128, Sec. 2, Academic Rd., Nankang, Taipei 115, Taiwan
e-mail: yingchih@gate.sinica.edu.tw

M.J.M. Magbanua, J.W. Park (eds.), *Isolation and Molecular Characterization of Circulating Tumor Cells*, Advances in Experimental Medicine and Biology 994,
DOI 10.1007/978-3-319-55947-6_2

2.1 Metastasis and Dissemination of Cancer Cells

Cancer is a leading cause of disease death worldwide. Cancer metastasis is believed to responsible for the recurrence of cancer as well as the mortality of cancer patients. Metastasis starts with the shedding of cancer cells from the primary tumor. Once the primary tumor established, the epithelial origin of the primary cancer cells will enable local migration and invasion, leading to dissemination of the tumor cells into the bloodstream through intravasation (Chaffer and Weinberg 2011). Despite continuous intravasation of the cancer cells into blood stream during cancer progression, not all of the disseminated cancer cells survive through the strong shear stress and escape from apoptosis/anoikis mediated cell death in circulation (Mehlen and Puisieux 2006; Mitchell and King 2013). The disseminated cancer cells present in circulating blood are known as circulating tumor cells (CTCs). Pre-metastasis CTCs from a primary tumor early in the progression of cancer progression present an opportunity for further investigation on the mechanism of early cancer progression and later metastasis establishment. The surviving CTCs will travel through the body and attach at a preferential site for further adaptation, after appropriate extravasation and migration, to form a secondary colonization as the malignant tumor. Whether the cancer cells disseminate early and lie dormant for metabolic adaptation and later proliferation, or disseminate late to accumulate sufficient mutations and facilitate further cancer progression is still under debate (Podsypanina et al. 2008; Klein 2008). Identification of CTCs in the bloodstream during cancer metastasis may provide an opportunity to investigate potential mechanisms participate in cancer progression, reveal early detection targets of cancer dissemination, and elucidate potential strategies for anti-cancer therapy development.

During the progression of cancer metastasis, the epithelial-to-mesenchymal transition (EMT) has been shown to correlate with the shedding of primary tumor cells into the bloodstream (Chaffer and Weinberg 2011). The epithelial-origin cancer cells from the primary tumor may undergo the EMT transition to facilitate cancer cell migration and invasion progression. Through EMT, cancer cells can invade surrounding tissues and finally escape from primary site into bloodstream. Further mesenchymal-to-epithelial transition (MET) of the metastatic cancer cells may re-express epithelial phenotypes after extravasation and enable colonization at a distant site. It has been reported that the expression of EMT markers on CTCs show dynamic inverse expression in between epithelial (ex: cytokeratin 5, 7, 8, 18, 19, and EpCAM) and mesenchymal markers (ex: fibronectin 1, cadherin 2, and SERPINE/PAI 1) in clinical breast cancer patients under chemotherapy treatment (Yu et al. 2013). It has also been reported that over 80% of the CTCs in patients with metastatic, castration-resistant prostate cancer and metastatic breast cancer express both epithelial and mesenchymal markers (Armstrong et al. 2011). Despite the dynamic expression of both epithelial and mesenchymal markers on the cancer cell surface, suggested basal level expression of the epithelial/mesenchymal markers presenting as major population on CTCs as a mixed-expression cell type and could be used as surface marker to distinguish cancer cells from blood cells.

2.2 Strategies for Enrichment of CTCs

Despite the very low concentration of CTCs observed in circulation, a variety of technologies have been disclosed for the identification and isolation of CTCs from blood samples of cancer patients. Due to the short half-life of the CTCs in bloodstream (estimated from 1 to 2.4 h) (Meng et al. 2004), CTC isolation devices must be efficient enough to preserve potential CTCs for further investigation. Because the CTCs are shed from the primary solid tumor, biological properties such as expression of cell surface adhesion molecule (ex: EpCAM) or deficiency in expression of blood-type surface antigen markers (ex: leukocyte marker CD45, granulocyte marker CD15) could be used to distinguish CTCs from blood cells. Also, physical properties, such as size, density, or electric charge, could be used as selection criteria for CTC isolation. The approaches in CTC-isolating devices include size-based filtration exclusion (Vona et al. 2000; Lee et al. 2014), density-based centrifugation isolation (Williams et al. 2015), biological affinity-based immuno-magnetic beads selection (Powell et al. 2012), antibody-functionalized microfluidic platforms (Nagrath et al. 2007; Kirby et al. 2012), surface-modified cell enrichment chips (Ke et al. 2015), acoustic-based cell selection devices (Antfolk et al. 2015), electric-charge-based electrophoresis (Adams et al. 2009), and a combination of multiple properties for CTC isolation (Ozkumur et al. 2013). Although there are different properties and advantages amongst the diverse platforms for capturing and isolating CTCs, size-based exclusion, density-based isolation, and antibody-based affinity capture remain the three major methods used for the isolation and identification of CTCs.

2.2.1 Size-Based Exclusion for CTCs Isolation

One of the first approaches to isolate CTCs from blood samples was based on the difference in size between tumor cells and blood cells. The average size of red blood cells (RBCs), white blood cells (WBCs), and monocytes is 6–8 μm, 10–15 μm, and 15–30 μm, respectively. Tumor cells have a high nuclear to cytoplasm ratio and higher stiffness, with an average size of 20 μm. Their larger size, compared to WBCs, led to the use of marker-free, size-based filtration for CTC isolation directly from blood. The size-based exclusion technology is featured in rapid separation and non-selected marker-free isolation for the CTCs, though the technology may not be able to distinguish monocytes from CTCs in blood samples. The early implementation of size-based exclusion used a commercially available, porous filter membrane to isolate the CTCs from blood samples (Seal 1964).

Problems that may need to be addressed to meet the critical utility for the size-based isolation and characterization approach include non-even pore sizes, low pore density, and the inability to isolate and hold the CTC. Recently, size-based CTC isolation using a microfabricated microfilter made by etching a polymer membrane with reactive ion etching to give precisely controlled pore sizes and density was demonstrated (Zhou et al. 2014). The isolation by size of epithelial tumor cells (ISET) technology is one of the earliest marker-free technologies to isolate CTCs based on the larger size of epithelial tumor cells by directly filtering blood through a calibrated, polycarbonate Track-Etch-type membrane with 8-μm-diameter pores. The ISET technology can detect CTCs in 80% of samples from stage III-IV in non-small cell lung cancer (NSCLC), and provides label-free CTC samples for further morphological, immunocytological, and genetic characterization of individual CTCs (Vona et al. 2000).

2.2.2 Density-Based Centrifugation for Isolation of CTCs

Blood contains various types of cells, including abundant RBCs, nucleated WBCs (including eosinophils, basophils, neutrophils, lymphocytes, and monocytes), and heterogeneous CTCs populations of varying number density in cancer patients. Density-based centrifugation technologies take advantage of the difference in cell density between blood cells to isolate nucleated cells directly from whole blood. By using mixtures of high molecular weight sucrose polymers and sodium diatrizoate, such as Ficoll-Paque, CTCs can be isolated from whole blood. Density-based separation provides rapid and non-selective methods, without additional processing, that enable obtaining viable cells directly from blood samples. But the density-based centrifugation methods show very low purity of the isolated CTCs due to the concomitant isolation of nucleated WBCs with the CTCs. Recently, Williams et al. have successfully established a patient-derived xenograft mouse model by using CTCs isolated from prostate cancer patients through density-based centrifugation accompanied with RBC lysis and additional CD45-depletion (Williams et al. 2015). The patient-derived mouse xenograft model provides a model platform for further investigation of CTCs in functional studies or molecular characterization*in vivo*.

2.2.3 Biological Affinity-Based Selection for Capture of CTCs

Most solid tumors derive from epithelial origin cells, which express EpCAM on the cell surface to facilitate cell-cell contact and adhesion. Identification of epithelial-origin tumor cells in the blood stream by using the anti-EpCAM antibody as an affinity-based method to capture CTCs provides good sensitivity and specificity in the isolation of CTCs from blood. However, selective capture of EpCAM-positive cells in the blood stream may result in a bias in the CTC population selection and may possibly lead to the loss of other CTC populations, such as those that have gone through EMT. It has been reported that most CTCs express both epithelial and mesenchymal markers on the cell surface (Armstrong et al. 2011), suggesting that EpCAM-based affinity capture could isolate the majority of the population of both epithelial and mesenchymal types of CTCs disseminated from solid tumors. The CellSearch® platform, the first CTC detection platform approved by FDA, uses anti-EpCAM to isolate CTCs and has been used as a standard for CTC studies in various types of cancers, including prostate, breast, ovarian, colorectal, lung, pancreatic, and head and neck cancer (Allard et al. 2004; Bidard et al. 2013; Grobe et al. 2014). Since the release of the CellSearch® platform, affinity-based devices for more sensitive and specific capture of CTCs have been developed.

The MagSweeper system was developed using 4.5 μm magnetic beads coated with antibody against human EpCAM for the isolation of CTCs directly from blood samples. The system shows higher CTC detection rates (70%) in metastatic breast cancer than the CellSearch® platform and is feasible for downstream molecular analysis such as single cell profiling (Powell et al. 2012; Deng et al. 2014). In addition, Nagrath et al. developed the CTC-chip for more efficient and selective separation of the CTCs from blood samples (Nagrath et al. 2007). The CTC-chip features as a microfluidic system consisting of anti-EpCAM-conjugated microspot arrays and is operated under predesigned laminar flow conditions without prelabeling of the blood samples. The platform reaches 99% identification rate in metastatic lung, prostate, pancreatic, breast, and colon cancer patients with high CTC capture number and approximately 50% purity. Although these devices demonstrated high efficiency in capturing CTCs directly from blood, releasing intact and viable cells from the devices is still a challenge.

In addition to the techniques describe above, Magbanua et al. have also reported a method that combines immunomagnetic enrichment and fluorescence-activated cell sorting (IE/FACS) for the specific isolation of CTCs using two independent EpCAM specific antibodies (Magbanua and Park 2013). The first EpCAM antibody is conjugated with magnetic beads for the initial separation of CTCs from blood cells. The initial separation is followed by the addition of fluorescence-conjugated EpCAM for secondary recognition and detection using FACS analysis. The CTCs isolated with IE/FACS has been used to isolate pure CTCs for molecular/genomic profiling such as RT-PCR, DNA sequencing, array-based comparative genomic hybridization (array-CGH), and microarray analysis for a variety of cancers, including liver and breast (Magbanua et al. 2013, 2015; Kelley et al. 2015; Lang et al. 2015). A wide range of copy number aberrations identified by array-CGH analysis confirmed primary tumor origin of CTCs. Gene expression array analysis of CTCs captured by IE/FACS revealed down-regulation in apoptosis signal and absence of immune signal in metastasized breast cancer. The assays further proved the feasibility of using CTC samples for clinical applications and the lineage diversity shared between the primary tumor and CTCs.

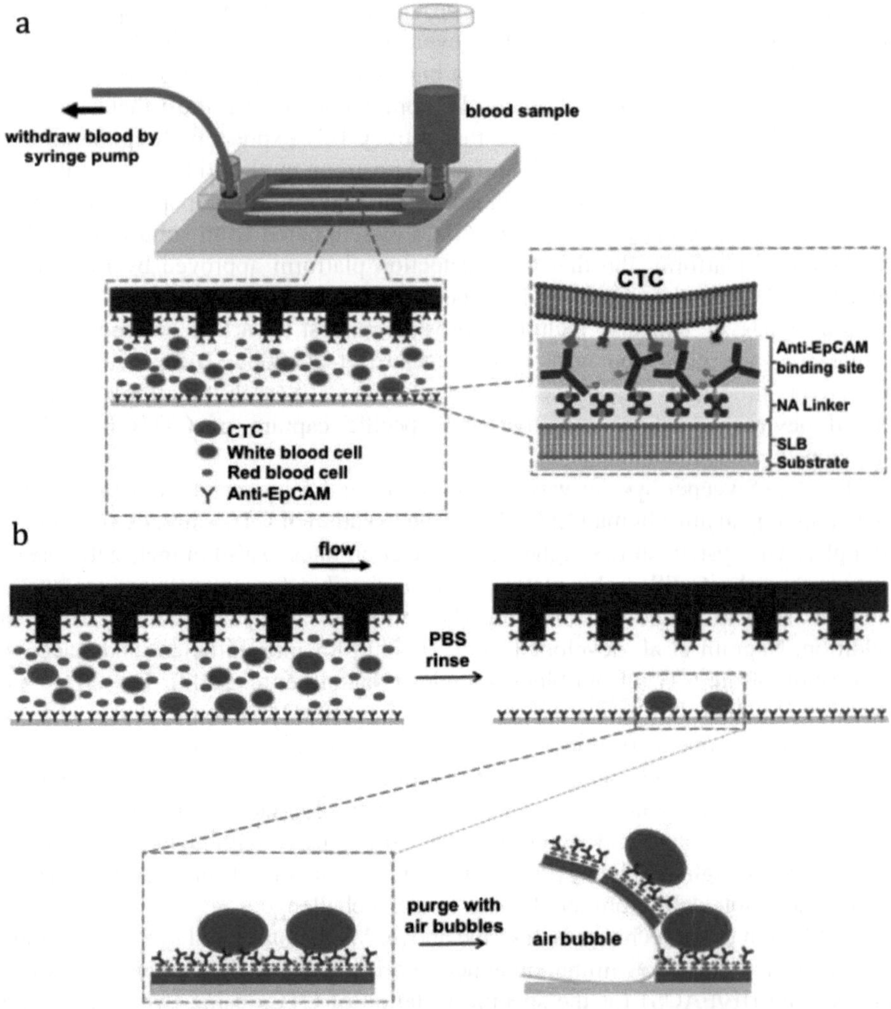

Fig. 2.1 Schematic of the CMx process for capturing and releasing circulating tumor cells (*CTCs*) (**a**) Blood is drawn through a microfluidic channel that is coated with a supported lipid bilayer (*SLB*) that is conjugated via NeutrAvidin (*NA*) to anti-EpCAM antibody. The anti-EpCAM antibody is able to capture CTCs directly from whole blood samples. (**b**) After the blood sample has been drawn through the microchannel, a phosphate buffered saline (*PBS*) rinse is used to flush out the red and white blood cells. The CTCs are then released with an air bubble, which disrupts the cohesion of the SLB to the substrate (Cancer Biology and Therapy (2016))

A recently developed system that enables effective release of viable CTCs is the CMx system. The CMx platform consists of a microfluidic chip through which a blood sample can be drawn with a syringe pump. The microchannels in the chip are coated with a supported lipid bilayer (SLB) that is conjugated to anti-EpCAM via a NeutrAvidin linker, as shown in Fig. 2.1a. The anti-EpCAM isolates any CTCs in the blood while other blood cells flow past. The release of CTCs is accomplished by introducing of air foam, which disrupts the hydrophobic interactions of the SLB with the substrate, as shown in Fig. 2.1b (Chen et al. 2016). The CMx platform sustains high cell capture efficiency (>95%) and releases viable cells for further molecular analysis and *in vitro* cultivation. The platform shows high sensitivity and specificity in identifying cancer patients from healthy individuals and is also able to distinguish early from late stage patients through CTC enumeration.

In another affinity-based microfluidic approach, Ke et al. have developed a thermo-responsive NanaVelcro CTC purification system, which integrates EpCAM-antibody-coated 3D poly(N-isopropyl acrylamide) brushes as a thermo-responsive substrate that can capture and release cells from the chip surface at 37 °C and 4 °C, respectively (Ke et al. 2015). Higher capture efficiency of NanoVelcro CTC capture platform compared to CellSearch® and capable in culture expansion and mutational analyses are opportunities created by using a microfluidic chip system for both clinical applications and disease monitoring (Ke et al. 2015; He et al. 2016).

Besides the positive EpCAM-based affinity capture of epithelial-origin CTC cells, negative selection by using blood cell-specific surface markers provides an alternative strategy for the population enrichment of CTCs without pre-selection of tumor markers. The multi-marker immune-magnetic negative depletion enrichment of CTCs (MINDEC) strategy takes advantage of using magnetic beads conjugated with multiple blood cell-markers including CD45 (pan-leukocytes), CD16 (natural killer cells and neutrophil granulocytes), CD19 (B-cells), CD163 (monocytes and macrophages), and CD235a (RBCs) to deplete the blood cells and enrich CTC population from blood samples (Lapin et al. 2016). The strategy shows good cell recovery rate (82 ± 10%) and depletion efficiency (437 ± 350 residual WBCs). The MINDEC strategy enables 71% positive detecting rate of CTCs in metastatic pancreatic cancer patients. Despite the effectiveness and marker-free selection of WBC-based negative selection for CTC isolation, aggregates of CTCs with WBCs such as CTC microembolisms (CTMs) may be eliminated from the major CTCs population selected by this strategy. Additionally, surface marker-based selection by using fluorescence activated cell sorting (FACS) screening also provides possibilities in analysis of marker-specific CTC populations in circulation (Reyes et al. 2014; Neves et al. 2014).

2.2.4 Combination of Multiple Properties for Purification of CTCs

The use of a combination of technologies for CTC separation provides an opportunity to capture and isolate CTCs with higher sensitivity, specificity, and efficiency. The CTC-iChip isolates CTCs based on a combination of several features including size exclusion, affinity-based negative selection, and magnetic separation to obtain a population of pure CTCs directly from whole blood samples (Ozkumur et al. 2013). The microspots in the first stage of the CTC-iChip provide hydrodynamic cell size sorting to separate the RBCs, platelets, plasma proteins, and free magnetic beads from WBCs and CTCs population. The second stage takes advantage of inertial focusing to order nucleated cells within the microfluidic channel. The final step involves the separation of any residual, tagged WBCs from the CTC population. This negative selection is accomplished by magnetic deflection of pre-mixed CD45 and CD15 immunomagnetic beads, with any residual WBCs attached to them. The CTC-iChip has demonstrated up to 95% cell recovery of various cell lines and identified 90% of cancer recurrence in prostate cancer patients based on triple stained CTC enumeration. The device shows efficient isolation with high purity of captured cells and enables further molecular characterization such as single cell RNA expression validation (Ozkumur et al. 2013). Similarly, Kirby et al. developed a geometrically enhanced differential immunocapture (GEDI) device for CTC isolation that features a combination of both size-based exclusion and affinity-based capture for the PSMA-positive CTCs from castration resistant prostate cancer blood samples (Kirby et al. 2012). In comparison with the CellSearch® system, the GEDI device shows a 2–400-fold increase in the number of CTCs captured in the same patient, indicating a remarkable improvement in the efficiency of CTC capture.

Although each CTC capturing technology has drawbacks in either CTC population bias or impurity in isolation of the cells, the count of isolated CTCs shows significant correlation with clinical outcome and prognosis prediction, as well as cancer progression and therapeutic treatment efficacy. The determination of more specific markers or isolation strategies for CTC isolation/purification will benefit the clinical utility of future application in blood-based cancer diagnosis.

2.3 Clinical Importance of CTCs and CTMs

As described above, CTCs can act as metastatic seeds spreading through circulation and colonizing at a preferential site for growth or dormant adaptation (Klein 2008; Podsypanina et al. 2008). CTCs were first identified by Thomas Ashworth in a male metastatic cancer patient. Ashworth postulated the existence of tumor cells in the blood that were similar with the primary tumor as the explanation of the formation of multi-tumor disease (Ashworth 1869). After Ashworth, Paget et al. brought out the seed-and-soil theory to describe their observation in breast cancer metastases, further suggesting the existence of tumor cells in circulation that have been shed from a primary tumor (Paget 1989). In the early 1990s, immunohistochemistry analyses identified micrometastasis in both lymph nodes and bone marrow (Smerage and Hayes 2008). At the same time molecular analyses, such as reverse-transcription polymerase chain reaction and fluorescence in situ hybridization techniques, were developed for the detection of metastatic cancer in circulation and correlated with tumor-positive patients (Katz et al. 1994; Smith et al. 1991).

A challenge in the detection of CTCs is that they are extremely rare in the bloodstream. The concentration of CTCs has been identified to be in the range of

1–10 cells per mL of blood, compared to 6×10^6 white blood cells, 2×10^8 platelets, and 4×10^9 erythrocytes per mL of blood (Allard et al. 2004; Coumans et al. 2012). Not until 2004, when Allard and colleagues used the CellSearch® system for specifically detecting CTCs in prostate, breast, ovarian, colorectal, and lung cancer patients from non-malignant patients and healthy donors, did translational research in CTC identification begin to be a possible tool for cancer detection and prognosis determination in cancer patients (Allard et al. 2004). Compared to traditional computer tomography (CT) and magnetic resonance imaging (MRI) scans, CTC enumeration is considered as a better marker for predicting overall survival in cancer patients (Budd et al. 2006).

Results from studies analyzing CTCs of a broad range of cancers indicate the potential benefits in screening of early cancer patients for CTCs and treatment efficacy of monitoring CTCs for future diagnosis. For example, it has been reported that an increase in the number of CTCs correlates with poor cancer prognosis and distant metastasis in multiple myeloma, colorectal, oral, and lung cancers (Gonsalves et al. 2014; Iinuma et al. 2011; Grobe et al. 2014; Tanaka et al. 2009). Elevated CTC numbers in breast, colon, oral, prostate, lung, and ovarian cancers show shorter overall survival (OS) and decreased progression-free survival (PFS) compared to patients with low CTC numbers (Cristofanilli et al. 2004; Hayes et al. 2006; Bidard et al. 2014; Aggarwal et al. 2013; de Bono et al. 2008; Iinuma et al. 2011; Grobe et al. 2014; Krebs et al. 2011; Poveda et al. 2011). Fluctuation of the number of CTCs in the blood tightly correlates with the progression and treatment efficacy in head and neck cancer (Qiao et al. 2015; Grisanti et al. 2014), showing the benefits of long-term real-time monitoring of disease progression after treatment. In addition, positive correlation of high CTC counts with a high risk of recurrence and poor prognosis has also been reported in a multi-institutional study of colorectal cancer patients (Iinuma et al. 2011). Furthermore, CTC counts in colorectal and lung cancers correlates with the stage of cancer progression (Chen et al. 2016; Lu et al. 2015; Nel et al. 2014), and correlates with after-treatment survival in castration-resistant prostate cancer (Scher et al. 2015). Additionally, CTC counts are higher in portal venous blood than in peripheral blood in pancreatic cancer patients, and portal CTC counts act as a significant indicator for liver metastasis within 6 months after adequate surgery (Tien et al. 2016). Similarly, higher CTC counts observed in central venous blood, compared with peripheral venous blood, in both breast and cervical cancers have also been observed (Peeters et al. 2015). By using the quantitative reverse transcription polymerase chain reaction (RT-qPCR) technique, they confirmed that there was no significant difference in the expression of 12 selected genes between central and peripheral venous CTCs. They also reported that a higher count of tumor cell emboli was observed in the microvasculature of the metastatic patient with higher CTC counts, suggesting that microvascular retention and cell-microenvironment interaction may contribute to the advancement of the metastasis of the cancer.

Recently, identification of CTC clusters and CTMs in the bloodstream has shown clinically to be significant associated with distant metastasis. The CTC clusters, defined as aggregates of more than 2 CTCs, have been identified in circulation from cancers including colorectal, prostate, beast, pancreas, and small cell lung cancers (Yu et al. 2013; Hou et al. 2012; Aceto et al. 2014; Molnar et al. 2001). CTMs represent one or more CTCs, accompanied with or without WBCs, including CTC clusters (Chen et al. 2016). Due to their extremely low concentration in circulating blood, only in the past few years have their been methods of CTC capture that were able to isolate and purify CTCs and CTMs from cancer patients including breast, prostate, colon, and pancreatic cancers (Aceto et al. 2014; Sarioglu et al. 2015; Chen et al. 2016; Chang et al. 2016). The presence of CTC clusters in circulation highly correlate with late stage and poor prognosis in lung, prostate, and metastatic breast cancers (Hou et al. 2012; Aceto et al. 2014). Because interactions between cancer cells and immune cells are required for immune response, cancer cells may take advantage of mutations acquired for immune contact to facilitate their dissemination and survival during the progression of metastasis (Iwai et al. 2002). Interactions between CTCs, WBCs, and endothelial cells will further give rise to CTMs containing CTCs combined with WBCs, and promote both the survival and the metastatic ability of CTCs through adhesion and ligand-receptor conjugations on the cell surface (Chen et al. 2011). The presence of both CTC clusters and CTC-WBC-combined CTMs have already been identified in various cancers including colorectal, breast, prostate, and lung cancer (Stott et al. 2010a; Molnar et al. 2001; Reategui et al. 2015; Sarioglu et al. 2015; Chen et al. 2016). In addition, unfavorable CTM counts of over 30 per 2 mL of blood are indicative prognostic markers for both disease-free survival and overall survival in pancreatic ductal adenocarcinoma (Chang et al. 2016).

Aggregates of CTCs, such as CTMs, in the bloodstream have been suggested to provide a cell-cell adhesion advantage against shear stress in the blood stream and to activate survival signaling toward apoptosis and protection from anoikis (Hou et al. 2012; Yu et al. 2013). Evidence in β-integrin-mediated collective movement of primary tumor cells may provide further opportunity for the shedding of CTMs into the bloodstream (Ilina and Friedl 2009; Duda et al. 2010; Hegerfeldt et al. 2002). Attenuation of plakoglobin-mediated cell-cell interaction resulted in the absence of CTMs in circulation, diminished secondary metastasis in an animal model, and correlated with distant metastasis-free survival in breast cancer patients (Aceto et al. 2014). In addition, it has been reported that WBCs are able to fuse with tumor cells in a primary tumor and thereby facilitate invasion and intravasation of the cancer cells into circulation as CTMs, subsequently triggering metastasis of the tumor (Jiang et al. 2013; Man 2010). Recently, Au*et al.* has demonstrated the ability of tightly joined CTC clusters to traverse through micro-vessels and resist dissociation under the treatment of FAK inhibitor or paclitaxel drugs designed to weaken cell-cell interactions (Au et al. 2016). Their results further support the metastatic role of the CTMs during cancer progression. In contrast, the EMT transition is considered to be a non-essential process in cancer progression but is involved in the chemoresistance of both pancreatic and lung cancer (Zheng et al. 2015; Fischer et al. 2015), suggesting that the EMT transition may not be necessary during WBC-mediated intravasation or collective-movement-mediated CTM cancer metastasis.

2.4 Clinical Utility of Molecular Characterization of CTCs

Currently, the detection and diagnosis of common solid tumors is based on imaging modalities such as CT and MRI scans. Therapeutic regimens are made based on the formal TNM classification system coupled with ultrasound-guided fine-needle aspiration (FNA) and pathologic assessment of tissue biopsy (Ludwig and Weinstein 2005). Although improvements in imaging technology have allowed more sensitive detection of small cancer lesions, an increase in false-positive diagnoses can occur during CT image scanning (Hanash et al. 2011). Positron emission tomography (PET), CT, or MRI imaging can determine anatomic delineation of primary tumor lesions, but there is insufficient resolution and accuracy for micrometastasis detection. The FNA cytology analysis is a standard diagnostic procedure for both breast and pancreatic cancers, but current diagnoses still suffered from low accuracy due to limited sensitivity (75–94%) and specificity (78–95%) such as in pancreatic cancer (Gerhard and Schmitt 2014; Court et al. 2015). In contrast, the TNM classification protocol is the most useful system for developing a therapy strategy but it requires invasive tissue assessment based on surgical procedures and is unable to validate further information from pre-metastatic lesions (e.g., disseminated cancer cells during cancer progression in circulation before secondary metastasis establishment) and follow-up evaluations. Non-invasive blood-based biomarkers, such as serum tumor markers, have been discovered to have potential in screening, treatment response monitoring, and recurrence evaluation of cancer patients. For example, carbohydrate antigen 125 (CA-125) is a membranous glycoprotein that is used for cancer screening, therapy monitoring, recurrence detection, and prognosis evaluation in ovarian cancer. The carbohydrate antigen 19–9 (CA19–9) is a sialyl-Lewis antigen was been found up-regulated in several cancers and is used in therapy monitoring of pancreatic cancer. Similarly, prostate-specific antigen (PSA) and prostate specific membrane antigen (PSMA), glycoproteins specifically expressed by prostate tissue that increase serum concentration through disruption of anatomic barriers during cancer progression, are used for prostate cancer screening and diagnosis (Kulasingam and Diamandis 2008). However, very few serum tumor markers have been used in clinical applications due to deficiencies in specific clinical validations and side-by-side studies. In spite of the routinely used CA-125 tests in combination with CT scans in ovarian cancer surveillance after treatment remission, an increase in the use of chemotherapy and decrease in the quality of life without improvement in ovarian cancer patients has recently been reported (Esselen et al. 2016). In addition, low sensitivity and specificity in early stage cancer detection and the inability to distinguish aggressive from indolent tumors limits the clinical diagnostic utility of serum markers (Hanash et al. 2011).

2.4.1 Clinical Utility of Liquid-Based CTC Enumeration

Recently, liquid biopsy based on the isolation of CTCs in blood provides an opportunity to detect and characterize cancer for patient stratification and treatment monitoring. The first intervention trial, SWOG S0500, used CTC enumeration in the study of chemotherapy treatment response and patient prognosis based on the change in CTC count. The results confirmed that the CTC count fluctuates during chemotherapy treatment and indicates high CTC counts reflect a poor prognosis and therapy response in metastatic breast cancer patients (Smerage et al. 2014). In addition, clinical trials COU-AA-301 and IMMC-38 identified a 30% decline in CTC count from baseline after 4 weeks of chemotherapy, which acted as an independent prognostic factor that was associated with better overall survival compared to stable CTC counts in advanced prostate cancer patients (Lorente et al. 2016). The eSCOUT clinical trial of advanced colorectal cancer patients verified shorter overall survival in patients with high CTC count and indicated possible benefits for avoiding high-toxicity regimens in patients with low CTC count patients (Krebs et al. 2015). Multivariate analysis of high portal venous CTC counts also provide a significant predictor of liver metastasis within 6 months after adequate surgery in pancreatic cancer (Tien et al. 2016). A similar result also identified in NSCLC that the presence of CTCs after surgery was significantly associated with shorter disease-free survival and early recurrence in stage I-III patients undergoing radical resection (Bayarri-Lara et al. 2016). A CTC subpopulation analysis showed that an increase in CD133/panCK ratio or N-cadherin-positive CTCs significantly correlated with progression-free survival in NSCLC (Nel et al. 2014). Besides CTC enumeration, CTCs taken from small cell lung cancer patients demonstrated their capacity for xenograft growth by using immunocompromised mice with preserved morphology and genetic characteristics, and faithfully recapitulated the treatment response toward anticancer therapies (Hodgkinson et al. 2014). Among the studies in CTC-based verification, enumeration, and characterization, CTCs show potential clinical utility in monitoring cancer treatment efficacy, responding to prognosis prediction, and screening drugs for cancer patients.

2.4.2 Clinical Utility of ARv7 Gene Transcript Variant Verification in Prostate Cancer CTCs

Targeting androgen receptor (AR) signaling in prostate cancer by AR inhibitor abiraterone or enzalutamide has been used as a first line treatment in prostate cancer. However AR castration resistance and relapse remains an important issue in prostate cancer treatment. Expression of androgen receptor splice isoform variant 7 (ARv7) transcript has recently been identified in association with formation of castration-resistant prostate cancer (CRPC). The ARv7 transcript protein acts as a constitutive active transcription factor after nucleus translocation due to a lack of an AR ligand-binding domain. Identification of an ARv7 transcription variant in CTCs of CRPC patients disclosed a significant correlation in ARv7 expression with lower PSA response rates, shorter PSA progression-free survival, shorter clinical or radiographic progression-free survival, and shorter overall survival in ARv7-positive prostate cancer patients (Antonarakis et al. 2014). Dynamic ARv7 expression may reflect selective pressure during AR-directed therapies and serve as a potential marker for real-time treatment monitoring and prognosis prediction using liquid biopsy of CTCs (Nakazawa et al. 2015). In addition, despite its primary resistance to taxanes chemotherapy, ARv7-positive CRPC patients appear to be responsive to taxanes treatment rather than AR-directed therapies and can be evaluated using liquid biopsy of CTCs (Antonarakis et al. 2015). Furthermore, next generation sequencing of CTCs from CRPC patients revealed that activation of noncanonical Wnt signaling participates in AR castration-resistancy of prostate cancer (Miyamoto et al. 2015). Ectopic expression of Wnt5a shows an increase resistance against AR-inhibition treatment through attenuation of the anti-proliferation effect in prostate cancer cells, whereas suppression of Wnt5a restores AR-treatment sensitivity in drug-resistant cell lines. The results provide solid evidence in elucidating mechanisms that participate in cancer progression and show the feasibility of using CTCs as non-invasive approach for further investigations.

2.4.3 *Clinical Utility of CTC-Based Liquid Biopsy in PD1/PDL1 Targeted Therapy*

In addition to ARv7 gene validation, a variety of genes have also been verified in CTCs for cancer detection, patient stratification, and treatment monitoring in cancer patients. Overexpression of PD1 ligands (PD-L1) has been discovered on the surface of a variety of cancer cells for immune-escape including melanoma, lung, and ovarian cancers (Pardoll 2012). The PD-L1 serves as strong inhibitory ligand for the PD-1 receptor (CD279), which expresses on the surface of an activated T-cell. Once the PD-L1 bonds with the PD-1 receptor through the ligand-receptor binding effect, the tumor cells will accomplish immune escape by inhibition of the T-cell activity and reduction of cytokine production accompanied with suppression of T-cell proliferation. Targeting PD-1/PD-L1 signaling with the PD-1/PD-L1 antibody has recently been approved by the FDA for the treatment of metastatic melanoma, lymphoma, metastatic renal carcinoma, NSCLC, and head and neck cancer (Chen and Han 2015). Although patients who do not express PD1 ligands can still respond to PD1/PD-L1 blockade therapy, a higher response rate in PD-L1-expressed tumors toward PD1/PD-L1 blockade therapy has been reported for multiple tumor types (Postow et al. 2015). Identification of PD1/PD-L1 ligand expression has been reported as potential biomarker in predicting PD1/PD-L1 blockade therapeutic response (Rossille et al. 2014). In this fashion, the identification of patients with PD-L1 expression will help with treatment guidance and increase the therapeutic response rate. Recently, Mazel et al. used liquid biopsy of CTCs to identify PD-L1-positive CTCs in breast cancer patients (Mazel et al. 2015). The results indicate the possibility of using liquid biopsy for patient stratification and treatment guidance based on PD1 ligand expression on CTCs.

2.4.4 Clinical Utility of Molecular Characterization of CTCs for TKIs/ALK Targeting Therapy in Lung Cancer Treatment

Lung cancer has long been a leading cause of cancer death worldwide. Various chemotherapeutic approaches have been developed for the treatment of lung cancer including tyrosine kinase inhibitors (TKIs) and anaplastic lymphoma kinase (ALK) targeting therapies. However, mutations in tyrosine kinases downstream of epidermal growth factor receptor (EGFR) signaling, including Kirsten rat sarcoma (KRAS), proto-oncogene BRAF, and EGFR itself, will give rise to treatment resistance after TKI therapies. The detection of exon 19 deletion and exon 21 mutation in L858R and T790 M of the EGFR gene has been used as a biomarker that imply treatment resistance toward EGFR-TKI therapies in lung cancer patients (Sun et al. 2015). In all of these cases, it is still difficult to obtain tissue biopsies from each time point during chemotherapy regiments and afterwards for follow-up analyses. Identification of both KRAS mutations (Tsao et al. 2010) and EGFR mutations (Marchetti et al. 2014; Ran et al. 2013) in CTCs represents potential clinical applications of CTC characterization for treatment efficacy monitoring, resistance detection, and treatment guidance. In addition, about 3–7% of NSCLC patients been identified with oncogenic gene fusion between ALK and echinoderm microtubule associated protein-like 4 (EML4). Rearrangement of the EML4-ALK gene results in constitutive kinase activity of the ALK and provides downstream survival and proliferation of the cancer cells. Identification of CTCs in NSCLC patients with ALK gene rearrangement has been detected with CTC-based liquid biopsy and confirmed by pathological tests (Ilie et al. 2012; Pailler et al. 2013; Faugeroux et al. 2014; He et al. 2016). The establishment of chemotherapy target-based verification assays, such as assays for ARv7 transcript, PD1 ligands, ALK rearrangement, and EGFR mutations, shows the possibility and feasibility of non-invasive liquid biopsy as a clinical utility in patient stratification, chemotherapeutic guidance, real time treatment monitoring, prognosis prediction, and personalized medicine treatment.

2.4.5 Clinical Utility of CTC Molecular Analysis for Identification of Primary Cancer of Origin

The 5-year survival rate of patients with all types of solid tumors decreases significantly with the stage progression (Siegel et al. 2016). Based on the statistical observation, early cancer detection provides better opportunities to treat and manage cancer when it may still be curable. Systematic spreading of breast cancer, occuring early in the cancer progression, into both bone and lung has been demonstrated in HER-2 and PyMT transgenic mice model (Husemann et al. 2008). Their results suggest the dissemination of cancer may start earlier than the establishment and histological invasion of the primary tumor. It has also been reported that the quantity of CTCs shows statistical correlation with the progression of the cancer, and accumulating publications have shown that CTCs could be detected in the early stage of a variety of cancers (Chen et al. 2016; Bayarri-Lara et al. 2016; Lu et al. 2016). NGS whole exon sequencing in prostate cancer patients detected 70% of mutation identity between CTCs and paired tumor samples (Lohr et al. 2014). Single-cell RNA analyses show that metastatic cancer cells derived from high-burden tissues have similar gene expression to the primary tumor (Lawson et al. 2015). A strong correlation between single CTC cells and their paired tumor origin using RNA sequencing in prostate cancer further confirmed the tissue origin of the CTC cells (Miyamoto et al. 2015). The results indicate that the tissue of origin of the metastatic CTCs was the primary tumor, with additional heterogeneity shown in circulation.

Unknown primary tumors (UPTs) represent 3–5% of all new cancer patients diagnosed each year and are one of the ten most frequent cancer cases worldwide (Massard et al. 2011). The high mortality of UPT is characterized by an early dissemination and usually aggressive phenotype accompanied with an unfavorable prognosis and without an identifiable primary tumor after diagnosis (Massard et al. 2011; van de Wouw et al. 2002). Identification of the origin of the cancer cell in both UPT patients and for early cancer screening may thus improve the overall therapeutic outcome due to early cancer identification and detection. Emerging evidence has shown that the phenotypes of CTCs represent the characteristics of its own origin (Lu et al. 2016; Kirby et al. 2012; Stott et al. 2010b; Wang et al. 2000). PSA and PSMA are two antigens that have been used for prostate cancer detection using plasma, and have also been used to identify CTCs in prostate cancer patients (Lu et al. 2016). Cytoplasmic-expressed CK7 is believed to be a potential marker for lung cancer cells and has been used in CTC identification. Thyroid transcription factor 1 (TTF-1) is a nuclear protein selectively expressed in lung, thyroid, and diencephalons tissues. The combination of CK7 and TTF-1 as markers with different cellular localization is a feasible method for detection of CTCs from lung cancer (Lu et al. 2016). In addition, the combination of CK20 and gastrointestinal tract specific marker caudal type homeobox 2 (CDX2) shows the capability for the specific identification of colorectal cancer origin CTCs (Lu et al. 2016; Chu and Weiss 2002; Welinder et al. 2015). By using CK7/TTF1, CK20/CDX2,

PSA/PSMA, and panCK/CK18 markers for immunocytochemistry staining of CTCs in mixed types of blood samples with all stages for cancer origin identification, origin of the three types of cancer including prostate, colorectal, and lung could be clearly distinguished using the immunostaining strategy (Lu et al. 2016). Through a diverse combination of antibodies designed for specific cancer type identification, it is possible to determine the origin of the cancer type for both early cancer screening and tumor origin identification in UPT patients. Identifying the origin of the cancer at an early stage using CTCs, before the cancer has been diagnosed, will have clinical utility during routine cancer screening.

2.5 Perspective and Conclusion

More and more devices and strategies have been developed for the identification and enrichment of CTCs from clinical samples. Growing evidence also indicates the significance of CTCs in prognosis prediction, survival evaluation, and treatment efficacy validation in various types of cancer patients. Non-invasive liquid biopsy based on CTCs provides an opportunity for high purity, multiple sampling, and easily obtained specimens, in contrast to the traditional single time point surgery for tissue that may have high cell-type heterogeneity. The evaluation of CTCs should have utility in clinical applications such as early cancer detection, real-time disease monitoring, post-treatment examination, and possible *ex vivo* drug screening for personalized medicine development. Because CTCs act as a pre-metastatic lesion during cancer progression, they might be the missing piece in elucidating mechanisms that participate in cancer metastasis. Investigation of CTCs may further evaluate potential markers for early cancer diagnosis, develop novel targeting for cancer therapy, and identify possible strategies to cure and prevent cancer.

References

Aceto N, Bardia A, Miyamoto DT, Donaldson MC, Wittner BS, Spencer JA, Yu M, Pely A, Engstrom A, Zhu H, Brannigan BW, Kapur R, Stott SL, Shioda T, Ramaswamy S, Ting DT, Lin CP, Toner M, Haber DA, Maheswaran S (2014) Circulating tumor cell clusters are oligoclonal precursors of breast cancer metastasis. Cell 158(5):1110–1122. doi:10.1016/j.cell.2014.07.013

Adams JD, Thevoz P, Bruus H, Soh HT (2009) Integrated acoustic and magnetic separation in microfluidic channels. Appl Phys Lett 95(25):254103. doi:10.1063/1.3275577

Aggarwal C, Meropol NJ, Punt CJ, Iannotti N, Saidman BH, Sabbath KD, Gabrail NY, Picus J, Morse MA, Mitchell E, Miller MC, Cohen SJ (2013) Relationship among circulating tumor cells, CEA and overall survival in patients with metastatic colorectal cancer. Ann Oncol 24 (2):420–428. doi:10.1093/annonc/mds336

Allard WJ, Matera J, Miller MC, Repollet M, Connelly MC, Rao C, Tibbe AG, Uhr JW, Terstappen LW (2004) Tumor cells circulate in the peripheral blood of all major carcinomas

but not in healthy subjects or patients with nonmalignant diseases. Clin Cancer Res 10 (20):6897–6904. doi:10.1158/1078-0432.CCR-04-0378
Antfolk M, Magnusson C, Augustsson P, Lilja H, Laurell T (2015) Acoustofluidic, label-free separation and simultaneous concentration of rare tumor cells from white blood cells. Anal Chem 87(18):9322–9328. doi:10.1021/acs.analchem.5b02023
Antonarakis ES, Lu C, Wang H, Luber B, Nakazawa M, Roeser JC, Chen Y, Mohammad TA, Chen Y, Fedor HL, Lotan TL, Zheng Q, De Marzo AM, Isaacs JT, Isaacs WB, Nadal R, Paller CJ, Denmeade SR, Carducci MA, Eisenberger MA, Luo J (2014) AR-V7 and resistance to enzalutamide and abiraterone in prostate cancer. N Engl J Med 371(11):1028–1038. doi:10.1056/NEJMoa1315815
Antonarakis ES, Lu C, Luber B, Wang H, Chen Y, Nakazawa M, Nadal R, Paller CJ, Denmeade SR, Carducci MA, Eisenberger MA, Luo J (2015) Androgen receptor splice variant 7 and efficacy of taxane chemotherapy in patients with metastatic castration-resistant prostate cancer. JAMA Oncol 1(5):582–591. doi:10.1001/jamaoncol.2015.1341
Armstrong AJ, Marengo MS, Oltean S, Kemeny G, Bitting RL, Turnbull JD, Herold CI, Marcom PK, George DJ, Garcia-Blanco MA (2011) Circulating tumor cells from patients with advanced prostate and breast cancer display both epithelial and mesenchymal markers. Mol Cancer Res 9(8):997–1007. doi:10.1158/1541-7786.MCR-10-0490
Ashworth TR (1869) A case of cancer in which cells similar to those in the tumours were seen in the blood after death. Aust Med J 14:146
Au SH, Storey BD, Moore JC, Tang Q, Chen YL, Javaid S, Sarioglu AF, Sullivan R, Madden MW, O'Keefe R, Haber DA, Maheswaran S, Langenau DM, Stott SL, Toner M (2016) Clusters of circulating tumor cells traverse capillary-sized vessels. Proc Natl Acad Sci U S A 113 (18):4947–4952. doi:10.1073/pnas.1524448113
Bayarri-Lara C, Ortega FG, Cueto Ladron de Guevara A, Puche JL, Ruiz Zafra J, de Miguel-Perez D, Ramos AS, Giraldo-Ospina CF, Navajas Gomez JA, Delgado-Rodriguez M, Lorente JA, Serrano MJ (2016) Circulating tumor cells identify early recurrence in patients with non-small cell lung cancer undergoing radical resection. PLoS One 11(2):e0148659. doi:10.1371/journal.pone.0148659
Bidard FC, Huguet F, Louvet C, Mineur L, Bouche O, Chibaudel B, Artru P, Desseigne F, Bachet JB, Mathiot C, Pierga JY, Hammel P (2013) Circulating tumor cells in locally advanced pancreatic adenocarcinoma: the ancillary CirCe 07 study to the LAP 07 trial. Ann Oncol 24 (8):2057–2061. doi:10.1093/annonc/mdt176
Bidard FC, Peeters DJ, Fehm T, Nole F, Gisbert-Criado R, Mavroudis D, Grisanti S, Generali D, Garcia-Saenz JA, Stebbing J, Caldas C, Gazzaniga P, Manso L, Zamarchi R, de Lascoiti AF, De Mattos-Arruda L, Ignatiadis M, Lebofsky R, van Laere SJ, Meier-Stiegen F, Sandri MT, Vidal-Martinez J, Politaki E, Consoli F, Bottini A, Diaz-Rubio E, Krell J, Dawson SJ, Raimondi C, Rutten A, Janni W, Munzone E, Carañana V, Agelaki S, Almici C, Dirix L, Solomayer EF, Zorzino L, Johannes H, Reis-Filho JS, Pantel K, Pierga JY, Michiels S (2014) Clinical validity of circulating tumour cells in patients with metastatic breast cancer: a pooled analysis of individual patient data. Lancet Oncol 15(4):406–414. doi:10.1016/S1470-2045(14)70069-5
Budd GT, Cristofanilli M, Ellis MJ, Stopeck A, Borden E, Miller MC, Matera J, Repollet M, Doyle GV, Terstappen LW, Hayes DF (2006) Circulating tumor cells versus imaging–predicting overall survival in metastatic breast cancer. Clin Cancer Res 12(21):6403–6409. doi:10.1158/1078-0432.CCR-05-1769
Chaffer CL, Weinberg RA (2011) A perspective on cancer cell metastasis. Science 331 (6024):1559–1564. doi:10.1126/science.1203543
Chang MC, Chang YT, Chen JY, Jeng YM, Yang CY, Tien YW, Yang SH, Chen HL, Liang TY, Wang CF, Lee EY, Chang YC, Lee WH (2016) Clinical significance of circulating tumor microemboli as a prognostic marker in patients with pancreatic ductal adenocarcinoma. Clin Chem 62(3):505–513. doi:10.1373/clinchem.2015.248260

Chen L, Han X (2015) Anti-PD-1/PD-L1 therapy of human cancer: past, present, and future. J Clin Invest 125(9):3384–3391. doi:10.1172/JCI80011

Chen Q, Zhang XH, Massague J (2011) Macrophage binding to receptor VCAM-1 transmits survival signals in breast cancer cells that invade the lungs. Cancer Cell 20(4):538–549. doi:10.1016/j.ccr.2011.08.025

Chen JY, Tsai WS, Shao HJ, Wu JC, Lai JM, Lu SH, Hung TF, Yang CT, Wu LC, Chen JS, Lee WH, Chang YC (2016) Sensitive and specific biomimetic lipid coated microfluidics to isolate viable circulating tumor cells and microemboli for cancer detection. PLoS One 11(3): e0149633. doi:10.1371/journal.pone.0149633

Chu PG, Weiss LM (2002) Keratin expression in human tissues and neoplasms. Histopathology 40 (5):403–439

Coumans FA, Ligthart ST, Uhr JW, Terstappen LW (2012) Challenges in the enumeration and phenotyping of CTC. Clin Cancer Res 18(20):5711–5718. doi:10.1158/1078-0432.CCR-12-1585

Court CM, Ankeny JS, Hou S, Tseng HR, Tomlinson JS (2015) Improving pancreatic cancer diagnosis using circulating tumor cells: prospects for staging and single-cell analysis. Expert Rev Mol Diagn 15(11):1491–1504. doi:10.1586/14737159.2015.1091311

Cristofanilli M, Budd GT, Ellis MJ, Stopeck A, Matera J, Miller MC, Reuben JM, Doyle GV, Allard WJ, Terstappen LW, Hayes DF (2004) Circulating tumor cells, disease progression, and survival in metastatic breast cancer. N Engl J Med 351(8):781–791. doi:10.1056/NEJMoa040766

de Bono JS, Scher HI, Montgomery RB, Parker C, Miller MC, Tissing H, Doyle GV, Terstappen LW, Pienta KJ, Raghavan D (2008) Circulating tumor cells predict survival benefit from treatment in metastatic castration-resistant prostate cancer. Clin Cancer Res 14 (19):6302–6309. doi:10.1158/1078-0432.CCR-08-0872

Deng G, Krishnakumar S, Powell AA, Zhang H, Mindrinos MN, Telli ML, Davis RW, Jeffrey SS (2014) Single cell mutational analysis of PIK3CA in circulating tumor cells and metastases in breast cancer reveals heterogeneity, discordance, and mutation persistence in cultured disseminated tumor cells from bone marrow. BMC Cancer 14:456. doi:10.1186/1471-2407-14-456

Duda DG, Duyverman AM, Kohno M, Snuderl M, Steller EJ, Fukumura D, Jain RK (2010) Malignant cells facilitate lung metastasis by bringing their own soil. Proc Natl Acad Sci U S A 107(50):21677–21682. doi:10.1073/pnas.1016234107

Esselen KM, Cronin AM, Bixel K, Bookman MA, Burger RA, Cohn DE, Cristea M, Griggs JJ, Levenback CF, Mantia-Smaldone G, Meyer LA, Matulonis UA, Niland JC, Sun C, O'Malley DM, Wright AA (2016) Use of CA-125 tests and computed tomographic scans for surveillance in ovarian cancer. JAMA Oncol. doi:10.1001/jamaoncol.2016.1842

Faugeroux V, Pailler E, Auger N, Taylor M, Farace F (2014) Clinical utility of circulating tumor cells in alk-positive non-small-cell lung cancer. Front Oncol 4:281. doi:10.3389/fonc.2014.00281

Fischer KR, Durrans A, Lee S, Sheng J, Li F, Wong ST, Choi H, El Rayes T, Ryu S, Troeger J, Schwabe RF, Vahdat LT, Altorki NK, Mittal V, Gao D (2015) Epithelial-to-mesenchymal transition is not required for lung metastasis but contributes to chemoresistance. Nature 527 (7579):472–476. doi:10.1038/nature15748

Gerhard R, Schmitt FC (2014) Liquid-based cytology in fine-needle aspiration of breast lesions: a review. Acta Cytol 58(6):533–542. doi:10.1159/000362805

Gonsalves WI, Morice WG, Rajkumar V, Gupta V, Timm MM, Dispenzieri A, Buadi FK, Lacy MQ, Singh PP, Kapoor P, Gertz MA, Kumar SK (2014) Quantification of clonal circulating plasma cells in relapsed multiple myeloma. Br J Haematol 167(4):500–505. doi:10.1111/bjh.13067

Grisanti S, Almici C, Consoli F, Buglione M, Verardi R, Bolzoni-Villaret A, Bianchetti A, Ciccarese C, Mangoni M, Ferrari L, Biti G, Marini M, Ferrari VD, Nicolai P, Magrini SM, Berruti A (2014) Circulating tumor cells in patients with recurrent or metastatic head and neck carcinoma: prognostic and predictive significance. PLoS One 9(8):e103918. doi:10.1371/journal.pone.0103918

Grobe A, Blessmann M, Hanken H, Friedrich RE, Schon G, Wikner J, Effenberger KE, Kluwe L, Heiland M, Pantel K, Riethdorf S (2014) Prognostic relevance of circulating tumor cells in blood and disseminated tumor cells in bone marrow of patients with squamous cell carcinoma of the oral cavity. Clin Cancer Res 20(2):425–433. doi:10.1158/1078-0432.CCR-13-1101

Hanash SM, Baik CS, Kallioniemi O (2011) Emerging molecular biomarkers–blood-based strategies to detect and monitor cancer. Nat Rev Clin Oncol 8(3):142–150. doi:10.1038/nrclinonc.2010.220

Hayes DF, Cristofanilli M, Budd GT, Ellis MJ, Stopeck A, Miller MC, Matera J, Allard WJ, Doyle GV, Terstappen LW (2006) Circulating tumor cells at each follow-up time point during therapy of metastatic breast cancer patients predict progression-free and overall survival. Clin Cancer Res 12(14 Pt 1):4218–4224. doi:10.1158/1078-0432.CCR-05-2821

He W, Xu D, Wang Z, Xiang X, Tang B, Li S, Hou M, Zhang Y, Chen JF, Lin M, Wang L, Hou S, Tseng HR, Kuang M, Ke ZF (2016) Detecting ALK-rearrangement of CTC enriched by nanovelcro chip in advanced NSCLC patients. Oncotarget. doi:10.18632/oncotarget.8305

Hegerfeldt Y, Tusch M, Brocker EB, Friedl P (2002) Collective cell movement in primary melanoma explants: plasticity of cell-cell interaction, beta1-integrin function, and migration strategies. Cancer Res 62(7):2125–2130

Hodgkinson CL, Morrow CJ, Li Y, Metcalf RL, Rothwell DG, Trapani F, Polanski R, Burt DJ, Simpson KL, Morris K, Pepper SD, Nonaka D, Greystoke A, Kelly P, Bola B, Krebs MG, Antonello J, Ayub M, Faulkner S, Priest L, Carter L, Tate C, Miller CJ, Blackhall F, Brady G, Dive C (2014) Tumorigenicity and genetic profiling of circulating tumor cells in small-cell lung cancer. Nat Med 20(8):897–903. doi:10.1038/nm.3600

Hou JM, Krebs MG, Lancashire L, Sloane R, Backen A, Swain RK, Priest LJ, Greystoke A, Zhou C, Morris K, Ward T, Blackhall FH, Dive C (2012) Clinical significance and molecular characteristics of circulating tumor cells and circulating tumor microemboli in patients with small-cell lung cancer. J Clin Oncol 30(5):525–532. doi:10.1200/JCO.2010.33.3716

Husemann Y, Geigl JB, Schubert F, Musiani P, Meyer M, Burghart E, Forni G, Eils R, Fehm T, Riethmuller G, Klein CA (2008) Systemic spread is an early step in breast cancer. Cancer Cell 13(1):58–68. doi:10.1016/j.ccr.2007.12.003

Iinuma H, Watanabe T, Mimori K, Adachi M, Hayashi N, Tamura J, Matsuda K, Fukushima R, Okinaga K, Sasako M, Mori M (2011) Clinical significance of circulating tumor cells, including cancer stem-like cells, in peripheral blood for recurrence and prognosis in patients with Dukes' stage B and C colorectal cancer. J Clin Oncol 29(12):1547–1555. doi:10.1200/JCO.2010.30.5151

Ilie M, Long E, Butori C, Hofman V, Coelle C, Mauro V, Zahaf K, Marquette CH, Mouroux J, Paterlini-Brechot P, Hofman P (2012) ALK-gene rearrangement: a comparative analysis on circulating tumour cells and tumour tissue from patients with lung adenocarcinoma. Ann Oncol 23(11):2907–2913. doi:10.1093/annonc/mds137

Ilina O, Friedl P (2009) Mechanisms of collective cell migration at a glance. J Cell Sci 122 (Pt 18):3203–3208. doi:10.1242/jcs.036525

Iwai Y, Ishida M, Tanaka Y, Okazaki T, Honjo T, Minato N (2002) Involvement of PD-L1 on tumor cells in the escape from host immune system and tumor immunotherapy by PD-L1 blockade. Proc Natl Acad Sci U S A 99(19):12293–12297. doi:10.1073/pnas.192461099

Jiang B, Mason J, Jewett A, Qian J, Ding Y, Cho WC, Zhang X, Man YG (2013) Cell budding from normal appearing epithelia: a predictor of colorectal cancer metastasis? Int J Biol Sci 9 (1):119–133. doi:10.7150/ijbs.5441

Katz AE, Olsson CA, Raffo AJ, Cama C, Perlman H, Seaman E, O'Toole KM, McMahon D, Benson MC, Buttyan R (1994) Molecular staging of prostate cancer with the use of an enhanced reverse transcriptase-PCR assay. Urology 43(6):765–775

Ke Z, Lin M, Chen JF, Choi JS, Zhang Y, Fong A, Liang AJ, Chen SF, Li Q, Fang W, Zhang P, Garcia MA, Lee T, Song M, Lin HA, Zhao H, Luo SC, Hou S, Yu HH, Tseng HR (2015)

Programming thermoresponsiveness of NanoVelcro substrates enables effective purification of circulating tumor cells in lung cancer patients. ACS Nano 9(1):62–70. doi:10.1021/nn5056282

Kelley RK, Magbanua MJ, Butler TM, Collisson EA, Hwang J, Sidiropoulos N, Evason K, McWhirter RM, Hameed B, Wayne EM, Yao FY, Venook AP, Park JW (2015) Circulating tumor cells in hepatocellular carcinoma: a pilot study of detection, enumeration, and next-generation sequencing in cases and controls. BMC Cancer 15:206. doi:10.1186/s12885-015-1195-z

Kirby BJ, Jodari M, Loftus MS, Gakhar G, Pratt ED, Chanel-Vos C, Gleghorn JP, Santana SM, Liu H, Smith JP, Navarro VN, Tagawa ST, Bander NH, Nanus DM, Giannakakou P (2012) Functional characterization of circulating tumor cells with a prostate-cancer-specific microfluidic device. PLoS One 7(4):e35976. doi:10.1371/journal.pone.0035976

Klein CA (2008) Cancer. The metastasis cascade. Science 321(5897):1785–1787. doi:10.1126/science.1164853

Krebs MG, Sloane R, Priest L, Lancashire L, Hou JM, Greystoke A, Ward TH, Ferraldeschi R, Hughes A, Clack G, Ranson M, Dive C, Blackhall FH (2011) Evaluation and prognostic significance of circulating tumor cells in patients with non-small-cell lung cancer. J Clin Oncol 29(12):1556–1563. doi:10.1200/JCO.2010.28.7045

Krebs MG, Renehan AG, Backen A, Gollins S, Chau I, Hasan J, Valle JW, Morris K, Beech J, Ashcroft L, Saunders MP, Dive C (2015) Circulating tumor cell enumeration in a phase II trial of a four-drug regimen in advanced colorectal cancer. Clin Colorectal Cancer 14(2):115–122 e111-112. doi:10.1016/j.clcc.2014.12.006

Kulasingam V, Diamandis EP (2008) Strategies for discovering novel cancer biomarkers through utilization of emerging technologies. Nat Clin Pract Oncol 5(10):588–599. doi:10.1038/ncponc1187

Lang JE, Scott JH, Wolf DM, Novak P, Punj V, Magbanua MJ, Zhu W, Mineyev N, Haqq CM, Crothers JR, Esserman LJ, Tripathy D, van't Veer L, Park JW (2015) Expression profiling of circulating tumor cells in metastatic breast cancer. Breast Cancer Res Treat 149(1):121–131. doi:10.1007/s10549-014-3215-0

Lapin M, Tjensvoll K, Oltedal S, Buhl T, Gilje B, Smaaland R, Nordgard O (2016) MINDEC-an enhanced negative depletion strategy for circulating tumour cell enrichment. Sci Rep 6:28929. doi:10.1038/srep28929

Lawson DA, Bhakta NR, Kessenbrock K, Prummel KD, Yu Y, Takai K, Zhou A, Eyob H, Balakrishnan S, Wang CY, Yaswen P, Goga A, Werb Z (2015) Single-cell analysis reveals a stem-cell program in human metastatic breast cancer cells. Nature 526(7571):131–135. doi:10.1038/nature15260

Lee A, Park J, Lim M, Sunkara V, Kim SY, Kim GH, Kim MH, Cho YK (2014) All-in-one centrifugal microfluidic device for size-selective circulating tumor cell isolation with high purity. Anal Chem 86(22):11349–11356. doi:10.1021/ac5035049

Lohr JG, Adalsteinsson VA, Cibulskis K, Choudhury AD, Rosenberg M, Cruz-Gordillo P, Francis JM, Zhang CZ, Shalek AK, Satija R, Trombetta JJ, Lu D, Tallapragada N, Tahirova N, Kim S, Blumenstiel B, Sougnez C, Lowe A, Wong B, Auclair D, Van Allen EM, Nakabayashi M, Lis RT, Lee GS, Li T, Chabot MS, Ly A, Taplin ME, Clancy TE, Loda M, Regev A, Meyerson M, Hahn WC, Kantoff PW, Golub TR, Getz G, Boehm JS, Love JC (2014) Whole-exome sequencing of circulating tumor cells provides a window into metastatic prostate cancer. Nat Biotechnol 32(5):479–484. doi:10.1038/nbt.2892

Lorente D, Olmos D, Mateo J, Bianchini D, Seed G, Fleisher M, Danila DC, Flohr P, Crespo M, Figueiredo I, Miranda S, Baeten K, Molina A, Kheoh T, McCormack R, Terstappen LW, Scher HI, de Bono JS (2016) Decline in circulating tumor cell count and treatment outcome in advanced prostate cancer. Eur Urol. doi:10.1016/j.eururo.2016.05.023

Lu Y, Liang H, Yu T, Xie J, Chen S, Dong H, Sinko PJ, Lian S, Xu J, Wang J, Yu S, Shao J, Yuan B, Wang L, Jia L (2015) Isolation and characterization of living circulating tumor cells in patients by immunomagnetic negative enrichment coupled with flow cytometry. Cancer 121 (17):3036–3045. doi:10.1002/cncr.29444

Lu SH, Tsai WS, Chang YH, Chou TY, Pang ST, Lin PH, Tsai CM, Chang YC (2016) Identifying cancer origin using circulating tumor cells. Cancer Biol Ther 17(4):430–438. doi:10.1080/15384047.2016.1141839

Ludwig JA, Weinstein JN (2005) Biomarkers in cancer staging, prognosis and treatment selection. Nat Rev Cancer 5(11):845–856. doi:10.1038/nrc1739

Magbanua MJ, Park JW (2013) Isolation of circulating tumor cells by immunomagnetic enrichment and fluorescence-activated cell sorting (IE/FACS) for molecular profiling. Methods 64 (2):114–118. doi:10.1016/j.ymeth.2013.07.029

Magbanua MJ, Sosa EV, Roy R, Eisenbud LE, Scott JH, Olshen A, Pinkel D, Rugo HS, Park JW (2013) Genomic profiling of isolated circulating tumor cells from metastatic breast cancer patients. Cancer Res 73(1):30–40. doi:10.1158/0008-5472.CAN-11-3017

Magbanua MJ, Carey LA, DeLuca A, Hwang J, Scott JH, Rimawi MF, Mayer EL, Marcom PK, Liu MC, Esteva FJ, Park JW, Rugo HS, Translational Breast Cancer Research C (2015) Circulating tumor cell analysis in metastatic triple-negative breast cancers. Clin Cancer Res 21(5):1098–1105. doi:10.1158/1078-0432.CCR-14-1948

Man YG (2010) Aberrant leukocyte infiltration: a direct trigger for breast tumor invasion and metastasis. Int J Biol Sci 6(2):129–132

Marchetti A, Del Grammastro M, Felicioni L, Malatesta S, Filice G, Centi I, De Pas T, Santoro A, Chella A, Brandes AA, Venturino P, Cuccurullo F, Crino L, Buttitta F (2014) Assessment of EGFR mutations in circulating tumor cell preparations from NSCLC patients by next generation sequencing: toward a real-time liquid biopsy for treatment. PLoS One 9(8):e103883. doi:10.1371/journal.pone.0103883

Massard C, Loriot Y, Fizazi K (2011) Carcinomas of an unknown primary origin–diagnosis and treatment. Nat Rev Clin Oncol 8(12):701–710. doi:10.1038/nrclinonc.2011.158

Mazel M, Jacot W, Pantel K, Bartkowiak K, Topart D, Cayrefourcq L, Rossille D, Maudelonde T, Fest T, Alix-Panabieres C (2015) Frequent expression of PD-L1 on circulating breast cancer cells. Mol Oncol 9(9):1773–1782. doi:10.1016/j.molonc.2015.05.009

Mehlen P, Puisieux A (2006) Metastasis: a question of life or death. Nat Rev Cancer 6(6):449–458. doi:10.1038/nrc1886

Meng S, Tripathy D, Frenkel EP, Shete S, Naftalis EZ, Huth JF, Beitsch PD, Leitch M, Hoover S, Euhus D, Haley B, Morrison L, Fleming TP, Herlyn D, Terstappen LW, Fehm T, Tucker TF, Lane N, Wang J, Uhr JW (2004) Circulating tumor cells in patients with breast cancer dormancy. Clin Cancer Res 10(24):8152–8162. doi:10.1158/1078-0432.CCR-04-1110

Mitchell MJ, King MR (2013) Fluid shear stress sensitizes cancer cells to receptor-mediated apoptosis via trimeric death receptors. New J Phys 15:015008. doi:10.1088/1367-2630/15/1/015008

Miyamoto DT, Zheng Y, Wittner BS, Lee RJ, Zhu H, Broderick KT, Desai R, Fox DB, Brannigan BW, Trautwein J, Arora KS, Desai N, Dahl DM, Sequist LV, Smith MR, Kapur R, Wu CL, Shioda T, Ramaswamy S, Ting DT, Toner M, Maheswaran S, Haber DA (2015) RNA-Seq of single prostate CTCs implicates noncanonical Wnt signaling in antiandrogen resistance. Science 349(6254):1351–1356. doi:10.1126/science.aab0917

Molnar B, Ladanyi A, Tanko L, Sreter L, Tulassay Z (2001) Circulating tumor cell clusters in the peripheral blood of colorectal cancer patients. Clin Cancer Res 7(12):4080–4085

Nagrath S, Sequist LV, Maheswaran S, Bell DW, Irimia D, Ulkus L, Smith MR, Kwak EL, Digumarthy S, Muzikansky A, Ryan P, Balis UJ, Tompkins RG, Haber DA, Toner M (2007) Isolation of rare circulating tumour cells in cancer patients by microchip technology. Nature 450(7173):1235–1239. doi:10.1038/nature06385

Nakazawa M, Lu C, Chen Y, Paller CJ, Carducci MA, Eisenberger MA, Luo J, Antonarakis ES (2015) Serial blood-based analysis of AR-V7 in men with advanced prostate cancer. Ann Oncol 26(9):1859–1865. doi:10.1093/annonc/mdv282

Nel I, Jehn U, Gauler T, Hoffmann AC (2014) Individual profiling of circulating tumor cell composition in patients with non-small cell lung cancer receiving platinum based treatment. Transl Lung Cancer Res 3(2):100–106. doi:10.3978/j.issn.2218-6751.2014.03.05

Neves RP, Raba K, Schmidt O, Honisch E, Meier-Stiegen F, Behrens B, Mohlendick B, Fehm T, Neubauer H, Klein CA, Polzer B, Sproll C, Fischer JC, Niederacher D, Stoecklein NH (2014) Genomic high-resolution profiling of single CKpos/CD45neg flow-sorting purified circulating tumor cells from patients with metastatic breast cancer. Clin Chem 60(10):1290–1297. doi:10.1373/clinchem.2014.222331

Ozkumur E, Shah AM, Ciciliano JC, Emmink BL, Miyamoto DT, Brachtel E, Yu M, Chen PI, Morgan B, Trautwein J, Kimura A, Sengupta S, Stott SL, Karabacak NM, Barber TA, Walsh JR, Smith K, Spuhler PS, Sullivan JP, Lee RJ, Ting DT, Luo X, Shaw AT, Bardia A, Sequist LV, Louis DN, Maheswaran S, Kapur R, Haber DA, Toner M (2013) Inertial focusing for tumor antigen-dependent and -independent sorting of rare circulating tumor cells. Sci Transl Med 5(179):179ra147. doi:10.1126/scitranslmed.3005616

Paget S (1989) The distribution of secondary growths in cancer of the breast. 1889. Cancer Metastasis Rev 8(2):98–101

Pailler E, Adam J, Barthelemy A, Oulhen M, Auger N, Valent A, Borget I, Planchard D, Taylor M, Andre F, Soria JC, Vielh P, Besse B, Farace F (2013) Detection of circulating tumor cells harboring a unique ALK rearrangement in ALK-positive non-small-cell lung cancer. J Clin Oncol 31(18):2273–2281. doi:10.1200/JCO.2012.44.5932

Pardoll DM (2012) The blockade of immune checkpoints in cancer immunotherapy. Nat Rev Cancer 12(4):252–264. doi:10.1038/nrc3239

Peeters DJ, Brouwer A, Van den Eynden GG, Rutten A, Onstenk W, Sieuwerts AM, Van Laere SJ, Huget P, Pauwels P, Peeters M, Vermeulen PB, Dirix LY (2015) Circulating tumour cells and lung microvascular tumour cell retention in patients with metastatic breast and cervical cancer. Cancer Lett 356(2 Pt B):872–879. doi:10.1016/j.canlet.2014.10.039

Podsypanina K, Du YC, Jechlinger M, Beverly LJ, Hambardzumyan D, Varmus H (2008) Seeding and propagation of untransformed mouse mammary cells in the lung. Science 321 (5897):1841–1844. doi:10.1126/science.1161621

Postow MA, Callahan MK, Wolchok JD (2015) Immune checkpoint blockade in cancer therapy. J Clin Oncol 33(17):1974–1982. doi:10.1200/JCO.2014.59.4358

Poveda A, Kaye SB, McCormack R, Wang S, Parekh T, Ricci D, Lebedinsky CA, Tercero JC, Zintl P, Monk BJ (2011) Circulating tumor cells predict progression free survival and overall survival in patients with relapsed/recurrent advanced ovarian cancer. Gynecol Oncol 122 (3):567–572. doi:10.1016/j.ygyno.2011.05.028

Powell AA, Talasaz AH, Zhang H, Coram MA, Reddy A, Deng G, Telli ML, Advani RH, Carlson RW, Mollick JA, Sheth S, Kurian AW, Ford JM, Stockdale FE, Quake SR, Pease RF, Mindrinos MN, Bhanot G, Dairkee SH, Davis RW, Jeffrey SS (2012) Single cell profiling of circulating tumor cells: transcriptional heterogeneity and diversity from breast cancer cell lines. PLoS One 7(5):e33788. doi:10.1371/journal.pone.0033788

Qiao YY, Lin KX, Zhang Z, Zhang DJ, Shi CH, Xiong M, Qu XH, Zhao XH (2015) Monitoring disease progression and treatment efficacy with circulating tumor cells in esophageal squamous cell carcinoma: a case report. World J Gastroenterol 21(25):7921–7928. doi:10.3748/wjg.v21.i25.7921

Ran R, Li L, Wang M, Wang S, Zheng Z, Lin PP (2013) Determination of EGFR mutations in single cells microdissected from enriched lung tumor cells in peripheral blood. Anal Bioanal Chem 405(23):7377–7382. doi:10.1007/s00216-013-7156-y

Reategui E, Aceto N, Lim EJ, Sullivan JP, Jensen AE, Zeinali M, Martel JM, Aranyosi AJ, Li W, Castleberry S, Bardia A, Sequist LV, Haber DA, Maheswaran S, Hammond PT, Toner M, Stott SL (2015) Tunable nanostructured coating for the capture and selective release of viable circulating tumor cells. Adv Mater 27(9):1593–1599. doi:10.1002/adma.201404677

Reyes EE, VanderWeele DJ, Isikbay M, Duggan R, Campanile A, Stadler WM, Vander Griend DJ, Szmulewitz RZ (2014) Quantitative characterization of androgen receptor protein expression and cellular localization in circulating tumor cells from patients with metastatic castration-resistant prostate cancer. J Transl Med 12:313. doi:10.1186/s12967-014-0313-z

Rossille D, Gressier M, Damotte D, Maucort-Boulch D, Pangault C, Semana G, Le Gouill S, Haioun C, Tarte K, Lamy T, Milpied N, Fest T, Groupe Ouest-Est des Leucemies et Autres Maladies du S, Groupe Ouest-Est des Leucemies et Autres Maladies du S (2014) High level of soluble programmed cell death ligand 1 in blood impacts overall survival in aggressive diffuse large B-cell lymphoma: results from a French multicenter clinical trial. Leukemia 28 (12):2367–2375. doi:10.1038/leu.2014.137

Sarioglu AF, Aceto N, Kojic N, Donaldson MC, Zeinali M, Hamza B, Engstrom A, Zhu H, Sundaresan TK, Miyamoto DT, Luo X, Bardia A, Wittner BS, Ramaswamy S, Shioda T, Ting DT, Stott SL, Kapur R, Maheswaran S, Haber DA, Toner M (2015) A microfluidic device for label-free, physical capture of circulating tumor cell clusters. Nat Methods 12(7):685–691. doi:10.1038/nmeth.3404

Scher HI, Heller G, Molina A, Attard G, Danila DC, Jia X, Peng W, Sandhu SK, Olmos D, Riisnaes R, McCormack R, Burzykowski T, Kheoh T, Fleisher M, Buyse M, de Bono JS (2015) Circulating tumor cell biomarker panel as an individual-level surrogate for survival in metastatic castration-resistant prostate cancer. J Clin Oncol 33(12):1348–1355. doi:10.1200/JCO.2014.55.3487

Seal SH (1964) A sieve for the isolation of cancer cells and other large cells from the blood. Cancer 17:637–642

Siegel RL, Miller KD, Jemal A (2016) Cancer statistics, 2016. CA Cancer J Clin 66(1):7–30. doi:10.3322/caac.21332

Smerage JB, Hayes DF (2008) The prognostic implications of circulating tumor cells in patients with breast cancer. Cancer Investig 26(2):109–114. doi:10.1080/07357900701784204

Smerage JB, Barlow WE, Hortobagyi GN, Winer EP, Leyland-Jones B, Srkalovic G, Tejwani S, Schott AF, O'Rourke MA, Lew DL, Doyle GV, Gralow JR, Livingston RB, Hayes DF (2014) Circulating tumor cells and response to chemotherapy in metastatic breast cancer: SWOG S0500. J Clin Oncol 32(31):3483–3489. doi:10.1200/JCO.2014.56.2561

Smith B, Selby P, Southgate J, Pittman K, Bradley C, Blair GE (1991) Detection of melanoma cells in peripheral blood by means of reverse transcriptase and polymerase chain reaction. Lancet 338(8777):1227–1229

Stott SL, Hsu CH, Tsukrov DI, Yu M, Miyamoto DT, Waltman BA, Rothenberg SM, Shah AM, Smas ME, Korir GK, Floyd FP Jr, Gilman AJ, Lord JB, Winokur D, Springer S, Irimia D, Nagrath S, Sequist LV, Lee RJ, Isselbacher KJ, Maheswaran S, Haber DA, Toner M (2010a) Isolation of circulating tumor cells using a microvortex-generating herringbone-chip. Proc Natl Acad Sci U S A 107(43):18392–18397. doi:10.1073/pnas.1012539107

Stott SL, Lee RJ, Nagrath S, Yu M, Miyamoto DT, Ulkus L, Inserra EJ, Ulman M, Springer S, Nakamura Z, Moore AL, Tsukrov DI, Kempner ME, Dahl DM, Wu CL, Iafrate AJ, Smith MR, Tompkins RG, Sequist LV, Toner M, Haber DA, Maheswaran S (2010b) Isolation and characterization of circulating tumor cells from patients with localized and metastatic prostate cancer. Sci Transl Med 2(25):25ra23. doi:10.1126/scitranslmed.3000403

Sun W, Yuan X, Tian Y, Wu H, Xu H, Hu G, Wu K (2015) Non-invasive approaches to monitor EGFR-TKI treatment in non-small-cell lung cancer. J Hematol Oncol 8:95. doi:10.1186/s13045-015-0193-6

Tanaka F, Yoneda K, Kondo N, Hashimoto M, Takuwa T, Matsumoto S, Okumura Y, Rahman S, Tsubota N, Tsujimura T, Kuribayashi K, Fukuoka K, Nakano T, Hasegawa S (2009) Circulating tumor cell as a diagnostic marker in primary lung cancer. Clin Cancer Res 15 (22):6980–6986. doi:10.1158/1078-0432.CCR-09-1095

Tien YW, Kuo HC, Ho BI, Chang MC, Chang YT, Cheng MF, Chen HL, Liang TY, Wang CF, Huang CY, Shew JY, Chang YC, Lee EY, Lee WH (2016) A high circulating tumor cell count in portal vein predicts liver metastasis from periampullary or pancreatic cancer: a high portal venous CTC count predicts liver metastases. Medicine 95(16):e3407. doi:10.1097/MD.0000000000003407

Tsao DA, Yang MJ, Chang HJ, Yen LC, Chiu HH, Hsueh EJ, Chen YF, Lin SR (2010) A fast and convenient new technique to detect the therapeutic target, K-ras mutant, from peripheral blood in non-small cell lung cancer patients. Lung Cancer 68(1):51–57. doi:10.1016/j.lungcan.2009.05.023

van de Wouw AJ, Janssen-Heijnen ML, Coebergh JW, Hillen HF (2002) Epidemiology of unknown primary tumours; incidence and population-based survival of 1285 patients in Southeast Netherlands, 1984–1992. Eur J Cancer 38(3):409–413

Vona G, Sabile A, Louha M, Sitruk V, Romana S, Schutze K, Capron F, Franco D, Pazzagli M, Vekemans M, Lacour B, Brechot C, Paterlini-Brechot P (2000) Isolation by size of epithelial tumor cells : a new method for the immunomorphological and molecular characterization of circulatingtumor cells. Am J Pathol 156(1):57–63. doi:10.1016/S0002-9440(10)64706-2

Wang ZP, Eisenberger MA, Carducci MA, Partin AW, Scher HI, Ts'o PO (2000) Identification and characterization of circulating prostate carcinoma cells. Cancer 88(12):2787–2795

Welinder C, Jansson B, Lindell G, Wenner J (2015) Cytokeratin 20 improves the detection of circulating tumor cells in patients with colorectal cancer. Cancer Lett 358(1):43–46. doi:10.1016/j.canlet.2014.12.024

Williams ES, Rodriguez-Bravo V, Chippada-Venkata U, De Ia I-VJ, Gong Y, Galsky M, Oh W, Cordon-Cardo C, Domingo-Domenech J (2015) Generation of prostate cancer patient derived xenograft models from circulating tumor cells. J Vis Exp 105:53182. doi:10.3791/53182

Yu M, Bardia A, Wittner BS, Stott SL, Smas ME, Ting DT, Isakoff SJ, Ciciliano JC, Wells MN, Shah AM, Concannon KF, Donaldson MC, Sequist LV, Brachtel E, Sgroi D, Baselga J, Ramaswamy S, Toner M, Haber DA, Maheswaran S (2013) Circulating breast tumor cells exhibit dynamic changes in epithelial and mesenchymal composition. Science 339(6119):580–584. doi:10.1126/science.1228522

Zheng X, Carstens JL, Kim J, Scheible M, Kaye J, Sugimoto H, Wu CC, LeBleu VS, Kalluri R (2015) Epithelial-to-mesenchymal transition is dispensable for metastasis but induces chemoresistance in pancreatic cancer. Nature 527(7579):525–530. doi:10.1038/nature16064

Zhou MD, Hao S, Williams AJ, Harouaka RA, Schrand B, Rawal S, Ao Z, Brenneman R, Gilboa E, Lu B, Wang S, Zhu J, Datar R, Cote R, Tai YC, Zheng SY (2014) Separable bilayer microfiltration device for viable label-free enrichment of circulating tumour cells. Sci Rep 4:7392. doi:10.1038/srep07392

Chapter 3
Aptamer-Based Methods for Detection of Circulating Tumor Cells and Their Potential for Personalized Diagnostics

Anna S. Zamay, Galina S. Zamay, Olga S. Kolovskaya, Tatiana N. Zamay, and Maxim V. Berezovski

Abstract Cancer diagnostics and treatment monitoring rely on sensing and counting of rare cells such as cancer circulating tumor cells (CTCs) in blood. Many analytical techniques have been developed to reliably detect and quantify CTCs using unique physical shape and size of tumor cells and/or distinctive patterns of cell surface biomarkers. Main problems of CTC bioanalysis are in the small number of cells that are present in the circulation and heterogeneity of CTCs. In this chapter, we describe recent progress towards the selection and application of synthetic DNA or RNA aptamers to capture and detect CTCs in blood. Antibody-based approaches for cell isolation and purification are limited because of an antibody's negative effect on cell viability and purity. Aptamers transform cell isolation technology, because they bind and release cells on-demand. The unique feature of anti-CTC aptamers is that the aptamers are selected for cell surface biomarkers in their native state, and conformation without previous knowledge of their biomarkers. Once aptamers are produced, they can be used to identify CTC biomarkers using mass spectrometry. The biomarkers and corresponding aptamers can be exploited to improve cancer diagnostics and therapies.

A.S. Zamay (✉) • G.S. Zamay • O.S. Kolovskaya
Laboratory for Biomolecular and Medical Technologies, Krasnoyarsk State Medical University named after Professor V. F. Voyno-Yasenetsky, Krasnoyarsk, Russia

Federal Research Center, KSC Siberian branch of Russian Academy of Science, Krasnoyarsk, Russia
e-mail: annazamay@yandex.ru

T.N. Zamay
Laboratory for Biomolecular and Medical Technologies, Krasnoyarsk State Medical University named after Professor V. F. Voyno-Yasenetsky, Krasnoyarsk, Russia

M.V. Berezovski (✉)
Department of Chemistry and Biomolecular Sciences, University of Ottawa, 10 Marie Curie, Ottawa, ON K1N 6N5, Canada
e-mail: maxim.berezovski@uottawa.ca

M.J.M. Magbanua, J.W. Park (eds.), *Isolation and Molecular Characterization of Circulating Tumor Cells*, Advances in Experimental Medicine and Biology 994,
DOI 10.1007/978-3-319-55947-6_3

Keywords Aptamers • Biomarkers • Biosensors • Circulating tumor cells • CTCs • Cell isolation • Microfluidics

3.1 Introduction

Oncological diseases are the second leading cause of death after cardiovascular diseases. Early clinical diagnosis of pre-metastatic malignancy tumors could increase treatment efficiency and survival rate of cancer patients. One of promising tools for better lung cancer diagnosis and monitoring during treatment is evaluation and enumeration of circulating tumor cells (CTC) in blood (Punnoose et al. 2012). There are numerous methods for isolation and concentration of rare cancerous cells from blood, such as dielectrophoresis and stepping electric fields (Hatanaka et al. 2011; Chen et al. 2014), fluorescence-activated cell sorting (FACS), magnetic-activated cell sorting (Jacob et al. 2007). In general the methods for enriching CTCs can be divided into two categories: size-based and immunomagnetic approaches, the advantages and disadvantages of which have been addressed in the literature (Alunni-Fabbroni and Sandri 2010). Among immunomagnetic methods, the CellSearch system has been approved for clinical use by the U.S. FDA (Allard et al. 2004). It relies on antibody-based capture and staining of epithelial cell adhesion molecule (EpCAM) as well as Cytokeratins 8, 18, or 19.

Unfortunately, no single antibody is sufficient to capture and detect all rare CTCs. For instance, EpCAM is not a perfect marker for CTC detection due to the high variation in its gene expression between tumor subtypes (Lampignano et al. 2016). Many CTCs also express epithelial, mesenchymal, and stem-cell markers.

The CTC research has sparked considerable interest in the application of molecules that offer similar or enhanced functionalities to antibodies, but that can be easily synthesized with additional characteristics. Aptamers have enormous potential as such molecules. These small (5–30 kDa), single-stranded DNA and RNA molecules carry the blueprint for their own synthesis in their primary sequence, so they can be synthesized by pure chemical procedures. They fold into well-defined three-dimensional structures and show high affinity and specificity for their targets. In many respects, aptamers are superior to antibodies. They can be selected through an *in vitro* evolution process using live cancer cells or primary tumors in a few days without knowing beforehand cell specific biomarkers. The resulting aptamers are chemically synthesized in high purity at low cost (1000s times cheaper than the production of monoclonal antibodies), and are considered to be a synthetic chemical product, rather than a biological product. For isolation purposes aptamers can be easily removed from target cells washing out with chelators or nucleases (Jayasena 1999; Li et al. 2013; Shen et al. 2013; Wehbe et al. 2015) or DNA complementary sequences (Rusconi et al. 2002). In contrast antibody releasing from its targets requires harmful to cells harsh chemical or enzymatic treatments (Sheng et al. 2014).

3.2 Microfluidic Aptamer-Based Devices for CTC Capture

Currently, aptamer-based technologies are widely studied in various biomedical fields. Over 6000 published articles on aptamers are referenced in the PubMed database, and more than 1000 of them are related to cancer. The first microfluidic device utilizing the aptamer to EGFR for isolating cancer cells from a laminar flow of human mononuclear cells has been reported by Wan et al. (2011). Two following microfluidic devices have been shown in 2012. The first device utilized elliptical (30 μm × 15 μm) micropillars 32 μm in height and an interpillar distance of 80 μm in flow channels (Fig. 3.1) (Sheng et al. 2012). The micropillars were coated with DNA aptamers previously selected against the following cancer cell lines: CCRF-CEM cells, Ramos cells, HCT 116 cells, and DLD-1 cells (Martin et al. 2011; Sefah et al. 2010; Shangguan et al. 2006; Tang et al. 2007). Less than 30 min was enough to isolate as few as 10 colorectal tumor cells from 1 ml of unprocessed whole blood using this small device. The cancer cells captured with the micropillar flow chamber were viable and used for following cellular and molecular characterization.

The second Hele-Shaw microfluidic device with plain surface of the channel and with array of pits on the channel floor have been utilized for the efficient detection of rare cancerous cells (Fig. 3.2). The pits were filled with anti-EGFR aptamer functionalized glass beads. Cancer cells, flowing in solution through the channel, were captured by the beads with high specificity. Such design helped sorting cell sub-populations with varying EGFR expression. Cells were released from the beads by a complementary to oligonucleotide sequence. This approach isolated viable cells for further analysis (Wan et al. 2012).

A flat channel microfluidic device made of polydimethylsiloxane and functionalized with locked nucleic acid (LNA) aptamers targeting EpCAM and nucleolin has been developed by Maremanda et al. for quick and efficient capture of CTCs and cancer cells. The analysis of blood samples obtained from 25 head and neck cancer patients detected as small as 5 ± 3 CTCs in ml of blood. These microfluidic devices also maintained viability for *in vitro* culture and characterization (Maremanda et al. 2015).

Recently, another microfluidic assay has been developed using a cocktail of aptamers with a synergistic effect. When a single aptamer was employed in the chip composed of silicon nanowires and an overlaid PDMS chaotic mixer, the capture affinity of the device was relatively weak. Nevertheless, using several aptamers, the synergistic effects among individual aptamers lead to an enhanced capture affinity (Fig. 3.3). It has been shown that for the patients with nonsmall cell lung cancer (NSCLC) this method provided more comprehensive information in treatment monitoring (Zhao et al. 2016).

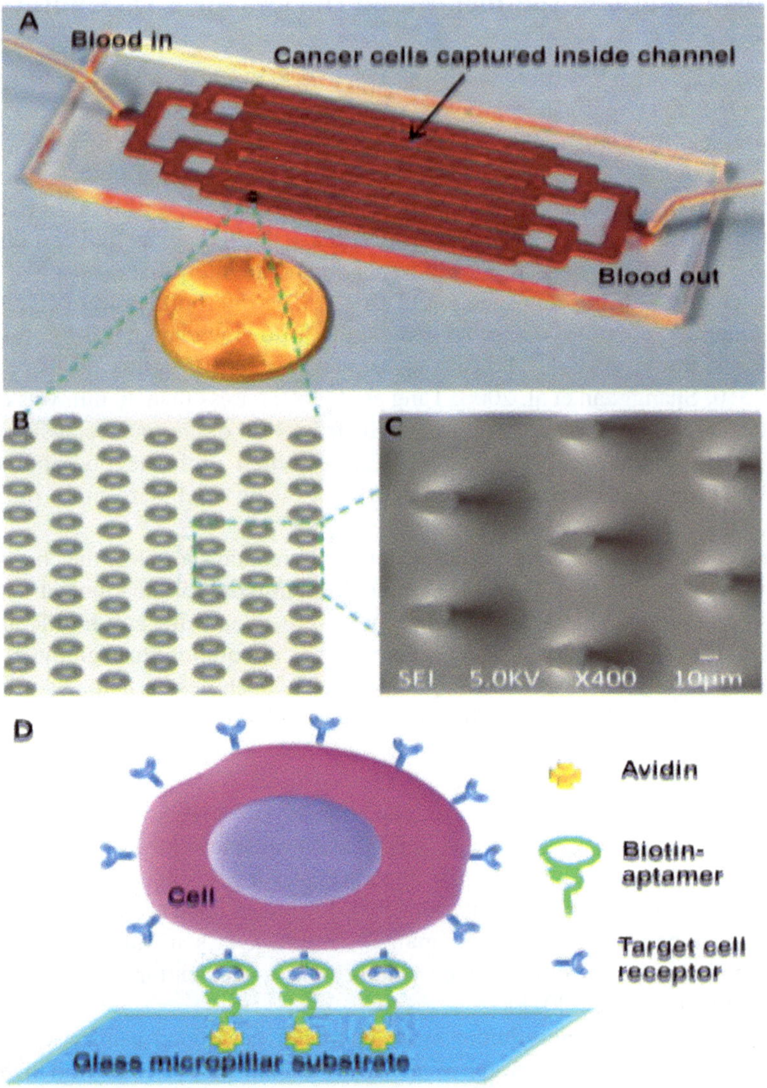

Fig. 3.1 Microfluidic micropillar device for cancer cell isolation (**a**) Optical micrograph (**b**) and scanning electron microscope images of a micropillar array in a channel in the glass substrate (**c**) Scanning electron microscopy image of elliptical micropillars (**d**) Scheme of capturing cancer cells in the device (From Sheng et al. 2012, with permission)

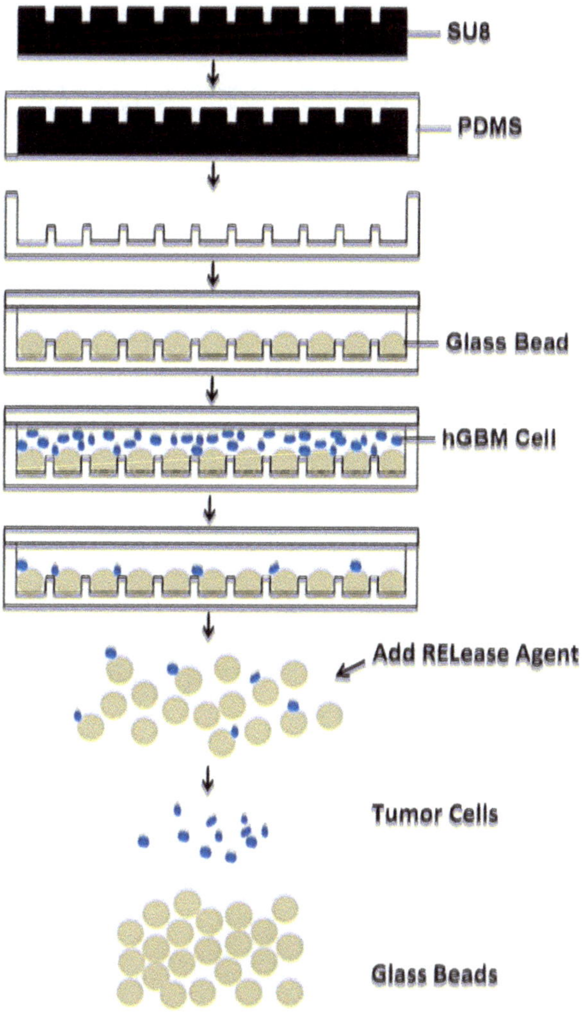

Fig. 3.2 Scheme of fabrication and application of Hele-Shaw microfluidic device. SU-8 photoresist is spin-cast on silicon wafer, exposed and wells are developed to form the desired pattern. PDMS is poured on SU-8 master, baked, and peeled off. 50 μm diameter glass beads (GBs) are loaded into 25 μm deep pits and the substrate is covered with a flat PDMS slab. Cancer cell suspension is flowed through the device, and cells are captured by aptamers-functionalized GBs. Captured cells are finally released from the GB surface after GBs are collected from the device (From Wan et al. 2012, with permission)

3.3 CTC Isolation with Aptamer-Functionalized Nanoparticles

Chitosan nanoparticle surface fabricated by electrospray was modified by polyethylene glycol and a DNA aptamer for a specific capture of viable rare CTCs from artificial white blood cell samples. Furthermore, an *in situ* culture strategy has been proposed (Fig. 3.4). This work provides a promising strategy for viable isolation and purification of rare CTCs and it has great potential for achieving clinical validity (Sun et al. 2015).

Aptamer-functionalized gold nanoparticles could be used to enrich and detect cancer cells using an aptamer-nanoparticle strip biosensor within a lateral flow

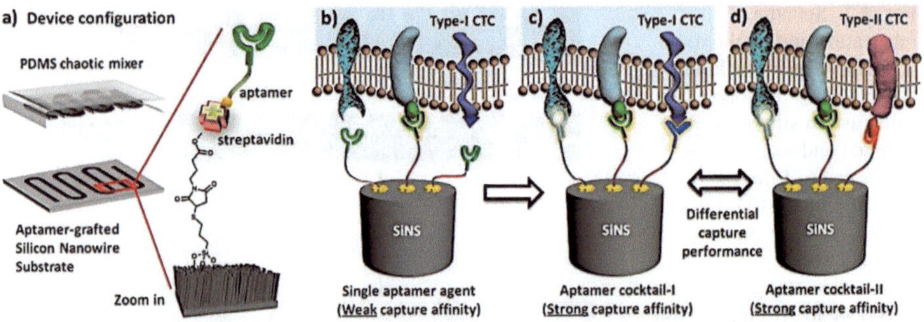

Fig. 3.3 Scheme of an aptamer cocktail based CTC assay. Microfluidic CTC chip is composed of an aptamer-grafted silicon nanowire substrate and an overlaid PDMS chaotic mixer (**a**) When a single aptamer capture agent was employed, the capture affinity of the device is relatively weak for the lack of synergistic binding (**b**) By using cocktail capture agents, the synergistic effects among individual aptamers lead to an enhanced capture affinity (**c**) Different cocktail capture agents are expected to have differential capture performance for CTC subpopulation recognition (From Zhao et al. 2016, with permission)

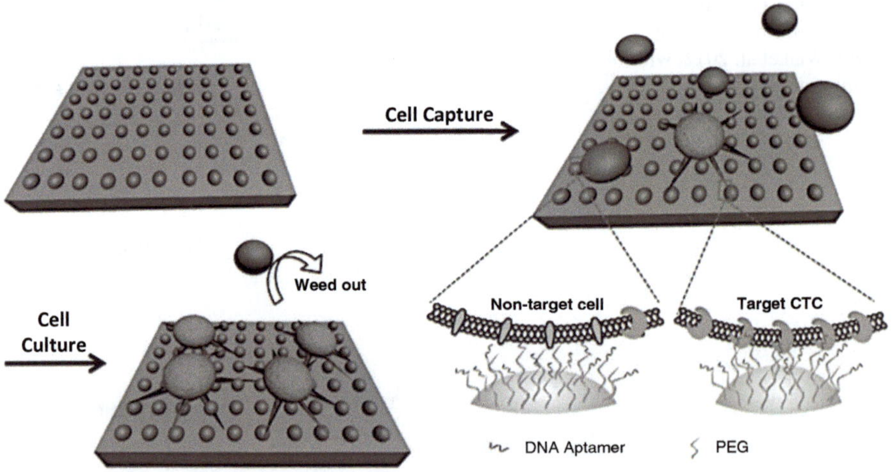

Fig. 3.4 Scheme of the chitosan nanoparticle substrate for rare number CTC isolation from non-target cells followed by the optimized in situ culture of captured cells (From Sun et al. 2015, with permission)

device (Fig. 3.5) (Liu et al. 2009). A pair of aptamers to Ramos cells – a thiolated aptamer (TD05) immobilized on gold nanoparticles and a biotinylated aptamer (TE02) immobilized in the test zone of a nitrocellulose membrane. The lateral flow strip device allowed cancer cells linked through TD05 aptamer with gold nanoparticles stay in the test zone. Accumulation of colloidal gold produced a visible red band. Unfortunately the large volumes of blood (more than 5 μL) masked the signal from the cancer cells because of the non-specific adsorption of

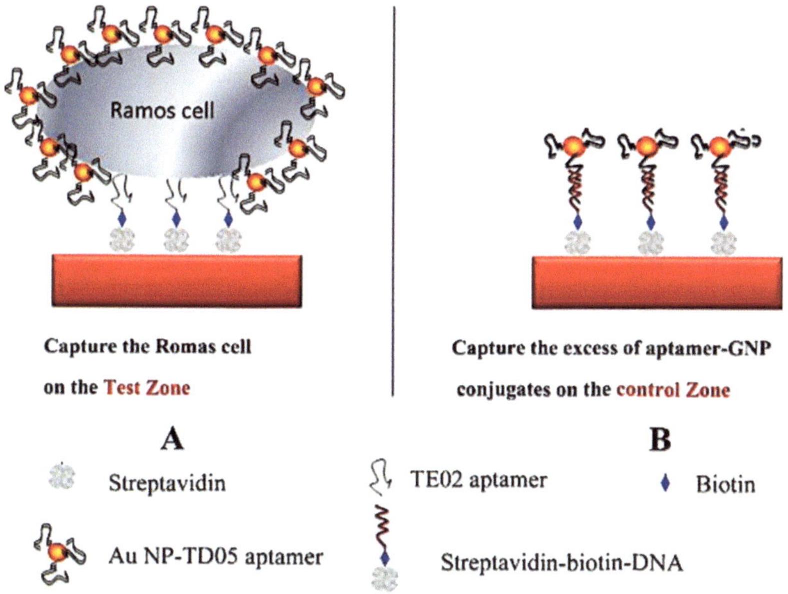

Fig. 3.5 Scheme of the detection of Ramos cells on aptamer-nanoparticle strip biosensor (**a**) Capturing Au-NP-aptamer-Ramos cells on the test zone through specific aptamer-cell interactions (**b**) Capturing the excess of Au-NP-aptamer on the control zone through aptamer-DNA hybridization reaction (From Liu et al. 2009, with permission)

erythrocytes on the membrane. The further optimization of this technology is required for the clinical implementation (Liu et al. 2009).

Technologies combining aptamer-functionalized nanoparticles with microfluidics can greatly enhance the robustness of aptamer-based CTC capture. A laminar flow flat channel microfluidic device allowed capture CCRF-CEM cells from blood due to the aptamer Sgc8 immobilized on gold nanoparticles (Sheng et al. 2013). The problem of the cancer cell diversity could be solved by using aptamer-functionalized barcode particles to capture and detect various types of CTCs (Fig. 3.6). Variations in reflection properties of different spherical colloidal crystal clusters each modified with an aptamer to a certain CTC type, act as a code for analyses. Dendrimers were used to amplify the effect of the aptamers, allowing for increased sensitivity, reliability, and specificity in CTC capture, detection and release (Zheng et al. 2014).

3.4 Electrochemical Aptasensors for CTC Detection

Another promising approach for potential CTC-related clinical applications is rather simple and ultrasensitive electrochemical sensor based on the cell-specific aptamer-modified glassy carbon electrode (GCE) detecting as few as a single BNL

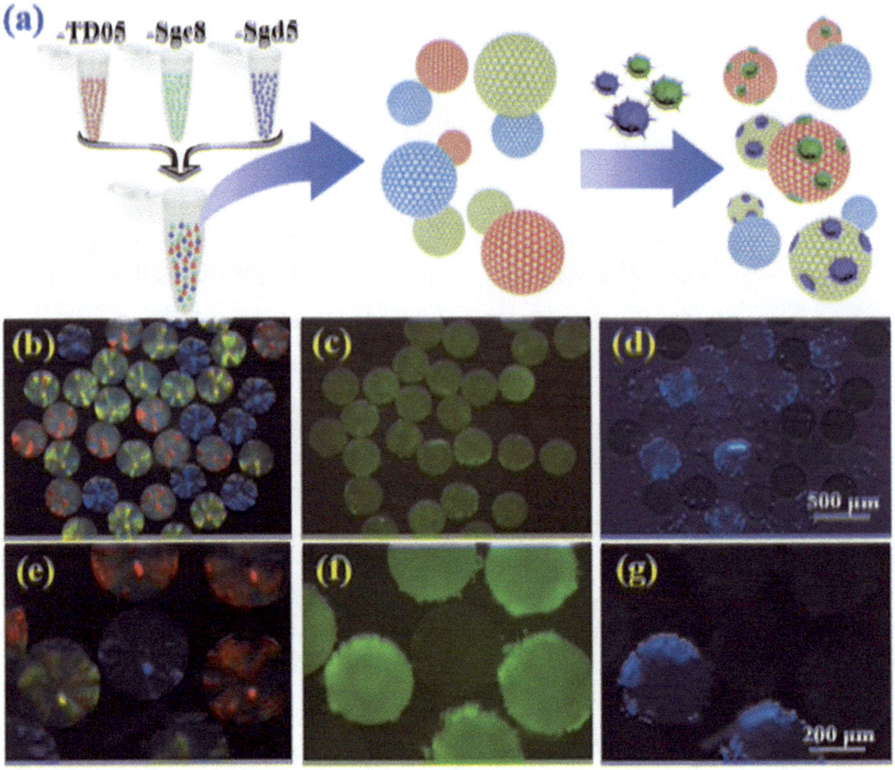

Fig. 3.6 Scheme showing the barcode particles capturing multiple types of CTCs. Various aptamers, TD05, Sgc8, and Sgd5, were used; and *green* and *blue*-stained cells were used as the target cells (From Zheng et al. 2014, with permission)

1ME A.7R.1 (MEAR) mouse hepatoma cell in 10^9 whole blood cells (Fig. 3.7) (Qu et al. 2014).

An RNA-aptamer biochip was developed for capturing and detecting a single tumor cell. The polydimethylsiloxane chip consisted of a cover containing a channel for introducing cells and sustaining their activity and microelectrode matrix on a silicon dioxide layer. The anti-EGFR RNA aptamers specifically bound the tumor cells, allowing the detection of a single cell due to the increase of ion current resistance between electrodes. This novel approach demonstrated the isolation of CTCs from peripheral blood, counting and follow-up gene or protein analysis (Wang et al. 2012).

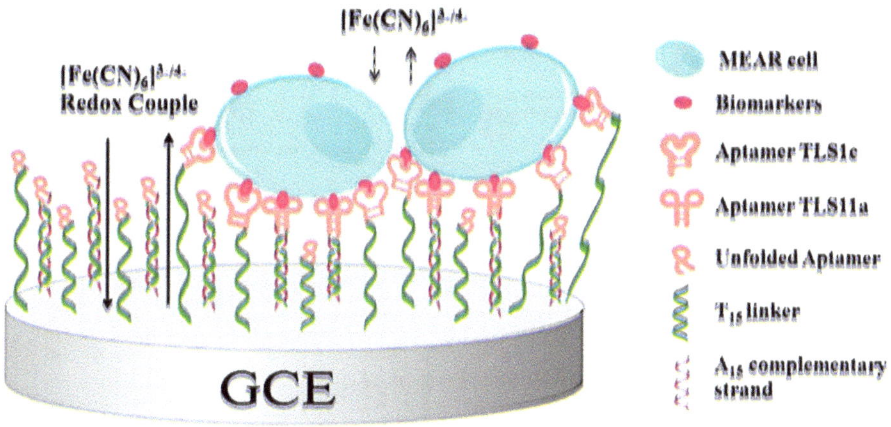

Fig. 3.7 Scheme of a dual modified electrode for specific and sensitive detection of tumor cells. Two MEAR cell-specific aptamers, TLS11a and TLS1c, conjugated to the surface of a glassy carbon electrode (GCE) via a rigid dsDNA linker (T15/A15) and a flexible ssDNA linker (T15), respectively. Specific binding brings a dramatic steric hindrance effect on the electron transfer of the redox couple $[Fe(CN)_6]^{3-/4-}$ through the GCE, while the electrostatic repulsion between negative charges of the cell surface and $[Fe(CN)_6]^{3-/4-}$ may further inhibit the electron transfer, thus significantly reducing the electron transfer speed (From Qu et al. 2014, with permission)

3.5 Aptamers for Fluorescent CTC Detection

One-step fluorochrome-quencher based strategy was described by Zeng et al. (2014) on the basis of an anti-CD30 RNA aptamer. In the absence of cells it did not emit fluorescence (Fig. 3.8), but when this aptamer-based probe interacted with a target cell, it was internalized and trafficked to the lysosome and where it was degraded. The quencher was separated from the fluorochrome, thereby allowing it to emit fluorescence. This was successfully used to identify CTCs in the whole blood of lymphoma patients, with a little background signal from the blood cells.

Another method for highly efficient capture and accurate identification of multiple types of blood CTCs using aptamer-modified porous graphene oxide membranes has been announced in 2015 by Ray group (Fig. 3.9). Aptamers to different cell types attached to 20–40 μm porous garphene oxide membranes were capable of capturing multiple types of tumor cells (SKBR3 breast cancer cells, LNCaP prostate cancer cells, and SW-948 colon cancer cells). The efficiency of graphene oxide membranes was about 95% for multiple types of tumor cells. Each aptamer had a different fluorescent dye conjugated at the 5′ end for multicolour fluorescence imaging (Nellore et al. 2015).

Another work opens up the possibility for personalized diagnostics, demonstrating advantages of using the aptamers over the antibodies, by allowing the detection of heterogenic biomarkers of tumor tissues from the individual patient. A novel in situ tissue slide-based SELEX strategy has been developed by Zhang et al. (2015). DNA aptamers that bind to formalin-fixed, paraffin-embedded breast infiltrating

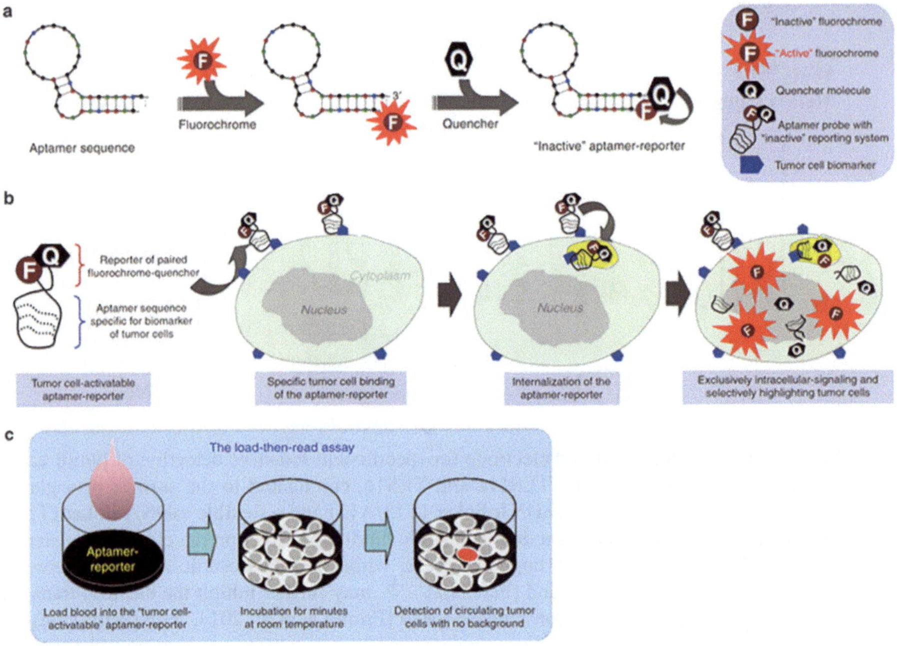

Fig. 3.8 Scheme of the tumor cell-activatable aptamer-reporter for one-step assay of CTCs in a whole blood sample (**a**) A biomarker-specific and tumor cell-activatable aptamer-reporter (**b**) Tumor cell-triggered intracellular activation of the aptamer-reporter. In assays containing tumor cells (**c**) Proposed one-step assay for rapid detection of CTCs (From Zeng et al. 2014, with permission)

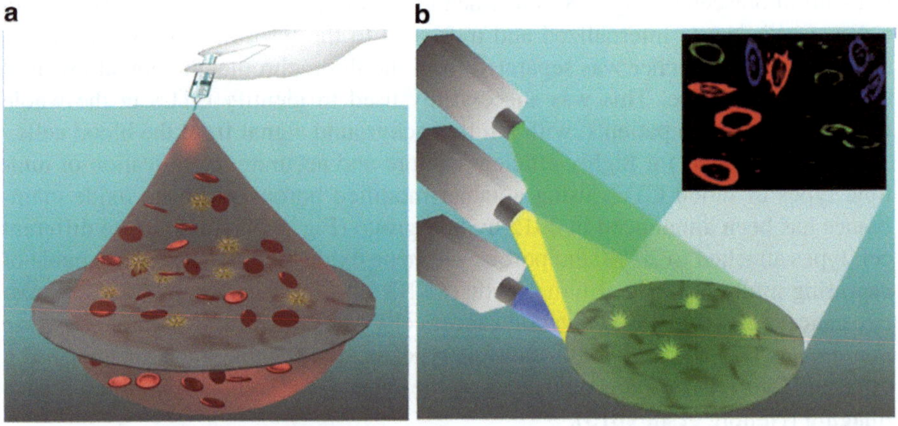

Fig. 3.9 Scheme of aptamer-conjugated porous graphene oxide membrane-based separation and (**a**) Scheme of aptamer-conjugated porous graphene oxide membrane-based capture of multiple CTC types from blood (**b**) fluorescence imaging of multiple types of CTCs captured by graphene oxide membranes using a dye-conjugated aptamer (From Nellore et al. 2015, with permission)

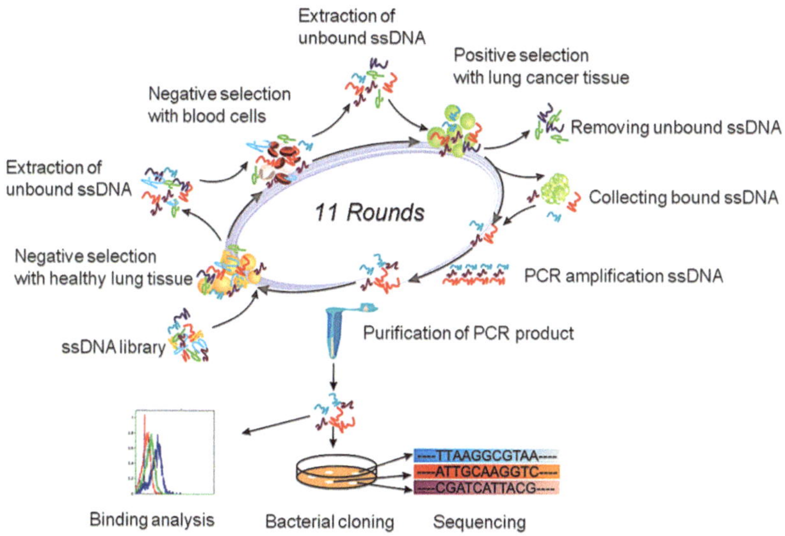

Fig. 3.10 Scheme of aptamer selection to lung adenocarcinoma postoperative tissues for producing of aptamers to intact heterogenic tumor cells (From Zamay et al. 2015, with permission)

ductal carcinomas showed fluorescence staining in the nuclei of the various human cancer cell lines as well as in CTCs isolated from pancreatic cancer patients. This aptamer method was compared with the well-established the anti-cytokeratin method on 15 pancreatic cancer patient blood samples, and enumeration indicated no difference between these two methods.

The unique feature of the work reported by Zamay et al. is the aptamer selection strategy for producing the aptamers for heterogenic lung cancer cell markers in their native state and conformation without previous knowledge of the biomarkers (Zamay et al. 2015). Tissue SELEX was used to select the aptamers with high selectivity to adenocarcinoma derived from postoperative tissues and cells capable to identify various cellular biomarkers (Fig. 3.10).

Interestingly the aptamers had very low affinity to A549 lung adenocarcinoma culture and did not bind to normal lung cells and lymphocytes. Aptamer-associated protein biomarkers for lung cancer for were identified using affinity purification with aptamer-coated magnetic beads followed by the mass-spectrometric identification. Thus anti-vimentin, anti-annexin A2, anti-annexin A5, anti-histone 2B, anti-neutrophil defensin, and anti-clusterin aptamers were used to detect CTCs in blood. These aptamers detected not only CTCs but also apoptotic bodies, and microemboli in clinical samples of peripheral blood of lung cancer and metastatic lung cancer patients. Due to the binding of multiple aptamers to different cell biomarkers, a pool of aptamer clones is more selective and efficient in CTC detection, than a single aptamer or a monoclonal antibody. Application of aptamers in combination with antibodies to tumor-specific antigens provides more reliable detection of rare CTCs. Such tumor-specific aptamers can be produced for individual patients and

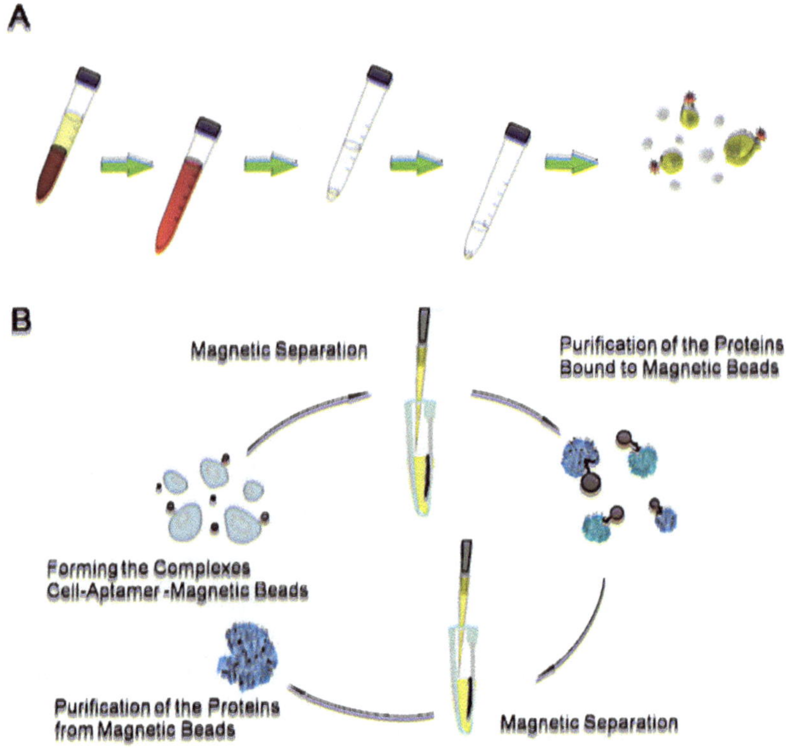

Fig. 3.11 Schemes of blood sample preparation and protein isolation (**a**) Red blood cells were lysed with hypotonic NH_4Cl solution followed by incubation with hypotonic NaCl (**b**) Aptamer-mediated affinity purification of proteins using magnetic separation for further mass spec identification (From Zamay et al. 2015, with permission)

synthesized many times during anticancer therapy, thereby opening up the possibility of personalized diagnostics.

Another valuable finding in this work was an improved blood preparation procedure reducing the time and labour required for the search of rare CTCs (Fig. 3.11). All red blood cells were lysed with NH_4Cl solution and the majority of white blood cells were lysed with hypotonic NaCl solution. Captured CTCs could be used for the following protein, genetic analyses, aptamer associated protein targets identification using aptamer-mediated affinity purification of the target proteins. Interestingly that aptamer-associated proteins identified from adenocarcinoma tissues were similar to the proteins from CTCs.

The captured CTCs pellet was visualized fluorescently labeled aptamers and/or antibodies. Live CTCs were analysed by confocal fluorescent microscopy immediately, or after fixation on glass slide. The additional Romanowsky-Giemsa staining on fixed smears allowed seeing the nuclei and aptamers (Fig. 3.12). Authors analysed blood smears from 105 individuals: 18 healthy people and 87 patients with various diagnosis including different types of primary lung cancer (52),

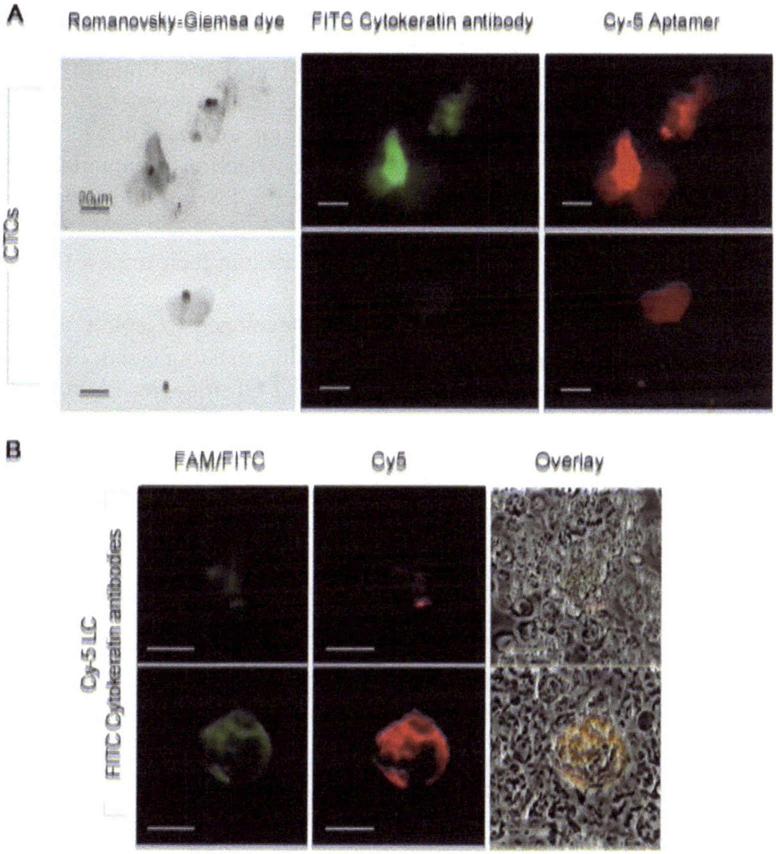

Fig. 3.12 (**a**) Co-staining of live CTCs from blood of a patient with squamous lung cancer by Cy-5 labeled LC-18 aptamer and FITC-labeled anti-pan cytokeratin antibodies (**b**) Fluorescent microscopy of blood smears of lung adenocarcinoma. Samples were pre-incubated with masking DNA, Cy-5 labeled LC-18 and FITC-labeled anti-pan cytokeratin antibodies. The samples were spread evenly on a glass slide. The smears were fixed in methanol for 5 min and then stained with Romanowsky-Giemsa dye. Magnification ×60 (From Zamay et al. 2015, with permission)

secondary lung cancer (1), other lung diseases (9), breast diseases (9), and glioblastoma (16). The sensitivity and specificity of the aptamer – based method was 86% and 76%, respectively (Zamay et al. 2015).

3.6 Conclusion

Tumor cells dissemination through the bloodstream is crucial for the metastasis formation and cancer progression. Therefore, analyses of CTC content in blood can be used after minimally invasive liquid biopsy for cancer diagnosis and prognosis.

Cytokeratins and epithelial cell adhesion molecules (EpCAM) are the most common CTC markers (Joosse and Pantel 2013). However, finding additional CTC markers and corresponding probes are in great demand due to high tumor diversity. Aptamers as synthetic affinity probes could be selected to cancer biomarkers in their native state and conformation without previous knowledge of them. These oncomarkers could be identified after the selection by aptamer-mediated affinity purification with magnetic separation and following mass spectrometry-based analysis. Aptamers that can be used for CTC capture and identification have been recently summarized by Dickey and Giangrande in their review (Dickey and Giangrande 2016).

Different methods and strategies have been developed to isolate and identify CTCs, but their efficacy needs to be validated against existing technologies such as antibody-based strategies (CellSearch) and PCR-based strategies (AdnaTest).

Acknowledgements This work was supported by Ministry of Education and Science of Russian Federation Federal Target Program # 14.604.21.0105.

References

Allard WJ, Matera J, Miller MC et al (2004) Tumor cells circulate in the peripheral blood of all major carcinomas but not in healthy subjects or patients with nonmalignant diseases. Clin Cancer Res 10(20):6897–6904

Alunni-Fabbroni M, Sandri M (2010) Circulating tumour cells in clinical practice: methods of detection and possible characterization. Methods 50(4):289–297

Chen G, Huang C, Wu H et al (2014) Isolating and concentrating rare cancerous cells in large sample volumes of blood by using dielectrophoresis and stepping electric fields. Biochip J 8 (2):67–74

Dickey D, Giangrande P (2016) Oligonucleotide aptamers: a next-generation technology for the capture and detection of circulating tumor cells. Methods 97:94–103

Hatanaka H, Yasukawa T, Mizutani F (2011) Detection of surface antigens on living cells through incorporation of immunorecognition into the distinct positioning of cells with positive and negative dielectrophoresis. Anal Chem 83(18):7207–7212

Jacob K, Sollier C, Jobodo N (2007) Circulating tumor cells: detection, molecular profiling and future prospects. Expert Rev Proteomics 4(6):741–756

Jayasena S (1999) Aptamers: an emerging class of molecules that rival antibodies in diagnostics. Clin Chem 45(9):1628–1650

Joosse S, Pantel K (2013) Biologic challenges in the detection of circulating tumor cells. Cancer Res 73(1):8–11

Lampignano R, Schneck H, Neumann M et al (2016) Detection of EpCAM-negative circulating tumor cells in metastatic breast cancer patients by using VyCAP filters technology. Oncol Res Treat 39:48–48

Li S, Chen N, Zhang Z et al (2013) Endonuclease-responsive aptamer-functionalized hydrogel coating for sequential catch and release of cancer cells. Biomaterials 34(2):460–469

Liu G, Mao X, Phillips J et al (2009) Aptamer-nanoparticle strip biosensor for sensitive detection of cancer cells. Anal Chem 81(24):10013–10018

Maremanda N, Roy K, Kanwar R et al (2015) Quick chip assay using locked nucleic acid modified epithelial cell adhesion molecule and nucleolin aptamers for the capture of circulating tumor cells. Biomicrofluidics 9(5):054110

Martin J, Phillips J, Parekh P et al (2011) Capturing cancer cells using aptamer-immobilized square capillary channels. Mol BioSyst 7(5):1720–1727

Nellore B, Kanchanapally R, Pramanik A et al (2015) Aptamer-conjugated graphene oxide membranes for highly efficient capture and accurate identification of multiple types of circulating tumor cells. Bioconjug Chem 26(2):235–242

Punnoose E, Atwal S, Liu W et al (2012) Evaluation of circulating tumor cells and circulating tumor DNA in non-small cell lung cancer: association with clinical endpoints in a phase II clinical trial of pertuzumab and erlotinib. Clin Cancer Res 18(8):2391–2401

Qu L, Xu J, Tan X et al (2014) Dual-aptamer modification generates a unique Interface for highly sensitive and specific electrochemical detection of tumor cells. ACS Appl Mater Interfaces 6 (10):7309–7315

Rusconi C, Scardino E, Layzer J et al (2002) RNA aptamers as reversible antagonists of coagulation factor IXa. Nature 419(6902):90–94

Sefah K, Meng L, Lopez-Colon D et al (2010) DNA aptamers as molecular probes for colorectal cancer study. PLoS One 5(12):e14269

Shangguan D, Li Y, Tang Z et al (2006) Aptamers evolved from live cells as effective molecular probes for cancer study. Proc Natl Acad Sci U S A 103(32):11838–11843

Shen Q, Xu L, Zhao L et al (2013) Specific capture and release of circulating tumor cells using aptamer-modified nanosubstrates. Adv Mater 25(16):2368–2373

Sheng W, Chen T, Katnath R et al (2012) Aptamer-enabled efficient isolation of cancer cells from whole blood using a microfluidic device. Anal Chem 84(9):4199–4206

Sheng W, Chen T, Tan W et al (2013) Multivalent DNA Nanospheres for enhanced capture of cancer cells in microfluidic devices. ACS Nano 7(8):7067–7076

Sheng W, Ogunwobi O, Chen T et al (2014) Capture, release and culture of circulating tumor cells from pancreatic cancer patients using an enhanced mixing chip. Lab Chip 14(1):89–98

Sun N, Wang J, Ji L et al (2015) A cellular compatible chitosan nanoparticle surface for isolation and in situ culture of rare number CTCs. Small 11(40):5444–5451

Tang Z, Shangguan D, Wang K et al (2007) Selection of aptamers for molecular recognition and characterization of cancer cells. Anal Chem 79(13):4900–4907

Wan Y, Tan J, Asghar W et al (2011) Velocity effect on aptamer-based circulating tumor cell isolation in microfluidic devices. J Phys Chem B 115(47):13891–13896

Wan Y, Liu Y, Allen P et al (2012) Capture, isolation and release of cancer cells with aptamer-functionalized glass bead array. Lab Chip 12(22):4693–4701

Wang L, Zheng Q, Zhang Q et al (2012) Detection of single tumor cell resistance with aptamer biochip. Oncol Lett 4(5):935–940

Wehbe M, Labib M, Muharemagic D et al (2015) Switchable aptamers for biosensing and bioseparation of viruses (SwAps-V). Biosens Bioelectron 67:280–286

Zamay G, Kolovskaya O, Zamay T et al (2015) Aptamers selected to postoperative lung adenocarcinoma detect circulating tumor cells in human blood. Mol Ther 23(9):1486–1496

Zeng Z, Tung C, Zu Y (2014) A cancer cell-activatable aptamer-reporter system for one-step assay of circulating tumor cells. Mol Ther Nucl Acid 3:e184

Zhang J, Li S, Liu F et al (2015) SELEX aptamer used as a probe to detect circulating tumor cells in peripheral blood of pancreatic cancer patients. PLoS One 10(3):e0121920

Zhao L, Tang C, Xu L et al (2016) Enhanced and differential capture of circulating tumor cells from lung cancer patients by microfluidic assays using aptamer cocktail. Small 12 (8):1072–1081

Zheng F, Cheng Y, Wang J et al (2014) Aptamer-functionalized barcode particles for the capture and detection of multiple types of circulating tumor cells. Adv Mater 26(43):7333–7338

Chapter 4
Development of a Protocol for Single-Cell Analysis of Circulating Tumor Cells in Patients with Solid Tumors

Carolina Reduzzi, Rosita Motta, Giulia Bertolini, Patrizia Miodini, Antonia Martinetti, Elisa Sottotetti, Maria Grazia Daidone, and Vera Cappelletti

Abstract Genomic characterization of circulating tumor cells (CTCs) enables the monitoring of tumor progression and of adaption occurring during treatment. CTC molecular characterization represents indeed a precious tool to implement in the clinical practice for better dealing with acquired resistance to systemic treatment and tumor evolution. Unfortunately CTCs are very rare and enrichments from blood samples and subsequent identification of these cells are technically very challenging. We describe here the main steps leading to the development of a technical protocol for visualization, enumeration and recovery of single CTCs exploiting the recently developed DEPArray™platform. Our description of the technical workflow starts with evaluation of pre-analytical aspects related to blood sample collection warning about the possible effects on immunoreactivity profiles which may bias the interpretation. Subsequently, other CTC-enrichment approaches are critically discussed and compared in relation to their performances with the DEPArray™. Identification of CTCs represents another critical point due to their heterogeneity and due to the still-to-be clarified role of different subpopulations, typically epithelial, mesenchymal or mixed. Finally, issues related to single cell analysis are illustrated. The chapter ends with an overview of results obtained on real clinical samples which support the reliability of the protocol and its transferability to the daily clinical routine.

C. Reduzzi • R. Motta • P. Miodini • M.G. Daidone • V. Cappelletti (✉)
Biomarker Unit, Department of Experimental Oncology and Molecular Medicine, Fondazione IRCCS Istituto Nazionale dei Tumori, Via Amadeo 42, 20133 Milano, Italy
e-mail: vera.cappelletti@istitutotumori.mi.it

G. Bertolini
Tumor Genomics Unit, Department of Experimental Oncology and Molecular Medicine, Fondazione IRCCS Istituto Nazionale dei Tumori, Via Venezian 1, 20133 Milano, Italy

A. Martinetti • E. Sottotetti
Medical Oncology Unit, Fondazione IRCCS Istituto Nazionale dei Tumori, Via Venezian 1, 20133 Milano, Italy

M.J.M. Magbanua, J.W. Park (eds.), *Isolation and Molecular Characterization of Circulating Tumor Cells*, Advances in Experimental Medicine and Biology 994,
DOI 10.1007/978-3-319-55947-6_4

Keywords Circulating tumor cells • CTC enrichment and identification • Single-cell analysis • Whole genome amplification • DEPArray™

4.1 Why Should We Study Single CTCs?

CTCs have been studied for a long time as prognostic and treatment response predictive biomarkers essentially focusing on their enumeration or more simply on their presence or absence (Paoletti and Hayes 2016; Bidard et al. 2016). More recently, many evidences have been collected over different tumor types indicating that CTCs represent the actual tumor mass as a whole (including primaries, metastases and possibly micrometastatic deposits) (Heitzer et al. 2013, Lohr et al. 2014, Ni et al. 2013, Yu et al. 2012). Furthermore, CTCs increasingly appear to even represent much more than just non-invasive surrogates for getting insight into the tumor molecular make-up.

In their pioneering study Heitzer et al. (2013) isolated 37 single CTCs from 6 patients with stage IV colorectal cancer and demonstrated that the copy number variations (CNV) detected in single CTC were present also in the primaries and that, whereas mutational profiles of single CTCs recapitulated the primary tumors, there were also some private CTC mutations. Intriguingly, such private mutations rather than represent technical artifacts due to DNA-amplification strategies were instead found to be present, although at subclonal level, also in the primaries by deeper sequencing. This amazing finding not only supports the ability of CTCs to represent the tumor from where they originate, but also holds the promise that the knowledge of the CTC genomic asset might lead to a reconsideration of a patient for a target treatment which was instead discarded based on the mutational profile of the primary tumor. If confirmed by other studies, such results support the concept that information derived from single CTCs might even represent a more reliable, and not only a more accessible, tumor sample.

In a prostate cancer study Dago and colleagues (Dago et al. 2014) revealed instead how characterization with respect to androgen receptor expression and CNV of single CTCs from blood draws longitudinally collected during treatment, allowed the reconstruction of the clonal evolution occurring during initial treatment response and subsequent progression. Their study provides a strong case for the clinical relevance of single CTC characterization during therapy cycles for a timely detection of clonal evolution and of genomic alterations driving the treatment resistance.

As highlighted by these examples, the possibility to molecularly characterize CTCs holds the potential for a real paradigm shift in the treatment of solid tumors by giving up the need to tailor treatments on molecular features of surgical samples or biopsies, which have been often obtained long times before treatment decision. CTC-derived molecular information could be unbiased by intra-tumor heterogeneity, by the temporal evolution resulting from selective pressure, but also by the subclonal nature of specific genomic alterations within the primary tumors which will eventually drive the resistance or evolution to a more aggressive phenotype.

Unfortunately, the translation into a framework for an analytically and clinically valid analysis of such CTC-based fluid biopsies is studded by technically difficulties. Indeed CTCs do not only represent rare events, but are also characterized by a marked heterogeneity which makes up their ability to survive in the circulation and to generate metastases. Hence, grasping the full informative content from CTCs would need the combination of enrichment methods able to avoid selection of specific CTC sub-populations with methods allowing the subsequent accurate sorting of specific single CTCs or of homogeneous groups of CTCs with well-defined characteristics.

In the next sections we describe the steps towards the definition of a methodological protocol suitable for enrichments, identification, sorting and isolation of single CTCs for downstream molecular interrogations considering pre-analytical issues and analytical validation.

The described protocol exploits the recently developed DEPArray™ system (SiliconBiosystems, Bologna, Italy). The DEPArray™ is an automated platform designed to isolate and recover single cells. The instrument is based on dielectrophoresis (DEP), an electrokinetic principle by which, creating a non-uniform electric field, it is possible to exert forces on neutral particles such as cells. The electric field is created inside a microfluidic chip (DEPArray™ cartridge) containing cells suspended in a liquid, where it forms DEP "cages" around cells trapping them. The DEPArray™ is also equipped with a six-channel fluorescent microscope and a CCD camera that captures images and identifies cells by their fluorescence labeling and morphological characteristics. The instrument offers the possibility to analyze the collected images with a software, chose the cells of interest and recover them in a tube for further analyses (Fuchs et al. 2006; Abonnenc et al. 2013).

4.2 First Things First: Pre-analytical Issues

In the context of best laboratory practice, optimal sample handling and storage are the first steps for reaching good analytical results (Elliott et al. 2008, Holland et al. 2003). Blood does not represent an exception to such a rule, and in the case of CTCs, which already *in vivo* have a short half life, rapid and accurate processing is essential to avoid cell lyses processes. Along with anticoagulants, addition of specific cell preservatives represents a frequently pursued way to retain the integrity of CTCs (Qin et al. 2014) and is often used also to avoid contamination of circulating tumor DNA by DNA released from peripheral blood mononucleated cells (PBMC) upon their lysis (Kang et al. 2016). Several blood collection tubes have been developed to such a purpose, starting from the CellSave Preservative Tubes specifically dedicated to blood collection of samples to be processed by the CellSearch® system, and which allow room temperature storage of samples for up to 96 h. (https://www.cellsearchctc.com/product-systems-overview/cellsave-preservative-tubes). Other commercially available tubes are the Cell-Free DNA™BCT (Streck, Omaha, NE) tubes containing a formaldehyde-free preservative which stabilizes nucleated blood cells, and extends the preservation of CTCs up to

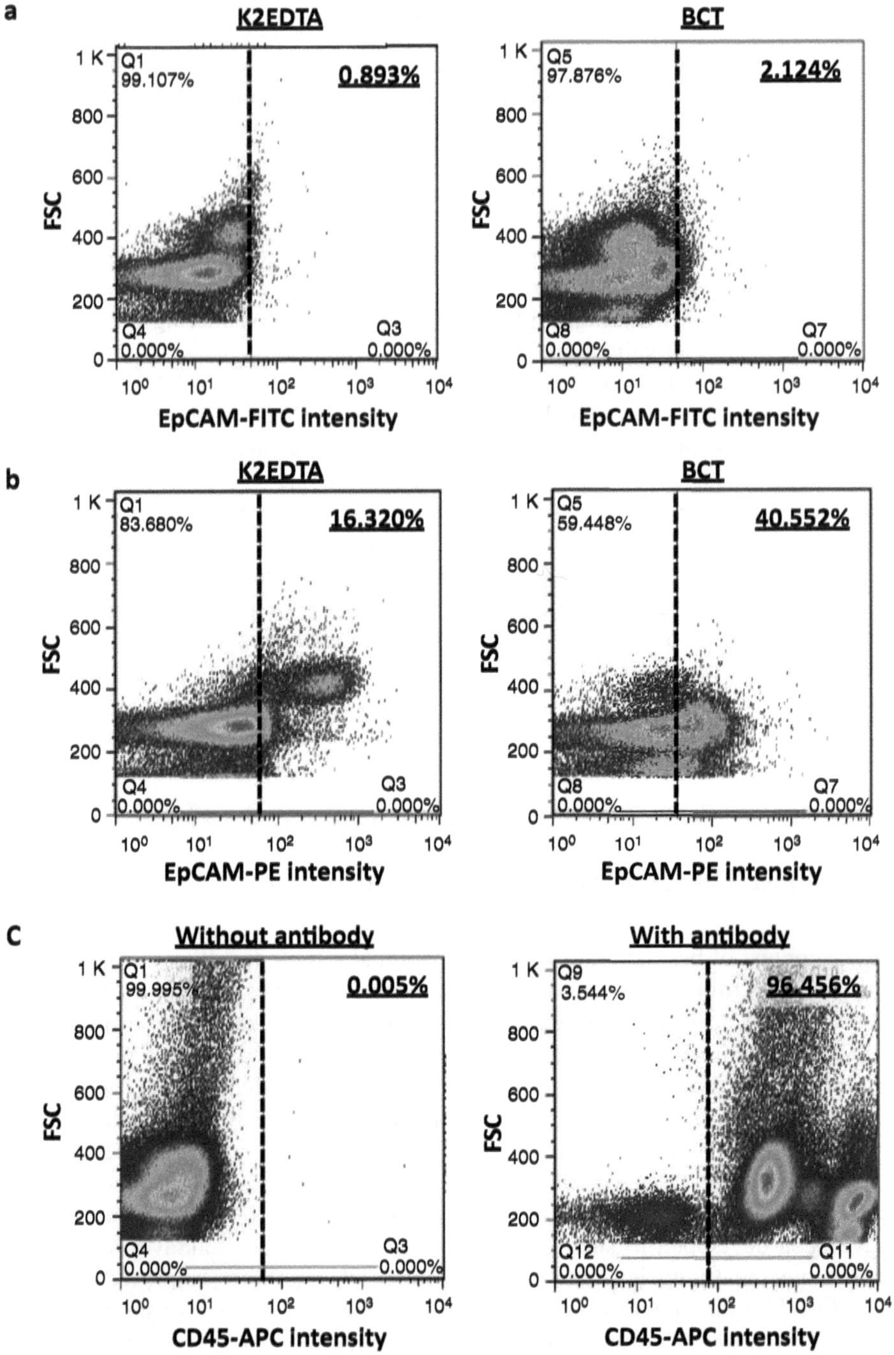

Fig. 4.1 Antibody specificity evaluated by flow cytometry. Flow cytometry analysis of PBMCs derived from HD blood samples collected in K_2EDTA or in BCT tubes and stained with distinct antibodies directed against EpCAM. *Panel a*: Miltenyi Biotec anti EpCAM-FITC antibody. No unspecific staining of PBMCs is observed, with both blood collection tubes. *Panel b*: Santa Cruz Biotechnology anti EpCAM-PE antibody. Variable fractions of HD PBMCs stain as EpCAM + ve

4-days (https://www.streck.com/product.aspx?p=cell-free%20dna%20bct), and the TransFix® (Cytomark, Buckingham, UK) tubes which stabilize cellular antigens for up to 10 days (http://www.biognost.be/files/cms1/TransFix%20Vacuum%20Blood%20Collection%20Tubes.pdf).

Notwithstanding the procedure chosen for CTC enrichments from blood samples, a crucial step in developing a CTC assay on intact cells is their identification which is necessarily done based on CTC or PBMC immunophenotyping, thus the effect of the chosen blood collection tube on immunorecognition must be carefully defined in preliminary experiments.

The specific molecular composition of the above mentioned preservatives is unknown, but we reasoned that, though designed to stabilize cells, the intrinsic fixation procedure still might modify cell surface antigen reactivity and interfere with CTC immunophenotyping. Literature data specifically addressing antibody specificity in the presence of preservatives are lacking, although Qin et al. (2014) report that BCT were in fact better preserving immunoreactivity after 4 days of blood storage at room temperature, compared to K_3EDTA tubes (BD Vacutainer®, Becton Dickinson, Franklin Lakes, NJ, USA) when tested with certain Anti CK8 and anti-EPCAM antibodies.

Therefore, since CTCs are commonly defined as nucleated cells expressing epithelial markers and lacking blood cells markers, we focused on the expression of EpCAM (an epithelial marker) and CD45 (a leukocyte marker), using fluorescently labeled antibodies. In particular we selected two antibodies directed against EpCAM (anti-human EpCAM PE-conjugated, clone O.N.276, Santa Cruz Biotechnology, Dallas, TX, USA and anti-human EpCAM FITC-conjugated, clone HEA-125, Miltenyi Biotec, Bergisch Gladbach, Germany) and one antibody against CD45 (anti-human CD45 APC-conjugated, clone 5B1, Miltenyi Biotec).

The specificity of the antibodies was preliminarily tested by flow cytometry analysis of PBMC collected using Ficoll from healthy donors (HD) blood samples by using staining conditions as recommended by the antibodies manufacturers. In particular, the effect of tubes used for blood collection on the immunoreactivity profile was evaluated comparing samples collected in K_2EDTA tubes and in the BCT. The anti-EPCAM antibody from Miltenyi Biotec showed a high specificity both in the sample collected using K_2EDTA tube and in the one collected with the BCT without any unspecific staining of blood cells, as shown in Fig. 4.1a. Conversely, the antibody from Santa Cruz Biotechnology unspecifically reacted with

Fig. 4.1 (continued) both in blood collected in K_2EDTA (*left panel*, 16%) and in BCT (*right panel*, 40%). *Panel c*: Flow cytometry analysis of MCF-7 cells spiked in PBMCs derived from HD blood samples collected in BCT tubes only. In the absence of the antibody (*left panel*) MCF-7 and WBC are distinguishable based on size (FSC axis) and are not APC-negative; addition of the antiCD45 antibody (*right panel*) shows a strong shift of staining towards positivity for both MCF7 and WBC. The *dotted lines* indicated the positivity thresholds of staining intensities defined on negative controls (omitting the antibody) (Abbreviations: *HD* healthy donor, *WBC* white blood cells, *PBMC* peripheral blood mononucleated cells)

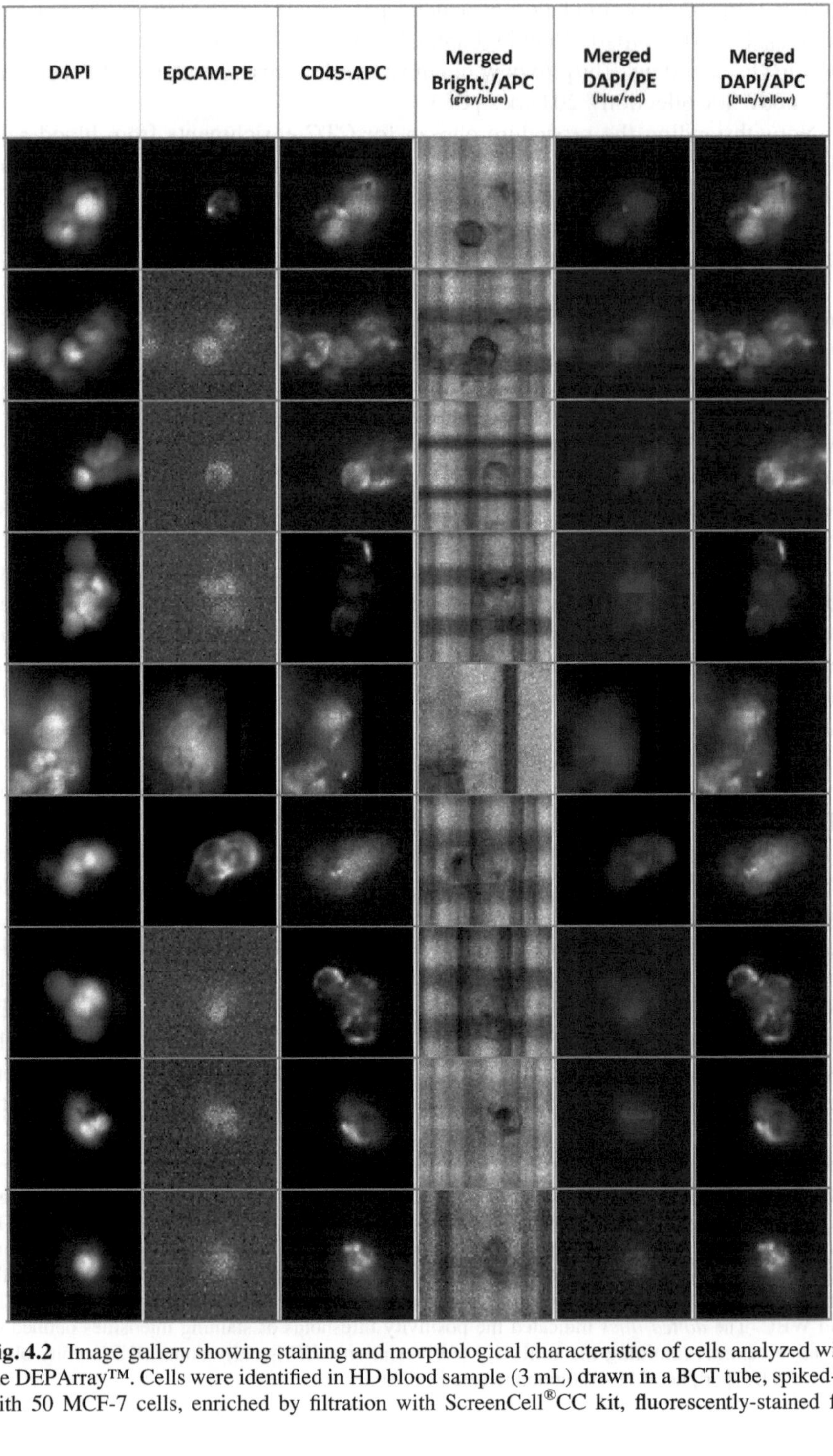

Fig. 4.2 Image gallery showing staining and morphological characteristics of cells analyzed with the DEPArray™. Cells were identified in HD blood sample (3 mL) drawn in a BCT tube, spiked-in with 50 MCF-7 cells, enriched by filtration with ScreenCell®CC kit, fluorescently-stained for

16% of blood cells collected with K_2EDTA tube, but also with 40% of blood cells when collection was performed using BCT (Fig. 4.1b). Finally, the specificity of the CD45 antibody was assessed using a breast cancer cell line negative for CD45 (MCF-7) spiked at a concentration of 15–20% into PBMCs isolated from HD blood using Ficoll density centrifugation: flow cytometry analysis surprisingly revealed an unspecific staining of all the MCF-7 cells by the anti-CD45 antibody in the blood sample collected with the BCT (Fig. 4.1c), which was about fourfold higher compared to that observed with K_2EDTA tubes (data not shown).

The above described data show that pre-analytical conditions, such as type of tubes used for blood collection, may definitely, depending on the antibody, affect its specificity. Preliminary tests must therefore be run before proceeding with CTC staining.

Following these results, which confirm the importance of pre-analytical issues, we decided to use the anti-EpCAM antibody characterized by higher specificity under our working conditions. The critical role played by blood collection tubes on immunoreactivity profiles, already described in flow cytometry experiments, was reconfirmed by DEPArray™ as shown in Figs. 4.2 and 4.3.

Blood collection in preservative-free tubes was further supported by morphological considerations, since tumor cells spiked into blood collected in BCT (Fig. 4.2) appeared as swollen compared to those collected in K_2 EDTA tubes (Fig. 4.3), a feature that might be rather confusing when trying to identify CTCs in clinical samples. Furthermore, collection of blood in BCT induced the formation of aggregates preventing the possibility to recover single cells from each DEP-cage. Finally, cells with a double staining for EpCAM and CD45 were observed impairing the distinction between tumor cells and white blood cells (WBC).

Therefore, due to the interference observed on immunoreactivity, cell morphology and stickiness when collecting blood in the presence of preservatives, we chose to draw blood in K_2EDTA tubes although this forced us to process samples within a short time from collection. To make the protocol more suitable for clinical samples analysis we introduced a stopping point after CTC-enrichment by adding a fixation step with 2% paraformaldehyde (PFA) for 20 min at room temperature.

Fig. 4.2 (continued) EpCAM, CD45 and nuclei and analyzed with the DEPArray™. The figure shows the presence of numerous cell-aggregates which prevent the correct visualization of cells by interfering with focus. Please note the cells positive for both tumor (PE-channel) and WBC (APC-channel) markers (*rows 1 and 6*) which cannot be identified as MCF-7 or WBCs by staining profiles nor can be distinguished by morphological characteristics, since all (including true CD45 + ve/EpCAM-ve WBCs) appear about the same size (*i.e.* larger than leukocytes observed in the blood sample drawn in K_2EDTA tube, Fig. 4.3). Overall, correct cell identification is biased by the poor quality of the sample and by the low staining specificity (Abbreviations: *HD* healthy donor, *WBC* white blood cell)

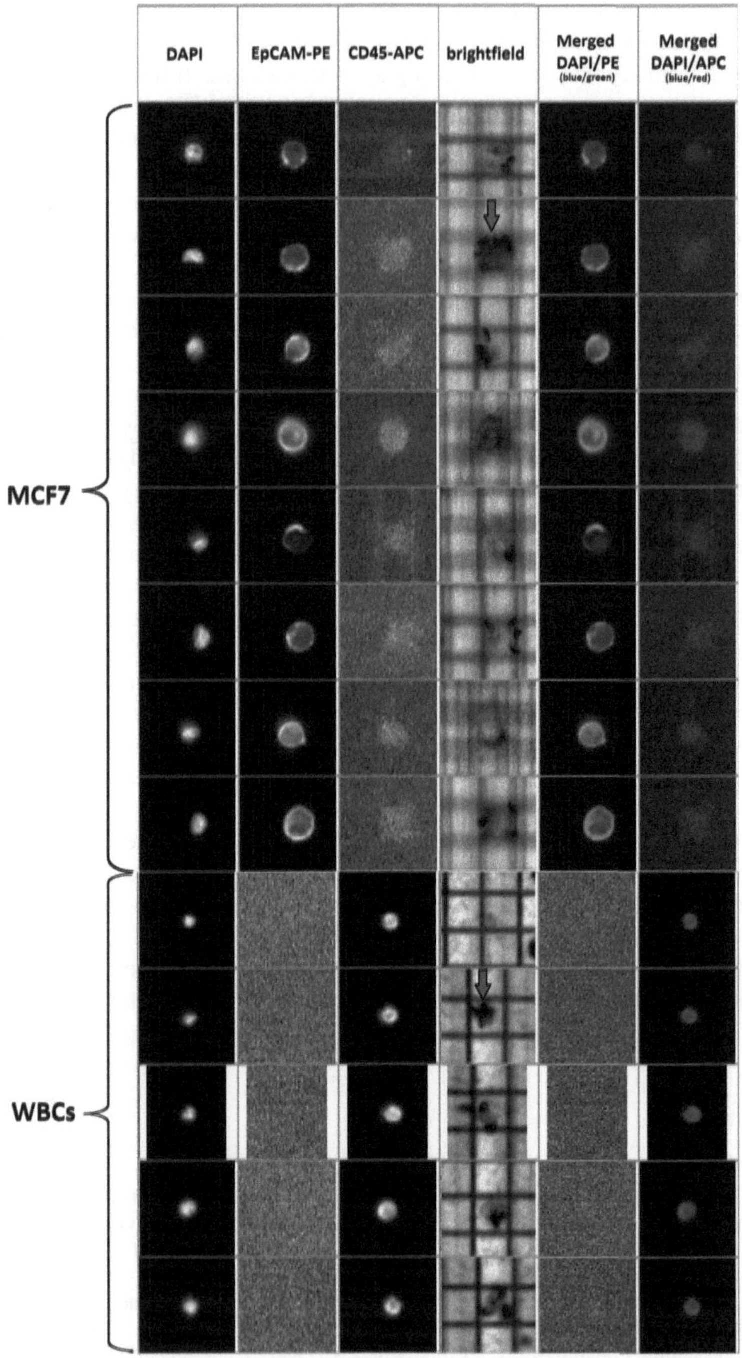

Fig. 4.3 Image gallery showing staining and morphological characteristics of cells analyzed with the DEPArray™. Cells were identified in a HD blood sample (3 mL) drawn in a K_2EDTA tube, spiked-in with 50 MCF-7 cells, enriched by filtration with ScreenCell®CC kit, fixed with 2% PFA,

4.3 Steps Towards Analytical Validation

4.3.1 Identifying CTCs by Classical Criteria

Experiments were performed by spiking the same number of MCF-7 (50 cells) into HD blood samples collected in K_2EDTA tubes, processed for CTCs enrichment and stained for EpCAM, CD45 and nucleus (Hoechst 33,342, Sigma Aldrich, St. Louis, MO, USA) either before or after the PFA fixation step. The number of MCF-7 recovered, defined as EpCAM-positive and CD45-ve nucleated cells, and the qualities of the staining were assessed with the DEPArray™. The numbers of recovered target cells were 11 and 13 respectively, and since no differences in the quality of the staining was observed we settled our workflow introducing the fixation step after enrichment and before staining for convenience.

Analysis of DEPArray™ image galleries obtained in the preliminary experiments highlighted a new issue, *i.e.* the presence of red blood cells interfering by masking the cells of interest and making their pictures rather unclear as can be seen from Fig. 4.3. To overcome this latter problem, the use of an RBC lysing buffer (BDPharm Lyse™, BD Biosciences, San Jose, CA, USA) was tested in spiking experiments with 50 MCF-7. The RBC lysis step (15 min at room temperature protected from light) was introduced before fixation and staining. Its use however, interfered with the recovery rates resulting in a fourfold lower number of recovered target cells compared to experiments without RBC lysis. This option was therefore abandoned.

Meanwhile the identification of CTCs was improved by adding the staining for cytokeratins (CK), another epithelial marker, but with an intracellular rather than cell membrane location. An anti-human pan Cytokeratin PE-conjugated antibody (clone C11, Abcam, San Francisco, CA, USA) was used strictly according to the manufacturers' instruction (dil 1:10, 10 min at room temperature) and its sensibility and specificity were tested. When MCF-7 cells were fixed with 2% PFA, stained for CK and observed under a fluorescent microscope, the antibody showed high sensibility since roughly 100% of the cells resulted CK+ve as expected. Its specificity was optimal as evidenced in following experiments in which 50 MCF-7 were spiked in HD blood samples, enriched, fixed with 2% PFA and stained for CK and CD45: no unspecific staining could be observed.

Interestingly, the staining protocol adopted for this intracellular antibody solved the problem of cellular image masking by RBC, as the required cell permeabilization step, performed using the detergent-containing reagent Inside

Fig. 4.3 (continued) fluorescently-stained for EpCAM, CD45 and nuclei and analyzed with the DEPArray™. Tumor cells (*top rows*) are well distinguishable from WBCs (*bottom rows*) both by marker expression (all MCF-7 cells are positive in the PE-channel and negative in the ACP-channel while all WBCs are EpCAM-ve and CD45 +ve) and by size (tumor cells appear larger than leukocytes). In some cases, the morphological evaluation in the brightfield channel is impaired by the presence of RBCs covering cells (indicated by *arrows*) (Abbreviations: *HD* healthy donor, *WBC* white blood cells, *RBC* red blood cell)

Perm (Miltenyi Biotech) effectively eliminated RBC without affecting the target cell yield which was maintained around 30%.

4.3.2 Optimizing CTC Enrichment

CTCs are extremely rare and their enrichment represents a technical challenge which we have addressed by comparing several technologies. However, there are much more different technologies available to this purpose compared to those tested here, and which are mainly subdivided into two categories: methods that enrich tumor cells by exploiting the expression of epithelial markers (positive enrichments) or blood cell markers (negative selection) and methods based on physical properties (size, density, deformability) (Joosse et al. 2014). Considering that CTCs are a heterogeneous population composed by different subclones which evolve during time and can undergo an epithelial to mesenchymal transition (Yu et al. 2013, Bulfoni et al. 2016), we decided to focus on technologies which are not based on the expression of epithelial markers, to include not only epithelial CTCs, but also cells with a mesenchymal phenotype (which could be associated with a higher metastatic potential, Yu et al. 2013).

Four technologies in particular have been tested: ScreenCell® CC kit (ScreenCell, Sarcelles, France), OncoQuick™ (Greiner Bio-One, Frickenhausen, Germany), AutoMACS® Pro separator (Miltenyi Biotec,) and Parsortix (Angle plc, Guildford, UK). To test their efficiency, blood samples from HD were spiked in with 50, 25 or 10 tumor cells derived from MCF-7 cell line and samples were processed by the different enrichment methods. The enriched fractions were analyzed to evaluate the number of recovered target cells. The identity of recovered cells was confirmed by mutational analysis of a specific mutation (p.E545K) using the Ampli1™ PIK3CA Seq kit (Silicon Biosystems) and Sanger sequencing.

4.3.2.1 ScreenCell® CC Kit

This technology is based on cell size: blood is filtered through an isolation support (IS) consisting in a membrane with pores of pre-defined size which traps larger cells and allows the passage of blood cells. Each IS allows processing of up to 3 mL of blood. Filtrations of spiked blood samples were done according to manufacturer's instructions, and cells were detached from IS essentially according to protocols furnished by ScreenCell, labeled according to our standard protocol (for EpCAM, CK, CD45, nuclei) and processed with the DEPArray™ for cell identification and counting. We performed independent spiking experiments using a cell line (MCF-7). Results, for samples spiked with 50 MCF-7 cells are reported in Table 4.1, and revealed a mean recovery rate of 32.5%. Spikes with lower cell numbers (25, 10) yielded more variable recoveries ranging from 22 to 56%.

Table 4.1 Recovery rates using cell-enrichment by ScreenCell®

	Independent spiking replicates with MCF-7 cell line (50 cells)					
EpCAM+/CK+/CD45-nucleated cells visualized by DEPArray™	11	13	8	13	14	11
% recovery corrected for DEPArray™ cartridge void volume[a]	31	37	22	37	39	31

[a]the DEPArray™ cartridge allows analysis of only part of the loaded sample

4.3.2.2 AutoMACS® Pro Separator

The AutoMACS® is a bench top instrument for rapid preparative cell sorting by immunomagnetic beads packed into separation columns and which allows positive/negative selection of cells expressing or lacking selected markers. We used the anti-CD45 microbeads (Miltenyi Biotec) to deplete leukocytes from HD blood samples spiked with 50 MCF-7 cells in two independent experiments. In both cases, the system was not able to recover any MCF-7 cell, and this approach was therefore discarded as CTC–enrichment method, although positive results have been recently published by investigators using this system in combination with the DEPArray™ in women with metastatic breast cancer (Bulfoni et al.2016).

4.3.2.3 OncoQuick™

This technology exploits a 50 mL-polypropylene tube containing a porous barrier inserted above a specially developed medium that enriches tumor cells by density gradient centrifugation. The system is designed to allow processing of up to 30 mL of whole blood without preliminary fixation. In nine spiking experiments, performed using 15 mL of HD blood and summarized in Table 4.2., it proved to have an overall mean recovery rate of 81%. The recovery rate was higher with lower number of target cells (10 cells) compared to samples containing 25–50 MCF-7 (100% and 71% respectively). The high recovery rates and the possibility to use large blood volumes make this enrichment system particularly attractive for clinical samples derived from patients with early disease where lower numbers of CTCs are expected.

However, despite its sensitivity, OncoQuick™ presented an important weakness when it was adopted for processing of clinical samples due to the high number of WBC contaminating the tumor target cells. The high number of contaminating WBC in samples processed with OncoQuick results into most (if not all) samples to exceed the maximum capacity of the DEPArray™ cartridges (40,000 cells) making the sorting of single cells impossible due to the presence of more than one cell in each dielectrophoretic cage (Fig. 4.4). This issue could be partially overcome by splitting the sample into multiple DEPArray™ cartridges, a solution which is very

Table 4.2. Recovery rates using cell-enrichment by OncoQuick™

	10 MCF-7 spiking triplicates			25 MCF-7 spiking triplicates			50 MCF-7 spiking triplicates		
EpCAM+/CK+/CD45-nucleated cells visualized by DEPArray™	7	8	7	11	14	10	26	30	27
% recovery corrected for DEPArray™ cartridge void volume[a]	100	100	100	61	78	56	72	83	75

[a]the DEPArray™ cartridge allows analysis of only part of the loaded sample

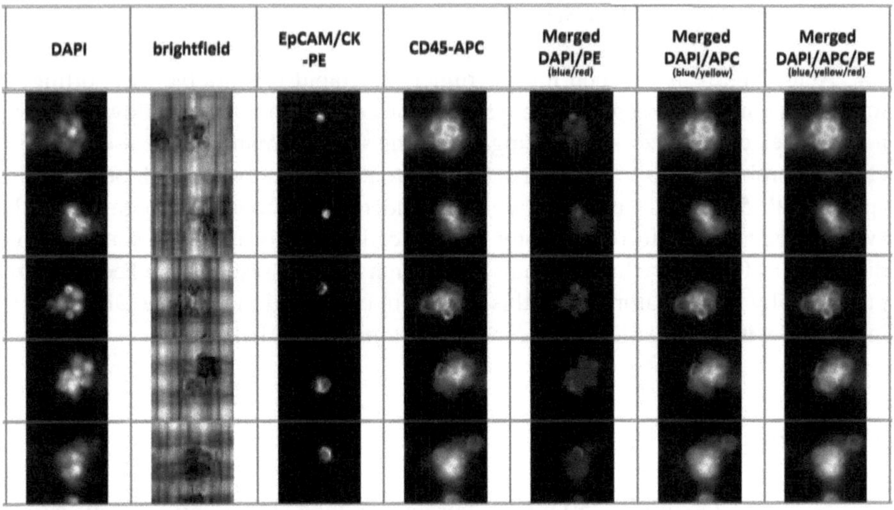

Fig. 4.4 CTCs identified in a metastatic breast cancer patient. A blood sample (13.7 mL) was collected from a metastatic breast cancer patient in K_2EDTA tube before starting chemotherapy. CTCs were enriched with OncoQuick™, fixed with 2% PFA, fluorescently-stained for EpCAM, CK, CD45 and nuclei and finally analyzed with the DEPArray™. Five of the 37 identified CTCs are reported in the Figure: their tumor phenotype is confirmed by expression of epithelial markers (EpCAM and CK, PE-channel) and by absence of CD45 staining (best evaluable in the last column merging DAPI, PE and APC channels). The high number of contaminating leukocytes present in the sample generates aggregates inside the DEP-cages interfering with correct routing and recovery of CTCs

time-consuming and expensive and does not represent the best choice for a protocol to be used for clinical samples.

4.3.2.4 Parsortix

This system uses a micro-fluidic technology to capture CTCs in a cassette, exploiting their less deformable nature and larger size compared to other blood components. Literature reports comparing this CTC-enrichment approach with classical EpCAM-based methods using different cell lines and a limited number of clinical samples, suggest its ability to detect larger numbers of cells (Xu et al. 2015; Chudziak et al. 2016; Hvichia et al. 2016).

The cell enrichment performance was initially explored using the MCF-7 cells for which comparative results with other enrichment approaches were available. Recovery rates were high ranging from 70 to 84% a performance which is comparable to that obtained with the OncoQuick™ approach, but with an important advantage in terms of specificity. Indeed, the total number of cells harvested with the use of Parsortix was on the average around 1500, almost 30-fold lower with respect to the DEPArray™ dielectrophoretic cartridges capacity, and allowing therefore true single-cell analyses, without the need to split the sample.

For these reasons, the Parsortix technology appeared in our hands as the best-suited one for developing a protocol to apply to clinical samples. This prompted us to extend our experiments also to other pathologies where CTC recovery and molecular characterization might be very useful.

Spiking experiments were run using the prostate cancer cell line PC3, and the cholangiocarcinoma cell lines EGI, HuCCT, HuH28. Cholangiocarcinoma cell lines were kindly provided by Prof. Strazzabosco (Università Milano-Bicocca, Monza, Italy) and cell authenticity was verified by STR analysis by our Institutional Genomics Core Facility.

Results for tumor cell recoveries with Parsortix are reported in Table 4.3 and refer to spiking 10, 25, 50 cells into 10 mL of HD blood using cells preliminarily labeled with a cell tracker (CellTracker™ Green CMFDA Dye, ThermoFisher Scientific, Waltham, MA, USA) and visualized under a fluorescent microscope after harvesting from the Parsortix cassette.

Table 4.3 Recovery rates using cell-enrichment by Parsortix

Cell line			
No. of spiked cells	No. of recovered cells	% recovery rate	Mean % recovery rate
PC3			
10	8	80	75.3 ± 4.2
25	18	72	
50	37	74	
EGI			
10	7	70	74.7 ± 5.0
25	20	80	
50	37	74	
HuCCT			
10	10	100	90.0 ± 11.1
25	23	92	
50	39	78	
HuH28			
10	8	80	87.0 ± 8.1
25	24	96	
50	43	86	

At difference to what observed with the OncoQuick™approach, the recovery rates did not change as a function of the number of spiked cells whereas there were differences in the number of recovered cells depending on the cell line. In particular, for the HuCCT and HuH28 cell lines the highest recovery rates were obtained (around 90%). Differences in recovery rates depending on the cell line are possible and are linked to differences in cell sizes among the different cell lines. Similar results have already been reported by others (Hvichia et al. 2016) and were demonstrated to directly correlate with the Feret diameter of cells. Overall, the mean recovery rate was 82%.

4.3.3 *Improving CTC Identification: Going Beyond Classical Epithelial CTCs*

As for the enrichment, also the identification step, which in our protocol was initially based on the expression of epithelial markers similarly to the majority of CTC isolation methods, had to be improved in order to include CTCs' heterogeneity. Therefore we proceeded by stepwise implementing the set of tumor markers used for CTC identification.

Since one of the most important and interesting aspects in CTCs detection and characterization is phenotype switching from epithelial to mesenchymal through EMT (Yu et al. 2013), we decided to add to the staining procedure an antibody directed against Vimentin, VIM (Santa Cruz Biotechnology, clone SC-6260, Alexa Fluor 488-conjugated), a protein expressed in mesenchymal cells. VIM is expressed also by blood cells and is not a CTC-specific marker, anyway it can be used to better characterize CTCs with a complete epithelial or mixed epithelial-mesenchymal phenotype.

Moreover, in a previous study in which AdnaGen technology was used to detect CTCs in patients with breast cancer by using immunomagnetic beads (Fina et al. 2015), we had observed that the addition of EGFR to the set of markers used for the enrichment, resulted in increased CTC detection; thus EGFR was introduced in our protocol as identification marker (anti-human EGFR PE-conjugated, clone 423,103, R&D Systems, Minneapolis, MN, USA). Both antibodies were essentially used according to the manufacturer's instructions.

Implementing positive selection markers is a possible strategy, but considering that it is impossible to predict which markers will be expressed by all the different subpopulation of CTCs, theoretically the best way to select CTCs would be to perform a negative selection of all blood cells. We tried to do so by using CD45 as negative selection marker but unfortunately all blood samples analyzed (including negative controls from HD) were characterized by the presence of many cells negative for both tumor markers and CD45, probably due to a non homogeneous expression of this antigen by different blood cell subpopulations or to insufficient sensitivity of the antibody. Consequently, the set of negative selection markers was implemented with CD14 and CD16, two proteins specifically expressed by some subpopulations of WBC (in particular CD14 by macrophages, neutrophils and dendritic cells; CD16 by natural killer cells, neutrophils polymorphonuclear leukocytes, monocytes and macrophages). The staining with the 3 antibodies against CD45, CD14 (clone M5E2, BD Biosciences Pharmigen, San Diego, CA) and CD16 (clone 3G8, BD Biosciences Pharmigen) together, dramatically reduced the number of double negative cells in the samples analyzed (0–20 double negative cells in most of the samples).

It is impossible to establish if these cells are effective tumor cells, since they do not express any of the tumor markers used for the identification of CTCs, and actually, while some of them are considerably larger than WBC, other have a morphology that closely resembles WBC, as shown in Fig. 4.5b. Nonetheless, the reduced number of double negative cells obtained with the improved staining allowed their recovery and consequently the possibility to perform molecular analyses in order to define their tumor/non-tumor nature.

After the reported considerations on CTC enrichment and identification our CTC detection protocol was modified as shown below.

- Blood collection in K_2EDTA tubes
- Enrichment with Parsortix (10 mL of blood)
- Fixation with 2% PFA (20 min at room temperature)
- Staining for positive-selection markers (PE-conjugated antibodies): EpCAM (1:11, 10 min at 4 °C), CK (1:10, 10 min at room temperature) and EGFR (1:11, 10 min at 4 °C); negative selection markers (APC-conjugated antibodies): CD45 (1:11, 10 min at 4 °C), CD14 (1:20, 10 min at 4 °C) and CD16 (1:20, 10 min at 4 °C); VIM (1:10, 10 min at room temperature) and nuclei (Hoechst 33,342, Sigma Aldrich, 1 µg/mL, 5 min at room temperature)
- Analysis with DEPArray™.

4.4 Stretching the Single Cell: Whole Genome Amplification (WGA)

Regardless the type of downstream molecular analysis, the DNA content of a single cell is definitely too scarce and therefore a whole genome amplification (WGA) step is mandatory. WGA, besides being essential, is also very tricky and critical, and its performance becomes the main factor determining the outcome of the following steps.

Some of the major problems connected to WGA are a partial coverage, the poor uniformity, allelic-dropouts and false positives. Consequently, preservation of the molecular complexity of the cells is at risk and, notwithstanding the specific type of platform adopted (microarrays, SNP arrays, NGS), the difficulty in the interpretation of results mainly lies in separating technical artifacts from genuine genetic variants. Many WGA kits, which can be divided into PCR-based and non

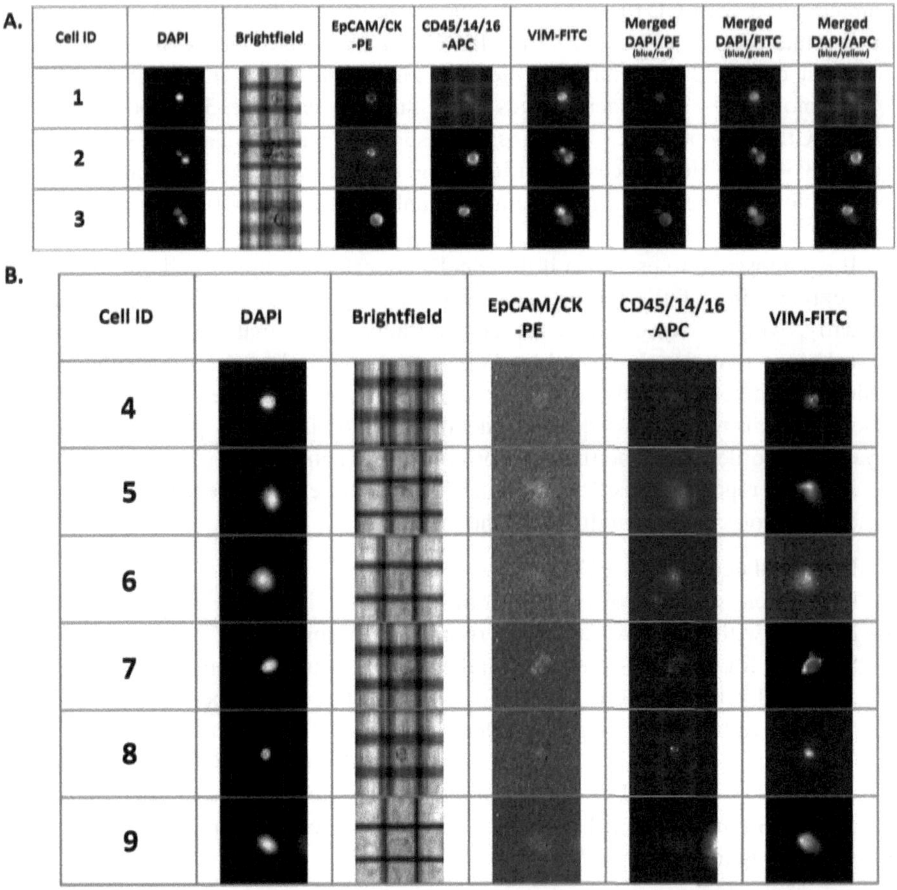

Fig. 4.5 CTCs and APC-ve cells identified in two cholangiocarcinoma patients. Blood samples (11 and 10 mL), drawn in K_2EDTA tube before starting chemotherapy, were enriched with OncoQuick™ (*panel A*) or Parsortix (*panel B*), fixed with 2% PFA, fluorescently-stained for EpCAM, CK, CD45, CD14, CD16 and VIM and subsequently analyzed with the DEPArray™. *Panel A*: three CTCs (PE +ve and APC −ve nucleated cells) identified based on the expression of epithelial/WBC markers (PE/APC channels). Please see the FITC channel for a further evaluation of the CTCs' phenotype ranging from more mesenchymal (*cell 1*) to more epithelial pattern (*cell 3*). *Panel B*: six cells negative for both tumor and WBC markers. Please note the heterogeneous morphology with sizes either similar to WBCs (*cell 8*) or to tumor cells (*cell 5 and 6*). In the FITC-channel the expression of VIM, similarly to the morphology, is very heterogeneous (*cell 7* shows the highest VIM expression, *cell 6* is VIM-ve) (Abbreviations: *WBC* white blood cell)

PCR-based (as typically multidisplacement amplification, MDA) are presently commercialized, but also mixed approaches have been described. A comprehensive dissection of all aspects of WGA from single-cells is beyond the scope of this chapter and readers can find most information on technical and biological aspects of single-cell genome analysis in excellent published reviews (Hou et al.2015; de Bourcy et al. 2014; Navin 2014; Wang and Navin 2015; Van Loo and Voet 2014).

We used in our protocol, an amplification method initially developed by Klein and colleagues (1999) and later adapted in a commercially available kit by Silicon Biosystems, the Ampli1 WGA (Polzer et al. 2014).

The manufacturer recommends its use in combination with the Ampli1 QC kit, a PCR-based assay useful for the evaluation of the WGA output product. A small aliquot from the WGA product obtained from cells isolated with the DEPArray™ during the previously described spiking experiments, was therefore processed with the QC multiplex PCR reaction which allows the simultaneous amplification of four human genomic targets of increasing length (91, 108–166, 299, 614 bp). The quality of the WGA products could this way be estimated by evaluating in a capillary gel-electrophoresis run the presence/absence of specific target amplicons. In particular, the absence of all of the amplicons suggests that a failure in WGA has occurred, whereas the presence of 1–2 targets corresponds to a low-quality WGA product limiting its downstream use to few gene-specific assays. Conversely, the presence of 3–4 of the amplicons testifies the good performance of the WGA and is a reliable predictor of success when performing downstream genome-wide analysis.

We have processed 286 samples including single cells or pools of few target cells, isolated with the DEPArray™ in spiking experiments. QC results were satisfying for 73% of samples, which were defined as high–quality (3–4 amplicons), whereas 21% were defined as low-quality with only 1 or 2 of the amplicons, but only 6% of samples presented no amplicons. Therefore, based on the predictions of the QC kit, this approach would allow genomic characterization of a high fraction of samples.

4.5 The Dark Side of the Moon: The Clinical Samples

Clinical samples obtained from patients with breast cancer, cholangiocarcinoma and renal cell carcinoma at different stages (early or metastatic) both at baseline or during treatment, were processed in parallel to the development of the technical protocol by stepwise introducing the protocol improvements in CTC-enrichments and in CTC-identification. At difference with spiking experiments, no direct technical comparison was run on the clinical samples.

As expected, CTC-enrichment represented a critical point also in the case of clinical samples. The two methods with the best cell recovery rates in spiking experiments, i.e. density based enrichment with OncoQuick™ and size/deformability enrichment with Parsortix performed very well also on clinical samples, although a matched comparison in the number of collected CTCs from the same samples is not possible since the two approached were not run in parallel. Using the OncoQuick™ we have processed 43 samples and have identified 101 cells defined as CTCs due to the positive PE staining (supporting their epithelial origin). Their visualization, sorting and recovery by DEPArray™ however, required processing the samples on 84 cartridges (an average of 2 cartridges for sample) due to the high number of contaminating WBCs which tended to saturate the capacity of the DEP-cages impairing single cell collection (see Fig. 4.4). Despite having split the samples into more than one run on the DEPArray™, only 49/101 (48.5%) of the identified PE+ve cells could be recovered for downstream analyses, a frustrating result when considering the additional time and costs for each sample. On the contrary, with Parsortix 18 samples have been so far processed, using a single DEPArray™ cartridge for each sample and allowing the recovery of 90% of the cells identified as PE+ve which represent CTCs with epithelial phenotype. The increased routing efficiency during the single cell recovery process from the DEPArray™ cartridge, is consequent to the lower number of cells in the cartridge due to the more efficient removal of WBC obtained with Parsortix compared to Oncoquick™.

As described in paragraph 4.3.3 our protocol was also developed for collection of non-epithelial CTCs defined as PE-ve/APC-ve cells. The procedure was used to process 48 patient-derived blood samples and 289 double negative cells were recovered. Since negative selection of CTCs is by definition not supported by the expression of CTC-specific markers, the actual tumoral nature of single cells collected under our protocol was uncertain and was therefore checked by evaluating chromosomal aneuploidies and copy number alterations (CNA) through a low pass whole genome sequencing using the PGM™system. To such a purpose multiplexed sequencing-ready libraries were generated using the Ampli1™ Low pass kit (Silicon Biosystems, Italy) which is specifically designed to process WGA products generated with the Ampli1 kits. Pools of ten leukocytes each, collected with the DEPArray™ as 'controls' from eight patients with choloangiocarcinoma and three patients with breast cancer, were all correctly classified as normal cells based on their diploid genome and on the absence of gains or losses of chromosomal regions. Preliminary results on the CNA of putative non-epithelial CTCs collected as PE-ve/APC-ve cells were encouraging as 11/32 cells recovered from cholangiocarcinoma patients and 4/10 recovered from breast cancer patients, were actually tumor cells with hyperdiploid genomes and numerous gains and losses of DNA regions along the entire genome. Interestingly, different CTCs from the same patients were characterized by genomic heterogeneity. These results support the validity of our protocol for isolation and recovery of non-epithelial CTCs.

Overall the developed protocol allowed us to build a bank of both epithelial CTCs and of non-epithelial CTCs with confirmed tumor nature isolated from blood samples of patients with different tumor types. All collected CTCs were stored as WGA products.

Quality control analysis of WGA performance is crucial for further downstream molecular analyses and was therefore run on clinical samples similarly to what done on spiking experiments. Results were super imposable with 73% of samples called as good-quality, 21% low-quality and only 6% of samples which failed amplification. This means that on the average three quarters of the cells isolated from patients with the described protocol qualify for downstream analysis of their genome. Indeed, the developed protocol allowed genotyping analysis of single CTCs. Ampli1 WGA kit products derived from CTCs and WBCs were processed using

Uniformity >75%
Depth 500-2000

	variants			effect	variant frequencies					
GENE	*aa*	*ref*	*var*	*type*	*sift*	*CTC1*	*CTC2*	*CTC3*		*WBC*
TP53 HotSpot	Arg273lHis	C	T	missense	deleterious			69.4		
PIK3CA novel	Trp105Leu	G	T	missense	deleterious			19.8		
PTPN11 novel	Ala509Ser	G	T	missense	deleterious	4.2	19.2			
	CTC heterogeneity				**new somatic heterozygous mutations**					

Fig. 4.6 Somatic single nucleotide variation in CTCs from a breast cancer patient. The panel reports the variant frequencies for three distinct single nucleotide variants (SNV) of *TP53, PIK3CA* and *PTPN11* genes detected in three CTCs isolated from a triple negative non metastatic breast cancer patient before the start of neoadjuvant treatment, using OncoQuick™ for CTC-enrichments. *Red boxes* (*dark grey*) indicate the presence of a SNV and report frequencies, *blue boxes* (*light grey*) indicate a wild-type genotype. CTCs were identified as nucleated PE +ve cells (*i.e.* either positive for EpCAM or panCK)/APC-ve cells (*i.e* negative for CD45). The reported SNV supports the presence of clonal heterogeneity among CTCs and acquisition of new somatic heterozygous mutations

the Ion AmpliSeq Custom Cancer Hotspot Panel v2 (50 genes) modified to take into account the enzymatic fragmentation with the restriction MseI enzyme on input DNA processed with the Ampli1 kit. Analyses were run using the TorrentSuite v 5.0 using the Variant Effect Predictor v83. Eleven CTCs and 6 WBC pools belonging to 5 distinct patients (4 women with breast cancer and one with renal cell cancer) have been analyzed. In one breast sample a somatic heterozygous mutation of TP53 (p.Arg273His) was observed in one of three CTCs, while in another sample 19 somatic mutations were present around 5 CTC with a prevalence in one of them. ERBB4 (p.Gln346His) and ATM (p.Arg3047Leu) missense variants were present with a heterozygous status with frequency deviations suggesting a possible copy-gain of the wild type allele. No biological or clinical interpretation of these results is so far possible, besides confirming that the data support the technical validity of the developed protocol. Results for one triple negative non-metastatic breast cancer patient are reported as an example in Fig. 4.6.

Finally, an interesting observation on clinical samples relates to the expression of VIM (FITC channel), which was in fact expressed at different intensities in PE + ve cells suggesting the presence of CTCs with a hybrid epithelial/mesenchymal phenotype (Fig. 4.5a). On the other hand, also some, though not all, of the PE-ve/APC-ve cells expressed VIM (Fig. 4.5b). In some cases VIM expression was accompanied by a less rounded morphology.

4.6 Conclusions

Single-cell analysis of CTCs is still in its infancy and much more work needs to be done to obtain technical protocols suitable for clinics, which can really impact the eagerly pursued precision medicine objectives. The described protocol should not be considered as one in its final stage, instead it represents a flexible technical approach open to additional improvements. Its analytical validity is supported by both results with spiking experiments, which have the advantage of allowing an accurate evaluation of data obtained with respect to expected results, but importantly is also confirmed by results with clinical samples. The next steps will necessarily deal with evaluation of its clinical validity, ideally within a well-defined clinical trial with target therapies.

Acknowledgments The study was supported by grants from the *Associazione Italiana per la Ricerca sul Cancro* (AIRC), grant IG 16900 to M.G.D and grant IG 15792 for supporting the fellowship of CR, from the *Italian Ministry of Health* (grant RF2013-02359692 to MGD) and from the *European Commission* under the 7th Framework Program, grant agreement n° 260791 Eurocan Platform.

RM, PM, MGD and VC are paid with funds from the *Italian Ministry of Health*.

References

Abonnenc M, Manaresi N, Borgatti M et al (2013) Programmable interactions of functionalized single bioparticles in a dielectrophoresis-based microarray chip. Anal Chem 85 (17):8219–8224

Bidard FC, Proudhon C, Pierga JY (2016) Circulating tumor cells in breast cancer. Mol Oncol 10 (3):418–430

Bulfoni M, Gerratana L, Del Ben F et al (2016) In patients with metastatic breast cancer the identification of circulating tumor cells in epithelial-to-mesenchymal transition is associated with a poor prognosis. Breast Cancer Res 18(1):30

Chudziak J, Burt DJ, Mohan S et al (2016) Clinical evaluation of a novel microfluidic device for epitope-independent enrichment of circulating tumour cells in patients with small cell lung cancer. Analyst 141(2):669–678

Dago AE, Stepansky A, Carlsson A et al (2014) Rapid phenotypic and genomic change in response to therapeutic pressure in prostate cancer inferred by high content analysis of single circulating tumor cells. PLoS One 9(8):e101777

de Bourcy CF, De Vlaminck I, Kanbar JN et al (2014) A quantitative comparison of single-cell whole genome amplification methods. PLoS One 9(8):e105585

Elliott P, Peakman TC, Biobank UK (2008) The UK Biobank sample handling and storage protocol for the collection, processing and archiving of human blood and urine. Int J Epidemiol 37(2):234–244

Fina E, Reduzzi C, Motta R et al (2015) Did circulating tumor cells tell us all they could? The missed circulating tumor cell message in breast cancer. Int J Biol Markers 30(4):e429–e433

Fuchs AB, Romani A, Freida D et al (2006) Electronic sorting and recovery of single live cells from microlitre sized samples. Lab Chip 6(1):121–126

Heitzer E, Auer M, Gasch C et al (2013) Complex tumor genomes inferred from single circulating tumor cells by array-CGH and next-generation sequencing. Cancer Res 73(10):2965–2975

Holland NT, Smith MT, Eskenazi B et al (2003) Biological sample collection and processing for molecular epidemiological studies. Mutat Res 543(3):217–234

Hou Y, Wu K, Shi X et al (2015) Comparison of variations detection between whole-genome amplification methods used in single-cell resequencing. GigaScience 4:37

Hvichia GE, Parveen Z, Wagner C et al (2016) A novel microfluidic platform for size and deformability based separation and the subsequent molecular characterization of viable circulating tumor cells. Int J Cancer 138(12):2894–2904

Joosse SA, Gorges TM, Pantel K (2014) Biology, detection, and clinical implications of circulating tumor cells. EMBO Mol Med 7(1):1–11

Kang Q, Henry NL, Paoletti C et al (2016) Comparative analysis of circulating tumor DNA stability In K3EDTA, Streck, and CellSave blood collection tubes. Clin Biochem. S0009-9120 (16)30040-6

Klein CA, Schmidt-Kittler O, Schardt JA (1999) Comparative genomic hybridization, loss of heterozygosity, and DNA sequence analysis of single cells. Proc Natl Acad Sci USA 96 (8):4494–4499

Lohr JG, Adalsteinsson VA, Cibulskis K et al (2014) Whole-exome sequencing of circulating tumor cells provides a window into metastatic prostate cancer. Nat Biotechnol 32(5):479–484

Navin NE (2014) Cancer genomics: one cell at a time. Genome Biol 15(8):452

Ni X, Zhuo M, Su Z et al (2013) Reproducible copy number variation patterns among single circulating tumor cells of lung cancer patients. Proc Natl Acad Sci USA 110(52):21083–21088

Paoletti C, Hayes DF (2016) Circulating tumor cells. Adv Exp Med Biol 882:235–258

Polzer B, Medoro G, Pasch S et al (2014) Molecular profiling of single circulating tumor cells with diagnostic intention. EMBO Mol Med 6(11):1371–1386

Qin J, Alt JR, Hunsley BA et al (2014) Stabilization of circulating tumor cells in blood using a collection device with a preservative reagent. Cancer Cell Int 14(1):23

Van Loo P, Voet T (2014) Single cell analysis of cancer genomes. Curr Opin Genet Dev 24:82–91

Wang Y, Navin NE (2015) Advances and applications of single-cell sequencing technologies. Mol Cell 58(4):598–609

Xu L, Mao X, Imrali A et al (2015) Optimization and evaluation of a novel size based circulating tumor cell isolation system. PLoS One 10(9):e0138032

Yu M, Ting DT, Stott SL et al (2012) RNA sequencing of pancreatic circulating tumour cells implicates WNT signalling in metastasis. Nature 487(7408):510–513

Yu M, Bardia A, Wittner BS et al (2013) Circulating breast tumor cells exhibit dynamic changes in epithelial and mesenchymal composition. Science 339(6119):580–584

Chapter 5
Flow Cytometric Methods for Circulating Tumor Cell Isolation and Molecular Analysis

Neha Bhagwat and Erica L. Carpenter

Abstract Circulating tumor cells provide a non-invasive source of tumor material that can be valuable at all stages of disease management, including screening and early diagnosis, monitoring response to therapy, identifying therapeutic targets, and assessing development of drug resistance. Cells isolated from the blood of cancer patients can be used for phenotypic analysis, tumor genotyping, transcriptional profiling, as well as for *ex vivo* culture of isolated cells. There are a variety of novel technologies currently being developed for the detection and analysis of rare cells in circulation of cancer patients. Flow cytometry is a powerful cell analysis platform that is increasingly being used in this field of study due to its relatively high throughput and versatility with respect to the large number of commercially available antibodies and fluorescent probes available to translational and clinical researchers. More importantly, it offers the ability to easily recover viable cells with high purity that are suitable for downstream molecular analysis, thus making it an attractive technology for cancer research and as a diagnostic tool.

Keywords Flow cytometry • Circulating tumor cells • Cell sorting • Acoustic focusing

5.1 Introduction

Circulating tumor cells (CTCs) are cells shed from solid tumors and found at extremely low frequency in the bloodstream of patients for most cancer types. A subset of these cells can seed distant organs in the body and give rise to metastatic

N. Bhagwat
Division of Gastroenterology, Department of Medicine, Perelman School of Medicine, University of Pennsylvania, Philadelphia, PA 19104, USA
e-mail: bhagwatn@mail.med.upenn.edu

E.L. Carpenter (✉)
Division of Hematology/Oncology, Department of Medicine, Perelman School of Medicine, Abramson Cancer Center, University of Pennsylvania, Philadelphia, PA 19104, USA
e-mail: erical@upenn.edu

M.J.M. Magbanua, J.W. Park (eds.), *Isolation and Molecular Characterization of Circulating Tumor Cells*, Advances in Experimental Medicine and Biology 994,
DOI 10.1007/978-3-319-55947-6_5

disease, which is the primary cause of cancer-related mortality. Isolation and characterization of these CTCs from patient blood can be a sensitive and non-invasive method for early cancer detection, disease monitoring while on therapy, and molecular analysis for detection of therapeutically targetable oncogenes.

5.2 Clinical Utility of CTCs

Several studies have demonstrated that the number of CTCs detected in patient blood correlates with lower survival and worse outcomes in solid tumors such as breast, lung, prostate, and colorectal (Cristofanilli et al. 2004; Cohen et al. 2008; de Bono et al. 2008). However, the focus on enumeration has limited the role of CTCs in clinical decision-making, and there is an increasing need to recover these cells in order to perform more sophisticated and detailed analysis, including the application of next-generation sequencing for detection of disease associated genetic variants, as well as specific molecular biomarkers of response or resistance to therapy (Smerage et al. 2014; Yee et al. 2016). A liquid biopsy offers minimally-invasive, repeat access to tumor material, which can be invaluable for early detection and real-time monitoring of acquired resistance to targeted therapies, especially when the tumor is surgically inaccessible (Maheswaran et al. 2008). Additionally, CTCs are thought to be shed by both primary and metastatic tumor, and are thus considered to more comprehensively represent the genetic heterogeneity of tumors and metastases as compared to single site tissue biopsies (Gerlinger et al. 2012; Ni et al. 2013). In metastatic castration resistant prostate cancer, detection of a nuclear androgen receptor splice variant, AR-V7 messenger RNA, in CTCs, was associated with resistance to inhibitors of androgen receptor signaling (Antonarakis et al. 2014; Scher et al. 2016). Another group recently found that PD-L1 was frequently expressed on breast cancer CTCs, leading to the development of a CTC/PD-L1 specific assay that can be used to stratify patients for immune checkpoint inhibitor therapy (Mazel et al. 2015). Nuclear expression of PD-L1 in CTCs was also associated with shorter overall survival in metastatic colon and prostate cancer, further supporting the prognostic role of this biomarker (Satelli et al. 2016). Several groups have recently reported that a high degree of genetic variation within a tumor is associated with enhanced response to immunotherapy (Rizvi et al. 2015; McGranahan et al. 2016), suggesting that development of a liquid biopsy to accurately measure tumor heterogeneity in CTCs could be used to select patients who would benefit most from such therapy.

Developing a molecular or protein signature that is indicative of distant organ metastases is another clinically relevant application of CTC molecular analysis. Two different studies conducted in breast cancer samples identified a set of protein biomarkers that enrich for cells that give rise to organ-specific metastasis (Zhang et al. 2013; Baccelli et al. 2013). Transcriptional profiling of CTCs, including single cells, has been successfully conducted in a number of cancer types (Miyamoto et al.

2015; Ramskold et al. 2012; Yu et al. 2012; Powell et al. 2012). Ting et al. demonstrated that a majority of CTCs isolated from mouse models and patients with pancreatic cancer exhibit high expression of extracellular matrix proteins such as SPARC. Further, suppression of SPARC resulted in a decrease in cell migration and invasion as well as reduction in metastatic burden in mouse models (Ting et al. 2014). Thus, transcriptomic analysis of CTCs can also be used to identify therapeutic vulnerabilities in the tumor, or to classify tumors into subtypes that have prognostic value (Bailey et al. 2016), or to predict response to targeted therapies (Guinney et al. 2015; Prat et al. 2015).

CTCs obtained from pre-clinical or clinical samples can be used as a source of tumor material for *ex vivo* profiling and functional analysis. CTCs isolated from late stage cancer patients have been successfully transplanted into and serially passaged in immunodeficient mice, and have been shown to recapitulate the donor patient tumor's molecular characteristics and response to therapy (Hodgkinson et al. 2014; Baccelli et al. 2013; Zhang et al. 2013). Long-term cultures of CTC-derived cell lines have also been generated from breast, prostate, melanoma, colorectal, and small cell lung cancer patients, including for patients whose primary or metastatic tissue was inaccessible or difficult to biopsy (Gao et al. 2014; Girotti et al. 2016; Cayrefourcq et al. 2015; Yu et al. 2014; Hamilton et al. 2016). While freshly isolated CTCs are extremely rare, these *ex vivo* models provide a renewable resource of cells with sufficient numbers to perform extensive phenotypic and molecular characterization, as well as functional assays to screen for drug sensitivity and predict response to therapy.

While the majority of studies over the last decade have focused on single CTCs, more recent reports have documented the presence of CTC clusters, also known as circulating tumor microemboli (CTM), in patient and mouse blood (Molnar et al. 2001; Stott et al. 2010; Khoja et al. 2012; Yu et al. 2013; Sarioglu et al. 2015; Aceto et al. 2014). In pre-clinical models, CTC clusters had increased metastatic potential as compared to single CTCs, with CTC clusters exhibiting clonal heterogeneity which decreased as disease progressed (Maddipati and Stanger 2015; Aceto et al. 2014). Further, in clinical studies, CTC clusters were associated with a lower progression free survival, suggesting that non-invasive monitoring of CTC clusters could have prognostic value (Hou et al. 2012; Jansson et al. 2016; Divella et al. 2014). Therefore, there is increasing interest to develop robust technologies for isolation of clusters along with single cells, and to promote a deeper understanding of the biology underlying the enhanced invasiveness and metastatic potential of CTC clusters.

Several major technical hurdles exist when isolating rare cells; one is the ability to isolate rare tumor cells from a sample that contains a background of billions of blood cells, and another is being able to do this in a high-throughput manner that would yield results within a clinically relevant timeframe. The only FDA approved platform for clinical enumeration of CTCs is CellSearch (Janssen). One key limitation of this methodology is that CTCs are enriched based on the expression of the epithelial marker EpCAM, which is not expressed on several tumor types, including melanoma and sarcomas (Momburg et al. 1987). Moreover CellSearch is likely to have low sensitivity for cells that have undergone epithelial to mesenchymal transition (EMT), a process known to be associated with metastasis (Ye and Weinberg 2015) in which EpCAM expression is lost or greatly reduced. CellSearch-enriched cells also undergo fixation, which can be incompatible with downstream molecular analysis or functional studies such as those described above. Antibody- and marker- independent technologies have been developed in the last decade that enrich CTCs based on cell size, density, or conductivity (Pailler et al. 2016; Gupta et al. 2012), while negative selection approaches, including immunomagnetic depletion of hematopoietic cells, also leave CTCs unlabeled (Issadore et al. 2012; Karabacak et al. 2014). Ferreira et al. provide an excellent and up-to-date review of the current platforms under development (Ferreira et al. 2016). In addition to new technologies, established methods of cell analysis such as flow cytometry are also increasingly being adapted for CTC isolation and characterization.

5.3 Flow Cytometric Methods of CTC Analysis

Flow cytometry is considered the gold standard of single cell phenotypic analysis and is extensively used in biological and clinical research, particularly for immunophenotyping a variety of biological samples including blood, bone marrow aspirate, and dissociated tumor tissue. In a flow cytometer, live or fixed cells in suspension are aligned in a single file, usually through hydrodynamic focusing with sheath fluid that creates laminar flow. This allows individual cells to intersect one at a time with a light source such as a laser. The scattered light is collected by the optics system and converted to a digital signal that can provide information on cell size, internal complexity, and other characteristics based on fluorescently labeled antibodies, probes, or dyes that can be used to tag cells. The latest flow cytometers can process thousands of events per second and measure tens of parameters on individual cells. This allows the investigator to multiplex different markers using non-overlapping fluorescent conjugates (Chattopadhyay et al. 2008). Thus, flow cytometry can provide *highly quantitative and detailed phenotypic information on individual cells in a high throughput manner*.

We and others have used flow cytometry to detect, enrich, or analyze CTCs in the blood of cancer patients (Table 5.1). One of the earliest studies used multiple pan-cytokeratin antibodies to identify tumor epithelial cells and a cocktail of hematopoietic lineage markers to exclude blood cells in a blood or bone marrow sample where they were able to detect tumor cells at a frequency as low as 10^{-7} (Gross et al. 1995). Racila et al. further modified this assay by performing immunomagnetic enrichment of EpCAM-positive cells prior to analysis by flow cytometry in a cohort of breast cancer patients. They were able to detect cytokeratin-positive, CD45-negative CTCs in 29/30 patients with a sensitivity of 1 cell in a tube of blood (Racila et al. 1998). We have more recently shown that flow-sorting can be used to enrich tumor cells disseminated to the bone marrow of

Table 5.1 List of key studies using flow cytometry for CTC analysis

References	Sample prep	Sample type	Markers used for analysis	Sensitivity	Downstream analysis
Gross et al. (1995)	NA	BT-20 cells spiked in PBMCs	pan-CK+; CD45-, CD42a-, CD61-, CD34-	1 in 10 million cells	Enumeration
Simpson et al. (1995)	NA	Peripheral blood, bone marrow and apheresis product from metastatic breast cancer patients (N = 44)	CK+, CD45-	1 in 200,000 cells	Enumeration
Racila et al. (1998)	Immunomagnetic enrichment of EPCAM+ cells	Peripheral blood from breast (N = 30) and prostate (N = 3) cancer patients	pan-CK+, CD45-,	1 in 1 ml of blood	Enumeration
Beitsch and Clifford (2000)	Immunomagnetic enrichment of EPCAM+ cells	Peripheral blood from breast cancer patients (N = 33)	pan-CK+, CD45-	NR	Enumeration
Allan et al. (2005)	Immunomagnetic depletion of CD45 + leukocytes	Mouse xenograft model of metastatic breast cancer	pan-CK+, CD45-, PI for aneuploidy	1 in 100,000 cells	Enumeration
Cruz et al. (2005)	NA	MCF-7 cells spiked in whole blood	CK18+; PI for aneuploidy	1 in 10 million cells	Enumeration
Wang et al. (2009)	NA	Peripheral blood from breast cancer patients (N = 48)	CK19+	1 in 10,000 cells	Enumeration
Hu et al. (2010)	NA	Peripheral blood from breast cancer patients (N = 45)	EPCAM+, pan-CK+, CD45-	1 in 100,000 cells	Enumeration
Takao and Takeda (2011)	Immunomagnetic enrichment of EPCAM+ cells	PC-3 and MCF-7 cells spiked in peripheral blood	EPCAM+, CD45-, viability dye	10 cells in 4 ml of blood	Enumeration and recovery for culture

(continued)

Table 5.1 (continued)

References	Sample prep	Sample type	Markers used for analysis	Sensitivity	Downstream analysis
Magbanua et al. (2012)	Immunomagnetic enrichment of EPCAM+ cells	Peripheral blood from prostate cancer patients (N = 20)	EPCAM+, CD45-	NR	Enumeration and recovery for array CGH
Watanabe et al. (2014)	Immunomagnetic depletion of CD45 + leukocytes	A549, KATO-III, PC-14, MCF-7, Hs578T cells spiked in peripheral blood	EPCAM+/−, CK+/−,Vim+/− CD45-, viability dye	10 cells in 1 ml of blood	Enumeration and recovery for culture
Magbanua et al. (2013)	Immunomagnetic enrichment of EPCAM+ cells	Peripheral blood from breast cancer patients (N = 181)	EPCAM+, CD45-	NR	Enumeration and recovery for array CGH
Lu et al. (2015)	Immunomagnetic depletion of CD45 + leukocytes	Peripheral blood from colorectal cancer patients (N = 18)	EPCAM+, CD45-, CD44+/−, CD47+/−	3 cells in 2 ml of blood	Enumeration and marker analysis
Hristozova et al. (2012)	NA	Peripheral blood from SCCHN patients (N = 33)	EPCAM+, pan-CK+, CD45-, EGFR/ pEGFR	NR	Enumeration and marker analysis
Gorner et al. (2015)	NA	Peripheral blood from pancreatic cancer patients (N = 8)	CD45-, EPCAM+, MUC1+, viability dye	1 in 1 million cells	Enumeration and recovery for qPCR
Carpenter et al. (2014)	NA	Bone marrow from neuroblastoma patients (N = 10)	CD45-, CD56+, GD2+, viability dye	1 in 1 million cells	Enumeration and recovery for targeted sequencing
Vishnoi et al. (2015)	NA	Peripheral blood from breast cancer patients (N = 38)	CD45-, EPCAM-, CD44+, CD24-, viability dye	NR	Recovery for genotyping, qPCR, functional assays

PBMCs Peripheral blood mononuclear cells, *CK* Cytokeratin, *PI* Propidium Iodide, *CGH* Comparative genomic hybridization, *SCCHN* Squamous cell carcinoma of head and neck, *qPCR* quantitative PCR, *NA* Not applicable, *NR* Not reported pediatric neuroblastoma patients prior to dielectrophoretic purification and sequencing of single cells (Carpenter et al. 2014). Other studies have utilized immunomagnetic depletion or negative selection of unwanted leukocytes in order to enrich for tumor cells prior to flow analysis (Allan et al. 2005; Watanabe et al. 2014; Lu et al. 2015; Rhim et al. 2012). More recently, Hristozova et al. described an 'electronic thresholding' protocol used during data acquisition that significantly improved sensitivity without prior enrichment or depletion (Hristozova et al. 2012).

Traditional flow cytometric techniques combined with high-speed microscopic imaging modalities have the ability to provide information on marker subcellular localization or colocalization, and other complex features such as DNA fragmentation. This platform, known as Imagestream^{X} (Amnis) has been used to study rare CTC populations in cancer patients in different tumor types (Dent et al. 2016; Ogle et al. 2016). Using image analysis, Catenacci et al. were able to confirm loss of expression of tumor-suppressors including *TP53, SMAD4,* and *P16/CDKN2A* in CTCs from pancreatic cancer patients, a finding that was correlated with worse outcome (Catenacci et al. 2015). The addition of high quality microscopic images can potentially reduce false-positives due to cell debris or antibody-aggregates that can occur in flow cytometric assays. This platform can also be useful for detailed characterization of non-tumor cells that could be present in CTC clusters.

In addition to complex phenotypic analysis, cell sorters also allow for the recovery of the cells of interest *at a very high purity*. Most modern cell sorters have the capability of simultaneously sorting multiple sub-populations as well as single cells. In addition, flow cytometric cell sorters can be modified with large nozzles and with the application of low sample pressure, can minimize shear forces and allow for recovery of intact circulating tumor clusters along with single cells. Magbanua et al. combined magnetic immunoenrichment and flow sorting to isolate tumor cells from blood in a cohort of metastatic prostate and breast cancer patients. They were further able to perform comparative genomic hybridization (array CGH) analysis on the isolated cells and observed similar frequencies of copy number alterations as previously published for primary tumors (Magbanua et al. 2012, 2013). In another study that highlights the versatility of flow cytometric analysis, Vishnoi et al. isolated four different subpopulations of EpCAM-negative CTCs from breast cancer patients with and without brain metastasis. CTCs were sorted based on presence or absence of urokinase plasminogen activator receptor (uPAR) and integrin β1, and comprehensive transcriptome and genotyping analyses were performed on each subset. Isolated cells were also cultured *in vitro* and used for functional assays where they found that the different CTC subsets had distinct proliferative and invasive properties that could potentially determine their ability to metastasize (Vishnoi et al. 2015).

5.4 Recent Developments in Flow Cytometry

5.4.1 New Methods of Cell Labeling

Fluorescent labeling of cells for flow cytometry is no longer limited to the use of validated antibodies. Aptamers are single-stranded nucleic acid molecules having unique secondary and tertiary structures that can be selected to recognize specific cell surface markers including EpCAM (Song et al. 2013). Aptamers are less susceptible than antibodies to aggregation, may have improved tissue penetration, and can be generated to recognize virtually any ligand through *in vitro* selection (Stoltenburg et al. 2007). They can also be easily conjugated to fluorescent dyes or other labels and have been used to detect CTCs in the blood of cancer patients (Sheng et al. 2012; Zhang et al. 2015; Zamay et al. 2015). Considerable progress has also been made in developing techniques to facilitate labeling of intracellular markers without fixation or membrane permeabilization, which can compromise cell viability and are not ideal for downstream molecular analysis. For example, a novel microfluidic platform uses gentle compression to transiently produce pores in the cell membrane through which macromolecules can rapidly (~1 min) pass, thereby minimizing effects on gene expression and cell viability. This method has been successfully used to introduce antibodies and nucleic acids into a number of cell types with high efficiency (Sharei et al. 2013). RNA probes can be introduced into cells using this gentle compression and used to detect intracellular gene transcripts by flow cytometry (Abe and Kool 2006; Hanley et al. 2013; Shi et al. 2016). In a recent study, oligonucleotide-modified gold nanoparticle probes hybridized to fluorophore complements, known as 'NanoFlares', were used to detect epithelial and mesenchymal gene transcripts in CTCs from a breast cancer xenograft model by flow cytometry (Halo et al. 2014). The labeled cells could be isolated and remained viable for downstream analysis and cell culture.

5.4.2 Acoustic Focusing

Flow cytometric analysis of CTCs from whole blood can be extremely time-consuming and cumbersome unless red blood cells (RBCs) are first removed. While this can be achieved by density gradient separation or osmotic buffer lysis, these processes can lead to significant loss of rare cells in the sample, particularly during the associated wash steps (Fritsch et al. 1997; Lara et al. 2004). Another limitation of flow cytometric sorting can be a low recovery rate particularly at the high sorting speeds necessary to analyze large blood volumes without RBC removal. However, there are several strategies that can be adopted to overcome these issues. Acoustophoresis, or acoustic focusing, is a powerful technique in which ultrasonic standing waves are used for particle separation based on their size, density, and compressibility (Lenshof et al. 2012; Li et al. 2015). This principle can be applied to separate smaller particles like cell debris, red blood cells, and platelets in whole blood from larger nucleated cells, which can then be directly analyzed by the flow cytometer. Additionally, the sample can be diluted and washed without centrifugation by flowing wash buffer during acoustic focusing thereby minimizing sample manipulation and cell loss during upstream processing. This effectively results in concentrating the cells of interest, thereby reducing sample analysis time. The volumetric throughput can be further increased by adding multiple channels in parallel (Laurell et al. 2007). This methodology has minimal effects on cell viability and is therefore conducive to downstream applications including *ex vivo* culture and molecular analysis (Burguillos et al. 2013). Overall, combining this methodology with conventional hydrodynamic flow sorting allows for rapid analysis of large blood volumes while maximizing cell recovery but without compromising sensitivity.

5.4.3 Analytic Tools

Due to the development of new markers and other advancements in flow cytometry, researchers are faced with analysis of enormous data sets. New algorithms such as Cytometric Fingerprinting (Rogers et al. 2008, 2015) and others (Aghaeepour et al. 2013) that allow for automated and unbiased detection of specific cell populations in complex multiparameter cytometric data have also been recently developed. A recent development in flow cytometry analysis is index sorting, in which all the phenotypic information from sorted single cells is retained and linked with their position in a multi-well plate. This can be used to correlate downstream analysis such as gene expression or functional assay readouts to phenotypic parameters measured by flow for individual cells. Index sorting has been previously used to characterize rare cell populations such as hematopoietic stem cells (Wilson et al. 2015), and would be particularly useful for the identification of specific markers on cells having distinct molecular profiles with prognostic or predictive value, or to identify functional phenotypes such as those associated with the ability to give rise to organ-specific metastasis. Index-sorted cells can then be used as input for single-cell molecular analysis pipelines, which are becoming increasingly scalable with the advent of sophisticated bioinformatic analysis (Lohr et al. 2014; Baslan et al. 2015), as well as barcoding, which allows multiple flow-sorted single cells to be pooled for library synthesis and sequencing, and with minimal effect on gene transcription (Fan et al. 2015; Macosko et al. 2015; Richardson et al. 2015). Single cell analysis of CTCs will be invaluable in deciphering intra-tumoral heterogeneity at both the genomic and transcriptional level and can help guide therapeutic intervention with high precision. For example, deep genotypic profiling of individual CTCs can detect development of therapy resistance with greater lead-time than standard clinical assays, thereby potentially improving clinical outcomes (Scher et al. 2016; Miyamoto et al. 2015).

These novel, recently developed technologies can be combined to enhance a workflow that is robust and compatible with detection, isolation, and molecular characterizationof CTCs.

5.5 Conclusions

Flow cytometry is a powerful, high-throughput, and versatile technology for rare cell analysis and is increasingly being used to isolate and characterize tumor cells in circulation. It is amenable to multiplexing both intracellular and cell surface markers and analysis of these markers can be incorporated or adapted to any tumor type. Importantly, this platform allows for integration of phenotypic analysis with downstream genomic or transcriptomic profiling. In addition, newer instruments have become increasingly automated thereby decreasing the dependence on highly skilled operators. Flow cytometry is already extensively being used in clinical settings for applications such as immunophenotyping of hematological malignancies (Cherian et al. 2005). Thus, similar approaches could be adapted in the future to extensively characterize the phenotype and molecular profile of CTCs.

References

Abe H, Kool ET (2006) Flow cytometric detection of specific RNAs in native human cells with quenched autoligating FRET probes. Proc Natl Acad Sci USA 103(2):263–268

Aceto N, Bardia A, Miyamoto DT et al (2014) Circulating tumor cell clusters are oligoclonal precursors of breast cancer metastasis. Cell 158(5):1110–1122

Aghaeepour N, Finak G, Hoos H et al (2013) Critical assessment of automated flow cytometry data analysis techniques. Nat Methods 10(3):228–238

Allan AL, Vantyghem SA, Tuck AB et al (2005) Detection and quantification of circulating tumor cells in mouse models of human breast cancer using immunomagnetic enrichment and multiparameter flow cytometry. Cytometry A 65(1):4–14

Antonarakis ES, Lu C, Wang H et al (2014) AR-V7 and resistance to enzalutamide and abiraterone in prostate cancer. N Engl J Med 371(11):1028–1038

Baccelli I, Schneeweiss A, Riethdorf S et al (2013) Identification of a population of blood circulating tumor cells from breast cancer patients that initiates metastasis in a xenograft assay. Nat Biotechnol 31(6):539–544

Bailey P, Chang DK, Nones K et al (2016) Genomic analyses identify molecular subtypes of pancreatic cancer. Nature 531(7592):47–52

Baslan T, Kendall J, Ward B et al (2015) Optimizing sparse sequencing of single cells for highly multiplex copy number profiling. Genome Res 25(5):714–724

Beitsch PD, Clifford E (2000) Detection of carcinoma cells in the blood of breast cancer patients. Am J Surg 180(6):446–448. discussion 448–449

Burguillos MA, Magnusson C, Nordin M et al (2013) Microchannel acoustophoresis does not impact survival or function of microglia, leukocytes or tumor cells. PLoS One 8(5):e64233

Carpenter EL, Rader J, Ruden J et al (2014) Dielectrophoretic capture and genetic analysis of single neuroblastoma tumor cells. Front Oncol 4:201

Catenacci DV, Chapman CG, Xu P et al (2015) Acquisition of portal venous circulating tumor cells from patients with pancreaticobiliary cancers by endoscopic ultrasound. Gastroenterology 149(7):1794–1803.e1794

Cayrefourcq L, Mazard T, Joosse S et al (2015) Establishment and characterization of a cell line from human circulating colon cancer cells. Cancer Res 75(5):892–901

Chattopadhyay PK, Hogerkorp CM, Roederer M (2008) A chromatic explosion: the development and future of multiparameter flow cytometry. Immunology 125(4):441–449

Cherian S, Moore J, Bantly A et al (2005) Peripheral blood MDS score: a new flow cytometric tool for the diagnosis of myelodysplastic syndromes. Cytometry B Clin Cytom 64(1):9–17

Cohen SJ, Punt CJ, Iannotti N et al (2008) Relationship of circulating tumor cells to tumor response, progression-free survival, and overall survival in patients with metastatic colorectal cancer. J Clin Oncol 26(19):3213–3221

Cristofanilli M, Budd GT, Ellis MJ et al (2004) Circulating tumor cells, disease progression, and survival in metastatic breast cancer. N Engl J Med 351(8):781–791

Cruz I, Ciudad J, Cruz JJ et al (2005) Evaluation of multiparameter flow cytometry for the detection of breast cancer tumor cells in blood samples. Am J Clin Pathol 123(1):66–74

de Bono JS, Scher HI, Montgomery RB et al (2008) Circulating tumor cells predict survival benefit from treatment in metastatic castration-resistant prostate cancer. Clin Cancer Res 14 (19):6302–6309

Dent BM, Ogle LF, O'Donnell RL et al (2016) High-resolution imaging for the detection and characterisation of circulating tumour cells from patients with oesophageal, hepatocellular, thyroid and ovarian cancers. Int J Cancer 138(1):206–216

Divella R, Daniele A, Abbate I et al (2014) The presence of clustered circulating tumor cells (CTCs) and circulating cytokines define an aggressive phenotype in metastatic colorectal cancer. Cancer Causes Control 25(11):1531–1541

Fan HC, Fu GK, Fodor SP (2015) Expression profiling. Combinatorial labeling of single cells for gene expression cytometry. Science 347(6222):1258367

Ferreira MM, Ramani VC, Jeffrey SS (2016) Circulating tumor cell technologies. Mol Oncol 10 (3):374–394

Fritsch G, Printz D, Stimpfl M et al (1997) Quantification of CD34+ cells: comparison of methods. Transfusion 37(8):775–784

Gao D, Vela I, Sboner A et al (2014) Organoid cultures derived from patients with advanced prostate cancer. Cell 159(1):176–187

Gerlinger M, Rowan AJ, Horswell S et al (2012) Intratumor heterogeneity and branched evolution revealed by multiregion sequencing. N Engl J Med 366(10):883–892

Girotti MR, Gremel G, Lee R et al (2016) Application of sequencing, liquid biopsies, and patient-derived Xenografts for personalized medicine in melanoma. Cancer Discov 6(3):286–299

Gorner K, Bachmann J, Holzhauer C et al (2015) Genetic analysis of circulating tumor cells in pancreatic cancer patients: a pilot study. Genomics 106(1):7–14

Gross HJ, Verwer B, Houck D et al (1995) Model study detecting breast cancer cells in peripheral blood mononuclear cells at frequencies as low as 10(−7). Proc Natl Acad Sci 92(2):537–541

Guinney J, Dienstmann R, Wang X et al (2015) The consensus molecular subtypes of colorectal cancer. Nat Med 21(11):1350–1356

Gupta V, Jafferji I, Garza M et al (2012) ApoStream(), a new dielectrophoretic device for antibody independent isolation and recovery of viable cancer cells from blood. Biomicrofluidics 6 (2):24133

Halo TL, McMahon KM, Angeloni NL et al (2014) NanoFlares for the detection, isolation, and culture of live tumor cells from human blood. Proc Natl Acad Sci USA 111(48):17104–17109

Hamilton G, Rath B, Klameth L et al (2016) Small cell lung cancer: recruitment of macrophages by circulating tumor cells. Oncoimmunology 5(3):e1093277

Hanley MB, Lomas W, Mittar D et al (2013) Detection of low abundance RNA molecules in individual cells by flow cytometry. PLoS One 8(2):e57002

Hodgkinson CL, Morrow CJ, Li Y et al (2014) Tumorigenicity and genetic profiling of circulating tumor cells in small-cell lung cancer. Nat Med 20(8):897–903

Hou JM, Krebs MG, Lancashire L et al (2012) Clinical significance and molecular characteristics of circulating tumor cells and circulating tumor microemboli in patients with small-cell lung cancer. J Clin Oncol 30(5):525–532

Hristozova T, Konschak R, Budach V et al (2012) A simple multicolor flow cytometry protocol for detection and molecular characterization of circulating tumor cells in epithelial cancers. Cytometry A 81(6):489–495

Hu Y, Fan L, Zheng J et al (2010) Detection of circulating tumor cells in breast cancer patients utilizing multiparameter flow cytometry and assessment of the prognosis of patients in different CTCs levels. Cytometry A 77(3):213–219

Issadore D, Chung J, Shao H et al (2012) Ultrasensitive clinical enumeration of rare cells ex vivo using a micro-hall detector. Sci Transl Med 4(141):141ra192

Jansson S, Bendahl PO, Larsson AM et al (2016) Prognostic impact of circulating tumor cell apoptosis and clusters in serial blood samples from patients with metastatic breast cancer in a prospective observational cohort. BMC Cancer 16:433

Karabacak NM, Spuhler PS, Fachin F et al (2014) Microfluidic, marker-free isolation of circulating tumor cells from blood samples. Nat Protoc 9(3):694–710

Khoja L, Backen A, Sloane R et al (2012) A pilot study to explore circulating tumour cells in pancreatic cancer as a novel biomarker. Br J Cancer 106(3):508–516

Lara O, Tong X, Zborowski M et al (2004) Enrichment of rare cancer cells through depletion of normal cells using density and flow-through, immunomagnetic cell separation. Exp Hematol 32(10):891–904

Laurell T, Petersson F, Nilsson A (2007) Chip integrated strategies for acoustic separation and manipulation of cells and particles. Chem Soc Rev 36(3):492–506

Lenshof A, Magnusson C, Laurell T (2012) Acoustofluidics 8: applications of acoustophoresis in continuous flow microsystems. Lab Chip 12(7):1210–1223

Li P, Mao Z, Peng Z et al (2015) Acoustic separation of circulating tumor cells. Proc Natl Acad Sci USA 112(16):4970–4975

Lohr JG, Adalsteinsson VA, Cibulskis K et al (2014) Whole-exome sequencing of circulating tumor cells provides a window into metastatic prostate cancer. Nat Biotechnol 32(5):479–484

Lu Y, Liang H, Yu T et al (2015) Isolation and characterization of living circulating tumor cells in patients by immunomagnetic negative enrichment coupled with flow cytometry. Cancer 121 (17):3036–3045

Macosko EZ, Basu A, Satija R et al (2015) Highly parallel genome-wide expression profiling of individual cells using Nanoliter droplets. Cell 161(5):1202–1214

Maddipati R, Stanger BZ (2015) Pancreatic cancer metastases harbor evidence of polyclonality. Cancer Discov 5:1086–1097

Magbanua MJM, Sosa EV, Scott JH et al (2012) Isolation and genomic analysis of circulating tumor cells from castration resistant metastatic prostate cancer. BMC Cancer 12(1):1–12

Magbanua MJ, Sosa EV, Roy R et al (2013) Genomic profiling of isolated circulating tumor cells from metastatic breast cancer patients. Cancer Res 73(1):30–40

Maheswaran S, Sequist LV, Nagrath S et al (2008) Detection of mutations in EGFR in circulating lung-cancer cells. N Engl J Med 359(4):366–377

Mazel M, Jacot W, Pantel K et al (2015) Frequent expression of PD-L1 on circulating breast cancer cells. Mol Oncol 9(9):1773–1782

McGranahan N, Furness AJS, Rosenthal R et al (2016) Clonal neoantigens elicit T cell immunoreactivity and sensitivity to immune checkpoint blockade. Science 351(6280):1463–1469

Miyamoto DT, Zheng Y, Wittner BS et al (2015) RNA-Seq of single prostate CTCs implicates noncanonical Wnt signaling in antiandrogen resistance. Science 349(6254):1351–1356

Molnar B, Ladanyi A, Tanko L et al (2001) Circulating tumor cell clusters in the peripheral blood of colorectal cancer patients. Clin Cancer Res 7(12):4080

Momburg F, Moldenhauer G, Hammerling GJ et al (1987) Immunohistochemical study of the expression of a Mr 34,000 human epithelium-specific surface glycoprotein in normal and malignant tissues. Cancer Res 47(11):2883–2891

Ni X, Zhuo M, Su Z et al (2013) Reproducible copy number variation patterns among single circulating tumor cells of lung cancer patients. Proc Natl Acad Sci USA 110(52):21083–21088

Ogle LF, Orr JG, Willoughby CE et al (2016) Imagestream detection and characterisation of circulating tumour cells – a liquid biopsy for hepatocellular carcinoma? J Hepatol 65 (2):305–313

Pailler E, Oulhen M, Billiot F et al (2016) Method for semi-automated microscopy of filtration-enriched circulating tumor cells. BMC Cancer 16:477

Powell AA, Talasaz AH, Zhang H et al (2012) Single cell profiling of circulating tumor cells: transcriptional heterogeneity and diversity from breast cancer cell lines. PLoS One 7(5): e33788

Prat A, Pineda E, Adamo B et al (2015) Clinical implications of the intrinsic molecular subtypes of breast cancer. Breast 24(Suppl 2):S26–S35

Racila E, Euhus D, Weiss AJ et al (1998) Detection and characterization of carcinoma cells in the blood. Proc Natl Acad Sci USA 95(8):4589–4594

Ramskold D, Luo S, Wang YC et al (2012) Full-length mRNA-Seq from single-cell levels of RNA and individual circulating tumor cells. Nat Biotechnol 30(8):777–782

Rhim AD, Mirek ET, Aiello NM et al (2012) EMT and dissemination precede pancreatic tumor formation. Cell 148(1–2):349–361

Richardson GM, Lannigan J, Macara IG (2015) Does FACS perturb gene expression? Cytometry A 87(2):166–175

Rizvi NA, Hellmann MD, Snyder A et al (2015) Mutational landscape determines sensitivity to PD-1 blockade in non–small cell lung cancer. Science 348(6230):124–128

Rogers WT, Moser AR, Holyst HA et al (2008) Cytometric fingerprinting: quantitative characterization of multivariate distributions. Cytometry A 73(5):430–441

Rogers WT, Zhang L, Welden S, Krieger B, Rickels M, Moore JS, Mohler ER (2015) Vascular health profile predicts cardiovascular outcomes in patients with diabetes. Cytometry Part B 00B:000–000

Sarioglu AF, Aceto N, Kojic N et al (2015) A microfluidic device for label-free, physical capture of circulating tumor cell clusters. Nat Methods 12(7):685–691

Satelli A, Batth IS, Brownlee Z et al (2016) Potential role of nuclear PD-L1 expression in cell-surface vimentin positive circulating tumor cells as a prognostic marker in cancer patients. Sci Rep 6:28910

Scher HI, Lu D, Schreiber NA et al (2016) Association of AR-V7 on circulating tumor cells as a treatment-specific biomarker with outcomes and survival in castration-resistant prostate cancer. JAMA Oncol 2:1441–1449

Sharei A, Zoldan J, Adamo A et al (2013) A vector-free microfluidic platform for intracellular delivery. Proc Natl Acad Sci 110(6):2082–2087

Sheng W, Chen T, Kamath R et al (2012) Aptamer-enabled efficient isolation of cancer cells from whole blood using a microfluidic device. Anal Chem 84(9):4199–4206

Shi J, Zhou M, Gong A et al (2016) Fluorescence lifetime imaging of Nanoflares for mRNA detection in living cells. Anal Chem 88(4):1979–1983

Simpson SJ, Vachula M, Kennedy MJ et al (1995) Detection of tumor cells in the bone marrow, peripheral blood, and apheresis products of breast cancer patients using flow cytometry. Exp Hematol 23(10):1062–1068

Smerage JB, Barlow WE, Hortobagyi GN et al (2014) Circulating tumor cells and response to chemotherapy in metastatic breast cancer: SWOG S0500. J Clin Oncol 32(31):3483–3489

Song Y, Zhu Z, An Y et al (2013) Selection of DNA aptamers against epithelial cell adhesion molecule for cancer cell imaging and circulating tumor cell capture. Anal Chem 85 (8):4141–4149

Stoltenburg R, Reinemann C, Strehlitz B (2007) SELEX—A (r)evolutionary method to generate high-affinity nucleic acid ligands. Biomol Eng 24(4):381–403

Stott SL, Hsu CH, Tsukrov DI et al (2010) Isolation of circulating tumor cells using a microvortex-generating herringbone-chip. Proc Natl Acad Sci USA 107(43):18392–18397

Takao M, Takeda K (2011) Enumeration, characterization, and collection of intact circulating tumor cells by cross contamination-free flow cytometry. Cytometry A 79(2):107–117

Ting DT, Wittner BS, Ligorio M et al (2014) Single-cell RNA sequencing identifies extracellular matrix gene expression by pancreatic circulating tumor cells. Cell Rep 8(6):1905–1918

Vishnoi M, Peddibhotla S, Yin W et al (2015) The isolation and characterization of CTC subsets related to breast cancer dormancy. Sci Rep 5:17533

Wang L, Wang Y, Liu Y et al (2009) Flow cytometric analysis of CK19 expression in the peripheral blood of breast carcinoma patients: relevance for circulating tumor cell detection. J Exp Clin Cancer Res 28:57

Watanabe M, Uehara Y, Yamashita N et al (2014) Multicolor detection of rare tumor cells in blood using a novel flow cytometry-based system. Cytometry A 85(3):206–213

Wilson NK, Kent DG, Buettner F et al (2015) Combined single-cell functional and Gene expression analysis resolves heterogeneity within stem cell populations. Cell Stem Cell 16 (6):712–724

Ye X, Weinberg RA (2015) Epithelial-mesenchymal plasticity: a central regulator of cancer progression. Trends Cell Biol 25(11):675–686

Yee SS, Lieberman DB, Blanchard T et al (2016) A novel approach for next-generation sequencing of circulating tumor cells. Mol Genet Genomic Med 4(4):395–406

Yu M, Ting DT, Stott SL et al (2012) RNA sequencing of pancreatic circulating tumour cells implicates WNT signalling in metastasis. Nature 487(7408):510–513

Yu M, Bardia A, Wittner BS et al (2013) Circulating breast tumor cells exhibit dynamic changes in epithelial and mesenchymal composition. Science 339(6119):580–584

Yu M, Bardia A, Aceto N et al (2014) Cancer therapy. Ex vivo culture of circulating breast tumor cells for individualized testing of drug susceptibility. Science 345(6193):216–220

Zamay GS, Kolovskaya OS, Zamay TN et al (2015) Aptamers selected to postoperative lung adenocarcinoma detect circulating tumor cells in human blood. Mol Ther 23(9):1486–1496

Zhang L, Ridgway LD, Wetzel MD et al (2013) The identification and characterization of breast cancer CTCs competent for brain metastasis. Sci Transl Med 5(180):180ra148

Zhang J, Li S, Liu F et al (2015) SELEX aptamer used as a probe to detect circulating tumor cells in peripheral blood of pancreatic cancer patients. PLoS One 10(3):e0121920

Chapter 6
Enrichment and Detection of Circulating Tumor Cells and Other Rare Cell Populations by Microfluidic Filtration

Michael Pugia, Mark Jesus M. Magbanua, and John W. Park

Abstract The current standard methods for isolating circulating tumor cells (CTCs) from blood involve EPCAM-based immunomagnetic approaches. A major disadvantage of these strategies is that CTCs with low EPCAM expression will be missed. Isolation by size using filter membranes circumvents the reliance on this cell surface marker, and can facilitate the capture not only of EPCAM-negative CTCs but other rare cells as well. These cells that are trapped on the filter membrane can be characterized by immunocytochemistry (ICC), enumerated and profiled to elucidate their clinical significance. In this chapter, we discuss advances in filtration systems to capture rare cells as well as downstream ICC methods to detect and identify these cells. We highlight our recent clinical study demonstrating the feasibility of using a novel method consisting of automated microfluidic filtration and sequential ICC for detection and enumeration of CTCs, as well as circulating mesenchymal cells (CMCs), circulating endothelial cells (CECs), and putative circulating stem cells (CSCs). We hypothesize that simultaneous analysis of circulating rare cells in blood of cancer patients may lead to a better understanding of disease progression and development of resistance to therapy.

Keywords Circulating tumor cells • Circulating mesenchymal cells • Circulating endothelial cells • Circulating stem cells • Filtration • Immunocytochemistry • Filter membranes

M. Pugia (✉)
Siemens Healthcare Diagnostics, 3400 Middlebury Street, Elkhart, IN 46515, USA
e-mail: michael.pugia@siemens.com

M.J.M. Magbanua • J.W. Park
Division of Hematology & Oncology, University of California San Francisco, San Francisco, CA 94115, USA

M.J.M. Magbanua, J.W. Park (eds.), *Isolation and Molecular Characterization of Circulating Tumor Cells*, Advances in Experimental Medicine and Biology 994,
DOI 10.1007/978-3-319-55947-6_6

6.1 Introduction

Filtration offers an alternative approach to antigen-dependent methods for enrichment of non-hematopoietic rare cells in blood. Using filter membranes to isolate circulating tumor cells (CTCs) away from blood cells can potentially eliminate reliance on cell surface antigens, like EPCAM (Farace et al. 2011; Desitter et al. 2011; Huang et al. 2014; Coumans et al. 2013b; Williams et al. 2014). Filter-based systems facilitate the enrichment of circulating rare cells by exploiting the size disparities between these cells and cells of hematopoietic origin (Farace et al. 2011; Desitter et al. 2011; Huang et al. 2014; Coumans et al. 2013b; Williams et al. 2014). For example, CTCs whose typical diameter is about 10 μM or greater (Coumans et al. 2013a; Ligthart et al. 2013) can be purified away from smaller white blood and red blood cells (diameter = 3–8 μM) by using a filter membrane with an appropriate pore size. Consequently, CTCs and other large cells that are caught on the membrane can be identified, enumerated and molecularly characterized (Hofman et al. 2012; Cummings et al. 2014; El-Heliebi et al. 2013).

6.2 Recent Advances in Cell Filtration

Early demonstration of enrichment of CTCs by filtration was reported in the mid-1960s (Seal 1964). Since then, the field has grown and many devices and design variations have been developed. Filtration is of considerable interest in the field of rare cell analysis because of the ability to exclude cells by size in response to cellular deformability, and that cell size could potentially be a parameter that allows analysis of a heterogeneous group of cell phenotypes that better reflects disease states. Cell separation by size-exclusion can be readily accomplished by filtration through a variety of membranes or microfluidics devices. Blood samples can filtered vertically through membranes or laterally through microfluidic filters (McFaul et al. 2012). Both methods take advantage of the same cellular properties such as size and deformability to distinguish target rare cells from blood cells (Coumans et al. 2013a, b).

6.2.1 Microfluidic Filters

A number of new microfluidic filter approaches for isolation of CTCs have been reported (Karabacak et al. 2014; Thege et al. 2014; Jackson et al. 2014; Sollier et al. 2014; Ozkumur et al. 2013). Microfluidic filtration involves the application of pressure that pushes the cells and fluid through micron scale constrictions. Designs for constricting the path that cells in fluid have to pass through, include micron-sized post structures, weir-style structures, grooves or herringbone structures

(McFaul et al. 2012). In all these cases, the "microstructures" serve as resistance that causes disruption in the fluid flow. These constrictions are designed such that certain particles can pass through while others are blocked. Other microfluidic designs involve constrictions that are created by reducing capillary diameter to generate a micron-sized gap (Pugia et al. 2005; Chudziak et al. 2016). A ratio of 1–10 capillary diameter/cell diameter was identified as a key parameter for optimal cell filtration (Pugia et al. 2005).

Another important parameter for filtration of cells is the wall surfaces of the microfluidic devices, which can impact separation due to physical attraction between the surface and the cell. This principle relies on surface energy of the microfluidic walls relative to that of the bulk fluid and of the cells of interest (Pugia et al. 2005). Adhesion increases as the gap height approaches the cell diameter, or when the gap surface energy becomes higher relative to the cell and/or fluid surface energy. Excessive adhesion can cause cell lysis (which results in cell loss), while weak adhesion allows the cells to flow through the gap. Adhesion can be adjusted for certain cell types, bulk solutions, cell diameters, and cell surface energy (Pugia et al. 2005).

6.2.2 *Filter Membranes*

Novel membrane filter approaches have also been developed for isolation of CTCs (Coumans et al. 2013a, b; Lecharpentier et al. 2011). Traditionally, track-etched filters (Nucleopore™) are used with pore sizes from 5 to 8 mm and thicknesses from 6 to 11 mm, and are designed to be flexible with random pore pattern distribution. Biomedical microelectromechanical systems (Bio-MEMS) fabrication techniques have allowed new generations of membranes in both flexible and stiff formats with uniform pore patterns (Balic et al. 2012; de Wit et al. 2015). The pore size, membrane structure and other filter parameters can be optimized to maximize cell recovery (Coumans et al. 2013a, b; Vona et al. 2000; Hofman et al. 2011). For example, the presence of small blood clots increases the likelihood of the membrane clogging, especially if the pore sizes are small (~5 um diameter). Also, smaller pores require the application of vacuum pressure (−100 mbar) that is lower than what is typically used (around −30 mbar) for filtering blood samples. This added pressure can result in increased shear stress and ultimately lead to cell loss. On the other hand, membrane filters with larger pores (>8 um diameter) are impractical because they are non-selective, allowing cells of interest to pass through, thereby reducing recovery of target cells. Hence, prior to working with precious clinical samples, the optimal pore size and filtration pressure needs to be ascertained to reduce background and maximize yield.

In a recent study by our group, we combined both features of a filter membrane and microfluidic filter to create a novel filtration system to enrich for CTCs and other rare cells in the blood of cancer patients. The robotic filtration device involves a filter membrane that is mounted onto a microfluidic slide that allows for efficient

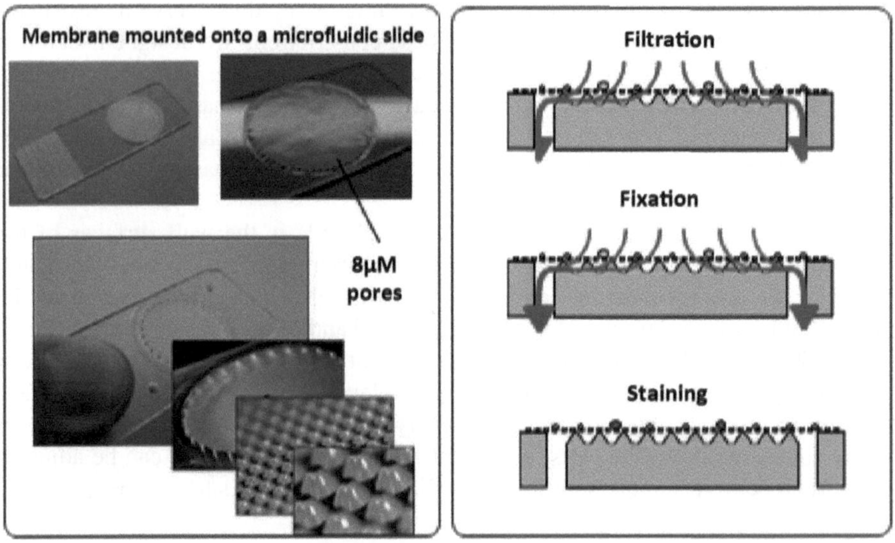

Fig. 6.1 Microfluidic filtration system. Design of the microfluidic filter device and the schematic overview of the processing steps for capture and detection of circulating rare cells (Reproduced from Magbanua et al. 2015)

cell capture and downstream processing of cells for imaging. The system includes an automated pipetting system that allowed for sequential and multiplexed ICC to identify different circulating rare cell populations (Fig. 6.1) (Magbanua et al. 2015).

6.3 Isolation of Rare Cells from Blood by Filtration

The analytical performance of filtration methods is often evaluated in pre-clinical studies using cancer cell lines spiked into healthy blood to evaluate cell yield. Unlike cells in culture, which are generally spherical and more uniform in size, cancer cells in clinical blood specimens are more likely to have a wide range of sizes and shapes, and may also be present as cell clusters. Interestingly, rare cells of 3–5 um in diameter have been captured from filtered clinical samples even when the mean pore diameter was 8 um (Magbanua et al. 2015). This may be due to cross-linking effect of the paraformaldehyde fixation or association with fibrin present in the sample, which allows the retention of smaller cells on the membrane, even though they are small enough to pass through the pores. That said, the isolation of these small non-hematopoietic cells raises the concern of whether spike-in experiments using cultured cells truly reflect cell recovery rates in clinical samples. Despite this potential confounder, the use spiked cell lines to test the analytical performance of filter-based assays provides a good model systems for selection of proper pore size and optimization of other filter parameters before clinical sample testing.

6.4 Identification of Captured Rare Cells by ICC

Once filtration is done, the cells that are retained on the membrane (also referred to as "captured" and/or "isolated" cells) can be stained via ICC and analyzed by fluorescence microscopy. Multiplexed immunocytochemical staining methods using specific antibody-based labels or probes have been developed to identify specific rare cell populations (Magbanua et al. 2015). Steps to prepare cells for imaging, which include fixation, washing, permeabilization, and incubation with antibodies/probes, can be done *in situ* (on the membrane). Automation, controlled filtration rates and precise addition of liquid volumes during this multi-step process can help achieve consistent staining results. In addition, staining parameters (such as antibody concentration and proper selection of fluorescent labels for conjugation) can be optimized to minimize the detection of false positive cells in healthy blood, and maximize the detection of true non-hematologic rare cells in cancer patient's blood. Moreover, the reagents used for washing and blocking during the cell preparation steps are also critical in obtaining reproducible signals. In some cases when the protein marker is expressed at very low levels, direct immunoassay staining can be replaced with higher sensitivity immunoassay methods. For example, using Tyramide Signal Amplification (TSA™, Life Technologies) has increased the detection limit for rarely expressed cell markers by 10–50 fold (Wang et al. 1999). Use of secondary antibodies, biotin-streptavidin labels, and enzyme amplification has all shown to enhance the detection of CTC by 2–5 fold (Pugia et al. unpublished data). In our study, we demonstrated the feasibility of performing up to three separate staining protocols on the same cells, while producing quality cellular images after each step (Magbanua et al. 2015).

6.5 Markers for Rare Cell Typing

Non-filtration methods, such as immunomagnetic-based approaches, use EpCAM to enrich for CTCs and are usually followed by ICC staining of cytokeratins to detect these cells (Magbanua and Park 2014; Alix-Panabieres and Pantel 2014). While these methods have facilitated reliable CTC detection, they can miss CTCs that do not express EpCAM. Recent studies have identified mesenchymal-like CTCs with down-regulated EPCAM expression and therefore may not be detected by epithelial-based assays (Sieuwerts et al. 2009; Yokobori et al. 2013). On the other hand, filtration methods allows for the enrichment of circulating rare cells without pre-selection, and therefore not only capture epithelial cells but also endothelial, mesenchymal, and putative stem cells. Since this approach provides an opportunity to detect and characterize a wide range of cell types, it requires more optimization to select appropriate and reliable biomarkers (in addition to EpCAM and cytokeratins) that can distinguish these rare cells from normal blood cells. While the characterization of these heterogeneous cell populations is more complex, it allows greater understanding of the biology of cancer spread, and may help elucidate the clinical significance of circulating rare cells, beyond CTCs.

6.5.1 Circulating Tumor Cells

ICC methods to detect and enumerate CTCs in blood typically utilize multiple fluorescent antibodies that are combined into one cocktail. A typical cocktail used for CTC detection includes labeled antibodies against epithelial cancer cell markers such as cytokeratins (CK). The staining protocol also includes a fluorescent nuclear stain like 4′,6-diamidino-2-phenylindole (DAPI) to identify nucleated cells. Since filtration methods also captures approximately 10,000–100,000 white blood cells (WBCs) per tube of blood, a third marker that is specific for blood cells, like CD45, is needed to rule out normal cells of hematopoietic origin. Using this strategy, CTCs can be identified as nucleated cells that are CK-positive, and CD45-negative, and be distinguished from WBCs, which are nucleated cells that are CK-negative and CD45-positive (Fig. 6.2).

6.5.2 Circulating Endothelial Cells.

Patients with cancer have elevated numbers of CECs that are probably shed from tumor angiogenesis-related processes, activated or damaged tumor vessel walls, or from injury of normal blood vessels (Ilie et al. 2014; Beerepoot et al. 2004; Rowand et al. 2007). In addition to cancer, fluctuations in CEC levels have also been observed in patients with infections or those diagnosed with cardiovascular disease (Damani et al. 2012; Mehran et al. 2014; Lopez et al. 2012; Bidard et al. 2010; Boos et al. 2006). For reasons that remain unclear, CECs are also present in blood of disease-free individuals (Beerepoot et al. 2004; Rowand et al. 2007). To quantify the levels of CECs, many immunoassays use endothelial markers such as vimentin, CD144, CD31, CD34, CD146, CD105, and CD133 to detect CECs (Ronzoni et al. 2010; Calleri et al. 2009; Bidard et al. 2010; Magbanua et al. 2015). In our recent study, we used CD144 to detect CECs, and were defined as nucleated cells that are CD144-positive, VIM-positive, CK-negative, and CD45-negative. CD144, which is localized on the cell membrane, has a distinctive staining pattern and facilitated the identification of CECs (Fig. 6.2).

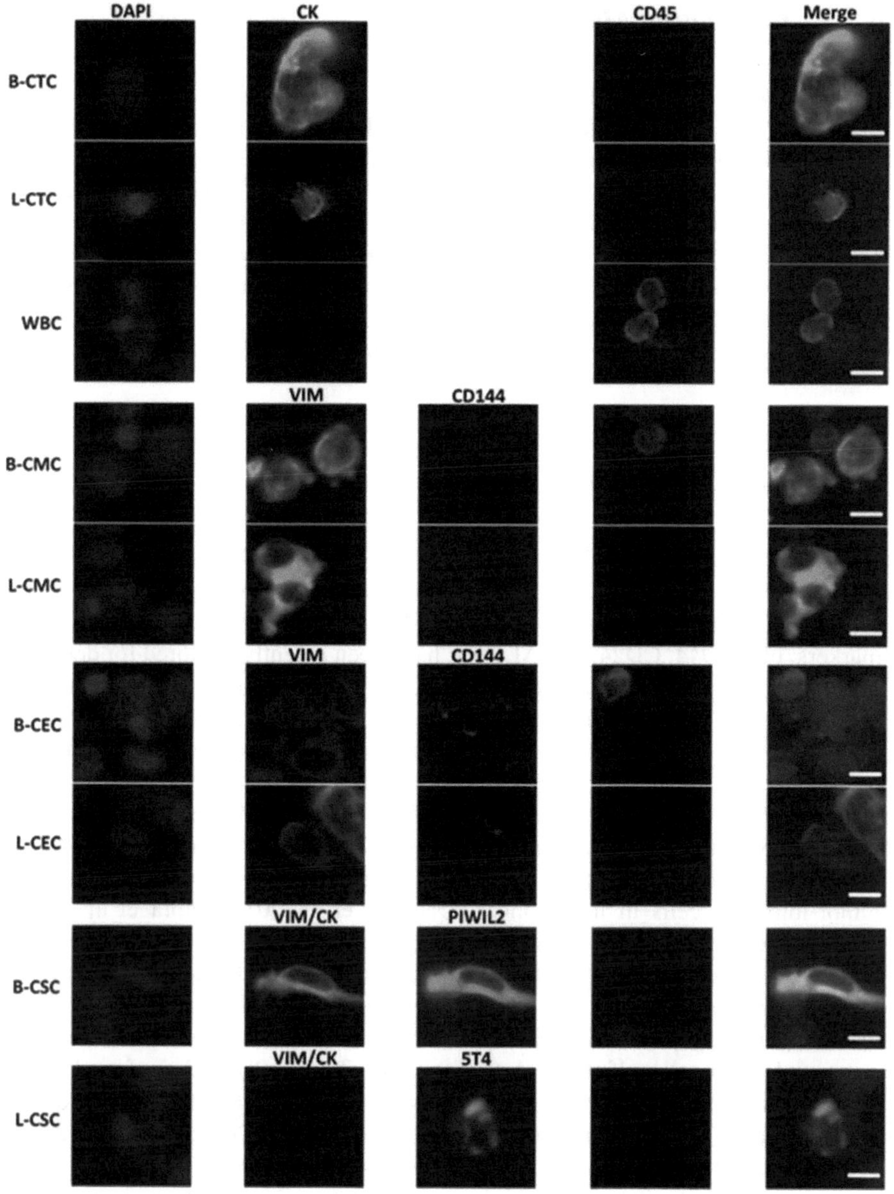

Fig. 6.2 Immunocytochemistry staining of circulating rare cells. Representative images of circulating tumor cells (*CTC*), white blood cells (*WBC*), circulating mesenchymal cells (*CMC*), circulating endothelial cells (*CEC*), and putative circulating stem cells (*CSC*) in metastatic breast (*B*) and lung (*L*) cancer patients. The scale bar represents 8 μM (Reproduced from Magbanua et al. 2015)

6.5.3 Circulating Mesenchymal Cells

During disease progression, tumor cells may undergo epithelial–mesenchymal transition (EMT). This process is accompanied by down-regulation of epithelial markers, like EPCAM (Hyun et al. 2016). A candidate marker for CMC detection is vimentin (VIM), a gene that is overexpressed during EMT process (Satelli et al. 2015). We recently have shown the feasibility of detecting CMCs using our filter-based approach (Magbanua et al. 2015). Since CECs may also express vimentin, the ICC staining cocktail should also include antibodies against CD144 to distinguish CMCs from CECs (Magbanua et al. 2015). CMCs were defined as nucleated, VIM-positive, CK-negative, CD144-negative, and CD45-negative (Fig. 6.2).

6.5.4 Circulating Stem Cells

The cancer stem cell hypothesis proposes that only a few distinct cells within the tumor (capable of self-renewal and multipotency) are responsible for tumor progression (O'Flaherty et al. 2012; Kasimir-Bauer et al. 2012). Cancer stem cell markers, like CD44, CD24, and ALDH1, have been recently explored for detection of putative cancer circulating stem cells (CSCs) in blood of cancer patients with solid tumors (Theodoropoulos et al. 2010; Sterlacci et al. 2014; Medema 2013). Recently, two novel candidate stem cell markers, trophoblast glycoprotein (TPGB/5 T4) (Damelin et al. 2011; Sapra et al. 2013) and piwi like RNA-mediated gene silencing 2 (PIWIL2) (Lee et al. 2010; Zhang et al. 2013) were used to detect putative CSCs in blood of cancer patients (Magbanua et al. 2015). TPBG/5 T4 is an oncofetal protein (Boyle et al. 1990) which has been shown to be expressed in tumor-initiating cells in lung cancer (Damelin et al. 2011; Sapra et al. 2013). Up-regulation of TPBG/5 T4 in different cancer types is correlated with poor patient outcome (Damelin et al. 2011; Naganuma et al. 2002; Starzynska et al. 1994; Wrigley et al. 1995). PIWIL2 is a member of the P-element-induced wimpy testis/Argonaute (PIWI/AGO) family and plays a vital role in germ cell development and stem-cell self-renewal (Qiao et al. 2002). PIWIL2 is found to be expressed in putative cancer stem cells, precancerous cells and tumor cells during different stages of breast cancer (Liu et al. 2010; Chen et al. 2007; Gao 2008; Zhang et al. 2013; Lee et al. 2010). In our previous work, we used our filtration system to detect putative CSCs in breast and lung cancer patients (Magbanua et al. 2015). We defined CSCs as nucleated, stem cell marker-positive, CK-positive/negative, VIM-positive/negative, CD144-negative, and CD45-negative. The TPBG/5T4 and PIWIL2 markers were used to identify putative lung and breast cancer CSCs, respectively (Fig. 6.2).

6.6 Detection of Rare Cells in Blood of Cancer Patients

Using fluorescence microscopy, we analyzed the staining patterns on cells captured on the filter membrane to detect different cell types. We enumerated rare cell populations, including CTCs, CMCs, CECs, and putative CSCs, using the definitions for each of the cell type as discussed above (Magbanua et al. 2015). CTCs were detected in almost a third of the cancer patients, but were largely absent from controls, except in one healthy donor where a single CTC was detected (Fig. 6.3). We detected CMCs in over half of cancer patients, but were also absent in healthy controls. Similarly, we found putative CSCs samples from cancer patients only, and none in healthy subjects. In contrast to other rare cell types, we detected CECs in both cancer patients and healthy individuals. Of note, CECs were usually found as cell clusters, while most other cell types were detected as single cells. CECs appeared to be the most abundant cell population captured, detected in approximately 50% of cancer patients and controls. This finding recapitulates previous observations from a study showing that CECs constitute majority of the rare cells isolated using a commercially-available filter system (El-Heliebi et al. 2013).

A major advantage of blood-based testing over tissue-based (biopsy) assays is the ease of performing serial analysis to monitor disease progression and treatment response. We conducted a proof-of-concept study to test the feasibility of analyzing blood samples collected at different points during therapy. Serial blood testing using our filtration/multiplex ICC method was performed in a small number of breast cancer patients. Results showed that the changes in the levels of circulating rare cells corresponded with the changes observed in established markers like such CA 15–3 and CTCs assayed by CellSearch®. In addition, we observed that patients who experienced an increase in the levels of circulating rare cells exhibited progressive disease. These observations are, however, preliminary and should be validated in a larger cohort of patients.

6.7 Conclusions

Cell isolation using filter membranes and microfluidic devices provide an antigen-independent approach for enrichment of circulating rare cells in blood of cancer patients. Unlike antibody-based enrichment methods, which can only capture specific antigen-expressing cells, size-based exclusion methods can ultimately yield cell populations that are highly heterogeneous. Another advantage of this system is that cells captured can be directly analyzed on the filter membrane, minimizing cell loss. In addition, multiplex immunostaining allows for the detection of different types of rare cells, in addition to CTCs. A major limitation of all filter-based method is that very small rare cells can to pass through the filter and will be missed by downstream analyses. Simultaneous detection of circulating rare cells

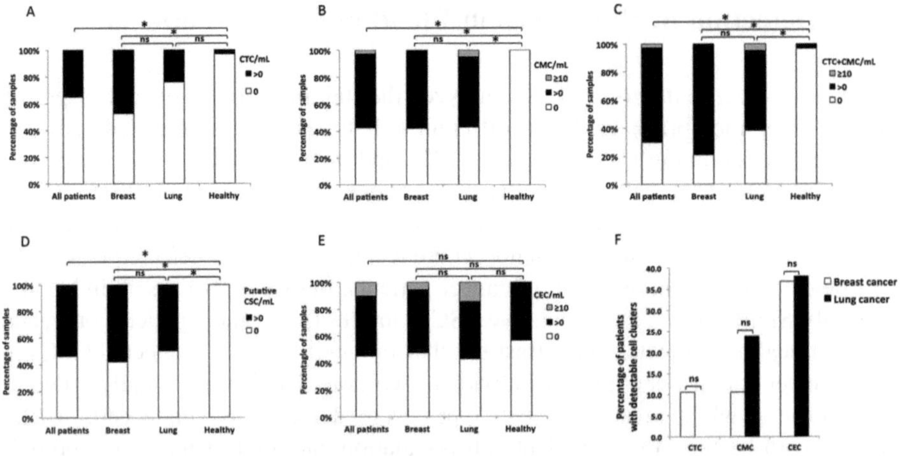

Fig. 6.3 Detection of circulating rare cells in metastatic breast and lung cancer patients and healthy controls. Percentage of samples with detectable rare cells: (**a**) circulating tumor cells (*CTC*), (**b**) circulating mesenchymal cells (*CMC*), (**c**) CTC and CMC, (**d**) putative circulating stem cells (*CSC*), and (**e**) circulating endothelial cells (*CEC*) in metastatic breast and lung cancer patients, and healthy controls. (**f**) Percentage of patients with detectable cell clusters. Percent detection between groups was compared using Fisher exact tests and was considered significant (*) when p-value was <0.05, otherwise, not significant (*ns*) (Reproduced from Magbanua et al. 2015)

in blood of cancer patients, in addition to CTCs, may lead to the discovery of novel biomarkers for monitoring disease progression and treatment efficacy.

Acknowledgements We acknowledge the research contributions by colleagues at Siemens Healthcare Diagnostics, namely, Mary Foltz, Karen Marfurt, Cathleen Hanau-Taylor, Julia Philps. We thank Jin Sun Lee, Marc Jabon, Victoria Wang, Matthew Gubens, and Hope S. Rugo at the University of California San Francisco for their assistance in the clinical work. MJM was supported in part by the Breast Cancer Research Foundation.

References

Alix-Panabieres C, Pantel K (2014) Challenges in circulating tumour cell research. Nat Rev Cancer 14(9):623–631

Balic M, Lin H, Williams A et al (2012) Progress in circulating tumor cell capture and analysis: implications for cancer management. Expert Rev Mol Diagn 12(3):303–312

Beerepoot LV, Mehra N, Vermaat JS et al (2004) Increased levels of viable circulating endothelial cells are an indicator of progressive disease in cancer patients. Ann Oncol 15(1):139–145

Bidard FC, Mathiot C, Degeorges A et al (2010) Clinical value of circulating endothelial cells and circulating tumor cells in metastatic breast cancer patients treated first line with bevacizumab and chemotherapy. Ann Oncol 21(9):1765–1771

Boos CJ, Lip GY, Blann AD (2006) Circulating endothelial cells in cardiovascular disease. J Am Coll Cardiol 48(8):1538–1547

Boyle JM, Grzeschik KH, Heath PR et al (1990) Trophoblast glycoprotein recognised by monoclonal antibody 5T4 maps to human chromosome 6q14-q15. Hum Genet 84(5):455–458

Calleri A, Bono A, Bagnardi V et al (2009) Predictive potential of Angiogenic growth factors and circulating endothelial cells in breast cancer patients receiving metronomic chemotherapy plus bevacizumab. Clin Cancer Res 15(24):7652–7657

Chen L, Shen R, Ye Y et al (2007) Precancerous stem cells have the potential for both benign and malignant differentiation. PLoS One 2(3):e293

Chudziak J, Burt DJ, Mohan S et al (2016) Clinical evaluation of a novel microfluidic device for epitope-independent enrichment of circulating tumour cells in patients with small cell lung cancer. Analyst 141(2):669–678

Coumans FA, van Dalum G, Beck M et al (2013a) Filter characteristics influencing circulating tumor cell enrichment from whole blood. PLoS One 8(4):e61770

Coumans FA, van Dalum G, Beck M et al (2013b) Filtration parameters influencing circulating tumor cell enrichment from whole blood. PLoS One 8(4):e61774

Cummings J, Sloane R, Morris K et al (2014) Optimisation of an immunohistochemistry method for the determination of androgen receptor expression levels in circulating tumour cells. BMC Cancer 14:226

Damani S, Bacconi A, Libiger O et al (2012) Characterization of circulating endothelial cells in acute myocardial infarction. Sci Transl Med 4(126):126ra133

Damelin M, Geles KG, Follettie MT et al (2011) Delineation of a cellular hierarchy in lung cancer reveals an oncofetal antigen expressed on tumor-initiating cells. Cancer Res 71(12):4236–4246

de Wit S, van Dalum G, Lenferink AT et al (2015) The detection of EpCAM(+) and EpCAM(−) circulating tumor cells. Sci Rep 5:12270

Desitter I, Guerrouahen BS, Benali-Furet N et al (2011) A new device for rapid isolation by size and characterization of rare circulating tumor cells. Anticancer Res 31(2):427–441

El-Heliebi A, Kroneis T, Zohrer E et al (2013) Are morphological criteria sufficient for the identification of circulating tumor cells in renal cancer? J Transl Med 11:214

Farace F, Massard C, Vimond N et al (2011) A direct comparison of CellSearch and ISET for circulating tumour-cell detection in patients with metastatic carcinomas. Br J Cancer 105 (6):847–853

Gao JX (2008) Cancer stem cells: the lessons from pre-cancerous stem cells. J Cell Mol Med 12 (1):67–96

Hofman V, Bonnetaud C, Ilie MI et al (2011) Preoperative circulating tumor cell detection using the isolation by size of epithelial tumor cell method for patients with lung cancer is a new prognostic biomarker. Clin Cancer Res 17(4):827–835

Hofman V, Long E, Ilie M et al (2012) Morphological analysis of circulating tumour cells in patients undergoing surgery for non-small cell lung carcinoma using the isolation by size of epithelial tumour cell (ISET) method. Cytopathology 23(1):30–38

Huang T, Jia CP, Jun Y et al (2014) Highly sensitive enumeration of circulating tumor cells in lung cancer patients using a size-based filtration microfluidic chip. Biosens Bioelectron 51:213–218

Hyun KA, Koo GB, Han H et al (2016) Epithelial-to-mesenchymal transition leads to loss of EpCAM and different physical properties in circulating tumor cells from metastatic breast cancer. Oncotarget 7(17):24677–24687

Ilie M, Long E, Hofman V et al (2014) Clinical value of circulating endothelial cells and of soluble CD146 levels in patients undergoing surgery for non-small cell lung cancer. Br J Cancer 110 (5):1236–1243

Jackson JM, Witek MA, Hupert ML et al (2014) UV activation of polymeric high aspect ratio microstructures: ramifications in antibody surface loading for circulating tumor cell selection. Lab Chip 14(1):106–117

Karabacak NM, Spuhler PS, Fachin F et al (2014) Microfluidic, marker-free isolation of circulating tumor cells from blood samples. Nat Protoc 9(3):694–710

Kasimir-Bauer S, Hoffmann O, Wallwiener D et al (2012) Expression of stem cell and epithelial-mesenchymal transition markers in primary breast cancer patients with circulating tumor cells. Breast Cancer Res 14(1):R15

Lecharpentier A, Vielh P, Perez-Moreno P et al (2011) Detection of circulating tumour cells with a hybrid (epithelial/mesenchymal) phenotype in patients with metastatic non-small cell lung cancer. Br J Cancer 105(9):1338–1341

Lee JH, Jung C, Javadian-Elyaderani P et al (2010) Pathways of proliferation and antiapoptosis driven in breast cancer stem cells by stem cell protein piwil2. Cancer Res 70(11):4569–4579

Ligthart ST, Coumans FA, Bidard FC et al (2013) Circulating tumor cells count and morphological features in breast, colorectal and prostate cancer. PLoS One 8(6):e67148

Liu JJ, Shen R, Chen L et al (2010) Piwil2 is expressed in various stages of breast cancers and has the potential to be used as a novel biomarker. Int J Clin Exp Pathol 3(4):328–337

Lopez M, San Roman J, Estrada V et al (2012) Endothelial dysfunction in HIV infection--the role of circulating endothelial cells, microparticles, endothelial progenitor cells and macrophages. AIDS Rev 14(4):223–230

Magbanua MJ, Park JW (2014) Advances in genomic characterization of circulating tumor cells. Cancer Metastasis Rev 33(2–3):757–769

Magbanua MJ, Pugia M, Lee JS et al (2015) A novel strategy for detection and enumeration of circulating rare cell populations in metastatic cancer patients using automated microfluidic filtration and multiplex immunoassay. PLoS One 10(10):e0141166

McFaul SM, Lin BK, Ma H (2012) Cell separation based on size and deformability using microfluidic funnel ratchets. Lab Chip 12(13):2369–2376

Medema JP (2013) Cancer stem cells: the challenges ahead. Nat Cell Biol 15(4):338–344

Mehran R, Nilsson M, Khajavi M et al (2014) Tumor endothelial markers define novel subsets of cancer-specific circulating endothelial cells associated with antitumor efficacy. Cancer Res 74 (10):2731–2741

Naganuma H, Kono K, Mori Y et al (2002) Oncofetal antigen 5T4 expression as a prognostic factor in patients with gastric cancer. Anticancer Res 22(2B):1033–1038

O'Flaherty JD, Barr M, Fennell D et al (2012) The cancer stem-cell hypothesis: its emerging role in lung cancer biology and its relevance for future therapy. J Thorac Oncol 7(12):1880–1890

Ozkumur E, Shah AM, Ciciliano JC et al (2013) Inertial focusing for tumor antigen-dependent and -independent sorting of rare circulating tumor cells. Sci Transl Med 5(179):179ra147

Pugia MJ, Blankenstein G, Peters RP et al (2005) Microfluidic tool box as technology platform for hand-held diagnostics. Clin Chem 51(10):1923–1932

Qiao D, Zeeman AM, Deng W et al (2002) Molecular characterization of hiwi, a human member of the piwi gene family whose overexpression is correlated to seminomas. Oncogene 21 (25):3988–3999

Ronzoni M, Manzoni M, Mariucci S et al (2010) Circulating endothelial cells and endothelial progenitors as predictive markers of clinical response to bevacizumab-based first-line treatment in advanced colorectal cancer patients. Ann Oncol 21(12):2382–2389

Rowand JL, Martin G, Doyle GV et al (2007) Endothelial cells in peripheral blood of healthy subjects and patients with metastatic carcinomas. Cytometry A 71(2):105–113

Sapra P, Damelin M, Dijoseph J et al (2013) Long-term tumor regression induced by an antibody-drug conjugate that targets 5T4, an oncofetal antigen expressed on tumor-initiating cells. Mol Cancer Ther 12(1):38–47

Satelli A, Mitra A, Brownlee Z et al (2015) Epithelial-mesenchymal transitioned circulating tumor cells capture for detecting tumor progression. Clin Cancer Res 21(4):899–906

Seal SH (1964) A sieve for the isolation of cancer cells and other large cells from the blood. Cancer 17:637–642

Sieuwerts AM, Kraan J, Bolt J et al (2009) Anti-epithelial cell adhesion molecule antibodies and the detection of circulating normal-like breast tumor cells. J Natl Cancer Inst 101(1):61–66

Sollier E, Go DE, Che J et al (2014) Size-selective collection of circulating tumor cells using vortex technology. Lab Chip 14(1):63–77

Starzynska T, Marsh PJ, Schofield PF et al (1994) Prognostic significance of 5T4 oncofetal antigen expression in colorectal carcinoma. Br J Cancer 69(5):899–902

Sterlacci W, Savic S, Fiegl M et al (2014) Putative stem cell markers in non-small-cell lung cancer: a clinicopathologic characterization. J Thorac Oncol 9(1):41–49

Thege FI, Lannin TB, Saha TN et al (2014) Microfluidic immunocapture of circulating pancreatic cells using parallel EpCAM and MUC1 capture: characterization, optimization and downstream analysis. Lab Chip 14(10):1775–1784

Theodoropoulos PA, Polioudaki H, Agelaki S et al (2010) Circulating tumor cells with a putative stem cell phenotype in peripheral blood of patients with breast cancer. Cancer Lett 288 (1):99–106

Vona G, Sabile A, Louha M et al (2000) Isolation by size of epithelial tumor cells : a new method for the immunomorphological and molecular characterization of circulatingtumor cells. Am J Pathol 156(1):57–63

Wang G, Achim CL, Hamilton RL et al (1999) Tyramide signal amplification method in multiple-label immunofluorescence confocal microscopy. Methods 18(4):459–464

Williams A, Chung J, Ou X et al (2014) Fourier ptychographic microscopy for filtration-based circulating tumor cell enumeration and analysis. J Biomed Opt 19(6):066007

Wrigley E, McGown AT, Rennison J et al (1995) 5T4 oncofetal antigen expression in ovarian carcinoma. Int J Gynecol Cancer 5(4):269–274

Yokobori T, Iinuma H, Shimamura T et al (2013) Plastin3 is a novel marker for circulating tumor cells undergoing the epithelial-mesenchymal transition and is associated with colorectal cancer prognosis. Cancer Res 73(7):2059–2069

Zhang H, Ren Y, Xu H et al (2013) The expression of stem cell protein Piwil2 and piR-932 in breast cancer. Surg Oncol 22(4):217–223

Chapter 7
Detection and Enumeration of Circulating Tumor Cells with Invasive Phenotype

Haizhen Wang and Xiangwei Wu

Abstract Circulating tumor cells (CTCs) disseminate from solid primary cancers into the peripheral blood and lymphatic vessels and can lead to metastatic tumor development; thus, CTC assays are an important clinical tool for monitoring progression and evaluating prognosis in cancer. However, CTCs are limited in number and heterogeneous in their biological and physical properties, making their detection, isolation, and enumeration a major challenge. To overcome these difficulties, novel techniques have been developed to detect and enumerate CTCs with an invasive phenotype. In this chapter, we will summarize these recently developed methods and detail two novel methods for capturing and enriching CTCs on the basis of their viability and their invasive properties.

Keywords CTCs • CTC detection • CTC enumeration • Invasive phenotype

7.1 CTCs Are Important Cancer Biomarkers

Circulating tumor cells (CTCs) are cells from a primary tumor that have shed into the vasculature and are circulating in the bloodstream (Plaks et al. 2013). Some of these cells are thought to be capable of spreading to distant organs and initiating metastatic tumor growth (Pantel et al. 2009; Yu et al. 2011). CTCs were first identified in the blood of a cancer patient in 1869, and significant advancements have been made in the detection and isolation of CTCs since then. During the past two decades, numerous studies have shown that CTCs can be used as a biomarker to monitor cancer treatment response and predict prognosis and overall survival in patients with metastatic colorectal (Cohen et al. 2008; Wong et al. 2009; Uen et al. 2008), lung (Maheswaran et al. 2008), prostate (Danila et al. 2007; Stott et al. 2010), ovarian (Fan et al. 2009; Pearl et al. 2014), breast (Cristofanilli et al. 2004; Lu et al. 2010), and pancreatic (Kulemann et al. 2015) cancers. It is now well

H. Wang • X. Wu (✉)
Department of Clinical Cancer Prevention, The University of Texas MD Anderson Cancer Center, 1515 Holcombe Blvd., Houston, TX 77030, USA
e-mail: hwang9@mdanderson.org; xwwu@mdanderson.org

M.J.M. Magbanua, J.W. Park (eds.), *Isolation and Molecular Characterization of Circulating Tumor Cells*, Advances in Experimental Medicine and Biology 994,
DOI 10.1007/978-3-319-55947-6_7

recognized that high CTC counts are correlated with aggressive disease, increased metastasis propensity, and relatively poor survival rate (Stott et al. 2010; Plaks et al. 2013; Chaffer and Weinberg 2011), making CTC detection and enumeration an important clinical tool.

7.2 Commonly Used Methods for CTC Detection

CTC analyses are considered a real-time "liquid biopsy" and are easy and safe to perform (Alix-Panabieres and Pantel 2013; Pantel and Alix-Panabieres 2012; Cai et al. 2014; Zhang et al. 2015; Marrinucci et al. 2009). CTC analyses have many advantages over tissue biopsy: blood collection is simpler, easer to perform, less invasive, easier to repeat, and more effective in monitoring disease progression and evaluating metastatic risk (Zhang et al. 2015; Hanssen et al. 2015; Pantel and Alix-Panabieres 2013). However, the concentration of CTCs in the blood of cancer patients is very low, from one to a few hundred CTCs per milliliter of whole blood containing millions of leukocytes and billions of red blood cells (erythrocytes) (Miller et al. 2010; Joosse and Pantel 2013; Coumans et al. 2012; Pantel and Alix-Panabieres 2015), making the identification of CTCs a major challenge (Coumans et al. 2012; Pantel and Alix-Panabieres 2015).

The most commonly used methods for detection of CTCs are based on their physical properties and protein markers on their surface (Carter et al. 2012; Harouaka et al. 2013; Esmaeilsabzali et al. 2013; Alix-Panabieres and Pantel 2014). For example, ScreenCell detects CTCs using a filtration-based device that separates CTCs from human whole blood on the basis of cell size, as CTCs are generally larger than leukocytes (Vona et al. 2000; Desitter et al. 2011). Some other methods of capture and selection are based on the expression of cell surface markers, such as epithelial cell adhesion molecule (EpCAM), on CTCs (Pantel et al. 2009; Kling 2012). One of these CTC detection methods, the CellSearch Assay from Veridex Inc., has been cleared by the U.S. Food and Drug Administration for use as a prognostic test in patients with metastatic breast cancer, colorectal cancer, and prostate cancer (Cristofanilli et al. 2005; de Bono et al. 2008; Cohen et al. 2008). This assay relies on the expression of EpCAM by epithelial cells and the capture of these cells by immuno-magnetic particles conjugated with anti-EpCAM antibodies. Other approaches detect and isolate CTCs from peripheral blood using Ficoll/Hypaque density centrifugation imaging (Pierga et al. 2004), immuno-affinity micropost (CTC-chip) (Pantel et al. 2008; Lu et al. 2010), flow cytometry (Georgakoudi et al. 2004), microfluidic imaging systems (Nagrath et al. 2007), high-throughput optical imaging systems, and real-time polymerase chain reaction for tumor-associated mRNA (Kraeft et al. 2004; Paterlini-Brechot and Benali 2007).

However, CTCs are a heterogeneous population of cells, and some undergo epithelial-to-mesenchymal transition (Chiang et al. 2016; Mitra et al. 2015; Lim et al. 2014), causing variation in cell marker expression and cell size (Yu et al.

2013; Wang et al. 2015). Therefore, these methods cannot detect all CTCs. More importantly, some CTCs may be derived from mechanical shedding rather than active invasion, and some of CTCs may lose their viability or functionality and thus become irrelevant to cancer metastasis (Wang et al. 2015). Therefore, the CTC counts generated by these methods may not accurately predict treatment response and cancer outcome.

7.3 Functional Assays for CTC Detection and Enumeration

It is well recognized that the dissemination of tumor cells from a primary tumor to form metastasis is a complex process involving a sequence of steps, including the local invasion of tissues surrounding the primary tumor cells, intravasation (tumor cells entering the bloodstream and lymphatic vessels), survival in the circulatory system, arrest at a secondary site, extravasation into a distant organ, and eventual seeding, proliferation, and development into metastatic tumors (Kim et al. 2012; Nguyen et al. 2009; Kang and Pantel 2013; Tsai and Yang 2013; van Zijl et al. 2011; Stoletov et al. 2010; Chambers et al. 2002). One of the hallmarks of metastasis is that tumor cells gain the ability to penetrate tissue barriers and migrate to other tissues (Martin and Jiang 2009; Liotta and Stetler-Stevenson 1991; Hujanen and Terranova 1985). Therefore, functional CTCs possess invasive ability to allow intravasation and extravasation. The following two techniques have been developed to detect and enumerate functional CTCs with invasive phenotypes (Paris et al. 2009; Wang et al. 2015; Friedlander et al. 2014).

7.3.1 CTC Identification by Collagen Adhesion Matrix Assay

One functional CTC identification method, called the collagen adhesion matrix (CAM) assay, was developed to detect viable CTCs with the ability to attach to and ingest CAM (Fan et al. 2009; Lu et al. 2010; Pearl et al. 2014). The unique feature of the CAM assay is that matrix mimics the tumor microenvironment to help distinguish CTCs from lymphocytes and erythrocytes in blood and enumerate the CTCs (Tulley et al. 2016). Only CTCs with high avidity for the extra-cellular matrix exhibit a proclivity to adhere to the CAM and to ingest the fluorescent CAM (Paris et al. 2009). The CAM assay has several advantages: CAM-captured CTCs are viable, as they are capable of ingesting the CAM. The assay also allows for direct visualization of CAM-ingesting CTCs, as the CAM fluoresce green and red; furthermore, the captured CTCs can be monitored in real time using fluorescence microscopy.

Owing to its high specificity and efficiency, the CAM assay has been used to detect and enumerate CTCs from blood samples of patients with breast cancer (Lu et al. 2010), ovarian cancer (Fan et al. 2009; Pearl et al. 2014), and prostate cancer (Paris et al. 2009) and has been successfully used for ex vivo drug-sensitivity testing of CTCs from patients with ovarian cancer (Tulley et al. 2016). In a small cohort of patients with breast cancer, CAM enrichment returned viable CTCs at a rate of nearly 100% ($99.9 \pm 0.1\%$) (Lu et al. 2010), which is a much higher rate than that of other CTC isolation methods, showing the high isolation efficiency of the CAM assay. Moreover, CTCs enriched by the CAM assay are capable of propagating into colonies and recovering the epithelial phenotype when cultured on the same CAM substrata for several days (Lu et al. 2010), indicating the high specificity of the assay for viable CTCs.

The CAM assay was also used in a pilot investigation of the prognostic significance of circulating epithelial cells with the collagen-invasive phenotype in patients with various stages of breast cancer. The results indicated a significant correlation between CTC counts and lymph node status: lymph node–positive cases showed a much higher CTC detection rate (65.7%) and higher mean CTC count (79/mL) than lymph node–negative cases (detection rate, 26.3%; mean CTC count, 14/mL) (Lu et al. 2010). When disease-free survival and overall survival were taken into consideration, survival status and CTC count were also significantly correlated: both overall survival and disease-free survival in the patients with high CTC counts (>10/mL) were significantly lower than in the patients with low CTC counts (≤10/mL) (Lu et al. 2010). None of the patients with low CTC counts (≤10/mL) had any disease recurrence or progression during the follow-up of 27.6 months (Lu et al. 2010). CTC detection rates and counts also varied significantly between different stages of the disease. CTCs were detectable in 27.3% of stage I and 28.6% of stage II cases, with mean CTC counts of 10/mL and 14/mL, respectively (Lu et al. 2010). Patients with stage III disease had much higher CTC counts; about 86.4% of stage III cases had at least one detectable CTC, with a mean CTC count of 119/mL (Lu et al. 2010).

The CAM assay also has been used to detect CTCs in patients with ovarian cancer and patients with castration-resistant prostate cancer (Paris et al. 2009). Like in breast cancer patients, CTCs were detectable in most epithelial ovarian cancer patients. Higher CTC counts reflected higher CA-125 levels and later stages of disease: significantly higher mean CTC counts were observed in stage III and IV cases (41.3/mL) than in stage I and II cases (6.0/mL). No detectable CTCs were found in benign control cases (Paris et al. 2009). Unlike in breast cancer patients, no significant difference in survival was observed between the ovarian cancer patients with high CTC counts (>31.5/mL) and those with low CTC counts (<31.5/mL) (Paris et al. 2009).

7.3.2 CTC Identification by InCTC

Although the purpose of the CAM assay is to detect and enumerate viable CTCs with the potential to invade, no migration or invasion is involved in the assay (Wang et al. 2015), so the invasiveness of CTCs detected by this assay is unknown.

A new assay named InCTC was developed to circumvent this shortcoming. InCTC detects and enumerates CTCs on the basis of their migration and invasion properties. The assay consists of three simple steps: mononuclear cell layer enrichment, a transwell Matrigel invasion assay, and immunostaining (Wang et al. 2015). The assay has been validated using mouse xenograft tumor models, and its utility was confirmed in a small cohort of patients with lung adenocarcinoma and esophageal squamous cell carcinoma, as described below. InCTC has several obvious advantages over other methods: it does not require special equipment and antigen expression for CTC selection, is less likely to be affected by the heterogeneity of the CTCs, and can be applied to virtually all kinds of cancers. Most importantly, only viable cancer cells with migratory properties and an invasive phenotype are detected and isolated by this method; thus, the CTC counts revealed by InCTC may correlate more strongly than CAM assay counts with treatment response and clinical outcome (Wang et al. 2015).

The InCTC assay was first validated in various xenograft tumor models in both athymic nude mice and C57BL/6 mice. CTC counts ranging from 28/mL to 70/mL were detected. No CTCs were detected in control mice or in tumor-bearing mice without metastasis (Wang et al. 2015). InCTC was then used to monitor tumor development in tumor-bearing mice. The CTC counts in these mice positively correlated with tumor growth, showing that InCTC can be used to monitor tumor development accurately, at least in xenograft tumor–bearing mice (Wang et al. 2015). InCTC was also used to detect CTCs in patients with lung and esophageal cancers. Blood samples from a small cohort of patients with stage II and III lung cancer and esophageal squamous cell carcinoma were collected and subjected to an invasion assay using InCTC. Invasive CTCs were detected in one of the four lung cancer patients and two of the two esophageal cancer patients. No CTCs were detected in control blood samples collected from healthy donors (Wang et al. 2015). Thus, InCTC can be used to detect invasive CTCs in human cancer patients.

The advantage of InCTC in detecting invasive CTCs was demonstrated with a head-to-head comparison between the InCTC assay and an EpCAM-based immuno-magnetic selection method. Although the immuno-magnetic selection detected more CTCs, fewer than half of those CTCs displayed the ability to invade. Moreover, the CTCs selected by the immuno-magnetic method included significantly fewer invasive cells compared with the invasive CTCs counts generated directly by InCTC. These results suggested that InCTC detects more viable cells with an invasive phenotype than the EpCAM antibody-based immunoselection method (Wang et al. 2015).

7.4 Conclusion

With the development of new techniques for CTC detection and isolation, CTC assays have been widely used in clinics for tracking cancer progression and metastasis and for evaluating prognosis (Zhang et al. 2015; Hanssen et al. 2015;

Pantel and Alix-Panabieres 2013; Ulivi 2016; Yin et al. 2016). CTC assays can also be used to monitor clinical response to treatment and to identify drug targets for personalized therapy (Lianidou 2014; Toss et al. 2014). Furthermore, the investigation of CTC biology has improved our understanding of cancer metastasis (Bidard et al. 2016; Wang et al. 2015). All these applications are better served by the detection and enumeration of functional and viable CTCs.

The two functional CTC assays discussed in this chapter are designed to detect and enumerate viable and invasive CTCs; as such, these techniques may track cancer progression and predict outcomes more accurately than CTC assays based on cell markers and physical properties. However, functional CTC assays remain to be directly compared with other CTC assays in patients. The CAM assay has been tested in several clinical studies and shown its ability to detect and enumerate CTCs in various cancer patients (Fan et al. 2009; Lu et al. 2010; Pearl et al. 2014). However, the ability of the CAM assay to isolate and propagate these CTCs is unclear, and whether CTCs detected by the CAM assay can actually invade is unknown. The InCTC assay, on the other hand, detects and enumerates CTCs with invasive ability. However, the development of the InCTC assay is still at an early phase, and more studies in cancer patients are needed to validate its clinical application. Despite these potential drawbacks, functional CTC assays will continue to improve, and patients will inevitably benefit from these new techniques.

References

Alix-Panabieres C, Pantel K (2013) Circulating tumor cells: liquid biopsy of cancer. Clin Chem 59 (1):110–118

Alix-Panabieres C, Pantel K (2014) Challenges in circulating tumour cell research. Nat Rev Cancer 14(9):623–631

Bidard FC, Proudhon C, Pierga JY (2016) Circulating tumor cells in breast cancer. Mol Oncol 10 (3):418–430

Cai LL, Ye HM, Zheng LM et al (2014) Circulating tumor cells (CTCs) as a liquid biopsy material and drug target. Curr Drug Targets 15(10):965–972

Carter L, Metcalf R, Blackhall FH et al (2012) Biology and clinical relevance of circulating tumour cells. J Thorac Dis 4(5):453–455

Chaffer CL, Weinberg RA (2011) A perspective on cancer cell metastasis. Science 331 (6024):1559–1564

Chambers AF, Groom AC, MacDonald IC (2002) Dissemination and growth of cancer cells in metastatic sites. Nat Rev Cancer 2(8):563–572

Chiang SP, Cabrera RM, Segall JE (2016) Tumor cell intravasation. Am J Physiol Cell Physiol 311 (1):C1–C14

Cohen SJ, Punt CJ, Iannotti N et al (2008) Relationship of circulating tumor cells to tumor response, progression-free survival, and overall survival in patients with metastatic colorectal cancer. J Clin Oncol 26(19):3213–3221

Coumans FA, Ligthart ST, Uhr JW et al (2012) Challenges in the enumeration and phenotyping of CTC. Clin Cancer Res 18(20):5711–5718

Cristofanilli M, Budd GT, Ellis MJ et al (2004) Circulating tumor cells, disease progression, and survival in metastatic breast cancer. N Engl J Med 351(8):781–791

Cristofanilli M, Hayes DF, Budd GT et al (2005) Circulating tumor cells: a novel prognostic factor for newly diagnosed metastatic breast cancer. J Clin Oncol 23(7):1420–1430
Danila DC, Heller G, Gignac GA et al (2007) Circulating tumor cell number and prognosis in progressive castration-resistant prostate cancer. Clin Cancer Res 13(23):7053–7058
de Bono JS, Scher HI, Montgomery RB et al (2008) Circulating tumor cells predict survival benefit from treatment in metastatic castration-resistant prostate cancer. Clin Cancer Res 14 (19):6302–6309
Desitter I, Guerrouahen BS, Benali-Furet N et al (2011) A new device for rapid isolation by size and characterization of rare circulating tumor cells. Anticancer Res 31(2):427–441
Esmaeilsabzali H, Beischlag TV, Cox ME et al (2013) Detection and isolation of circulating tumor cells: principles and methods. Biotechnol Adv 31(7):1063–1084
Fan T, Zhao Q, Chen JJ et al (2009) Clinical significance of circulating tumor cells detected by an invasion assay in peripheral blood of patients with ovarian cancer. Gynecol Oncol 112 (1):185–191
Friedlander TW, Ngo VT, Dong H et al (2014) Detection and characterization of invasive circulating tumor cells derived from men with metastatic castration-resistant prostate cancer. Int J Cancer 134(10):2284–2293
Georgakoudi I, Solban N, Novak J et al (2004) In vivo flow cytometry: a new method for enumerating circulating cancer cells. Cancer Res 64(15):5044–5047
Hanssen A, Loges S, Pantel K et al (2015) Detection of circulating tumor cells in non-small cell lung cancer. Front Oncol 5:207
Harouaka RA, Nisic M, Zheng SY (2013) Circulating tumor cell enrichment based on physical properties. J Lab Autom 18(6):455–468
Hujanen ES, Terranova VP (1985) Migration of tumor cells to organ-derived chemoattractants. Cancer Res 45(8):3517–3521
Joosse SA, Pantel K (2013) Biologic challenges in the detection of circulating tumor cells. Cancer Res 73(1):8–11
Kang Y, Pantel K (2013) Tumor cell dissemination: emerging biological insights from animal models and cancer patients. Cancer Cell 23(5):573–581
Kim YN, Koo KH, Sung JY et al (2012) Anoikis resistance: an essential prerequisite for tumor metastasis. Int J Cell Biol 2012:306879
Kling J (2012) Beyond counting tumor cells. Nat Biotechnol 30(7):578–580
Kraeft SK, Ladanyi A, Galiger K et al (2004) Reliable and sensitive identification of occult tumor cells using the improved rare event imaging system. Clin Cancer Res 10(9):3020–3028
Kulemann B, Pitman MB, Liss AS et al (2015) Circulating tumor cells found in patients with localized and advanced pancreatic cancer. Pancreas 44(4):547–550
Lianidou ES (2014) Molecular characterization of circulating tumor cells: holy grail for personalized cancer treatment? Clin Chem 60(10):1249–1251
Lim SH, Becker TM, Chua W et al (2014) Circulating tumour cells and the epithelial mesenchymal transition in colorectal cancer. J Clin Pathol 67(10):848–853
Liotta LA, Stetler-Stevenson WG (1991) Tumor invasion and metastasis: an imbalance of positive and negative regulation. Cancer Res 51(18 Suppl):5054s–5059s
Lu J, Fan T, Zhao Q et al (2010) Isolation of circulating epithelial and tumor progenitor cells with an invasive phenotype from breast cancer patients. Int J Cancer 126(3):669–683
Maheswaran S, Sequist LV, Nagrath S et al (2008) Detection of mutations in EGFR in circulating lung-cancer cells. N Engl J Med 359(4):366–377
Marrinucci D, Bethel K, Luttgen M et al (2009) Circulating tumor cells from well-differentiated lung adenocarcinoma retain cytomorphologic features of primary tumor type. Arch Pathol Lab Med 133(9):1468–1471
Martin TA, Jiang WG (2009) Loss of tight junction barrier function and its role in cancer metastasis. Biochim Biophys Acta 1788(4):872–891

Miller MC, Doyle GV, Terstappen LW (2010) Significance of circulating tumor cells detected by the cellsearch system in patients with metastatic breast colorectal and prostate cancer. J Oncol 2010:617421

Mitra A, Mishra L, Li S (2015) EMT, CTCs and CSCs in tumor relapse and drug-resistance. Oncotarget 6(13):10697–10711

Nagrath S, Sequist LV, Maheswaran S et al (2007) Isolation of rare circulating tumour cells in cancer patients by microchip technology. Nature 450(7173):1235–1239

Nguyen DX, Bos PD, Massague J (2009) Metastasis: from dissemination to organ-specific colonization. Nat Rev Cancer 9(4):274–284

Pantel K, Alix-Panabieres C (2012) The potential of circulating tumor cells as a liquid biopsy to guide therapy in prostate cancer. Cancer Discov 2(11):974–975

Pantel K, Alix-Panabieres C (2013) Real-time liquid biopsy in cancer patients: fact or fiction? Cancer Res 73(21):6384–6388

Pantel K, Alix-Panabieres C (2015) Cell lines from circulating tumor cells. Oncoscience 2 (10):815–816

Pantel K, Brakenhoff RH, Brandt B (2008) Detection, clinical relevance and specific biological properties of disseminating tumour cells. Nat Rev Cancer 8(5):329–340

Pantel K, Alix-Panabieres C, Riethdorf S (2009) Cancer micrometastases. Nat Rev Clin Oncol 6 (6):339–351

Paris PL, Kobayashi Y, Zhao Q et al (2009) Functional phenotyping and genotyping of circulating tumor cells from patients with castration resistant prostate cancer. Cancer Lett 277(2):164–173

Paterlini-Brechot P, Benali NL (2007) Circulating tumor cells (CTC) detection: clinical impact and future directions. Cancer Lett 253(2):180–204

Pearl ML, Zhao Q, Yang J et al (2014) Prognostic analysis of invasive circulating tumor cells (iCTCs) in epithelial ovarian cancer. Gynecol Oncol 134(3):581–590

Pierga JY, Bonneton C, Vincent-Salomon A et al (2004) Clinical significance of immunocytochemical detection of tumor cells using digital microscopy in peripheral blood and bone marrow of breast cancer patients. Clin Cancer Res 10(4):1392–1400

Plaks V, Koopman CD, Werb Z (2013) Cancer. Circulating tumor cells. Science 341 (6151):1186–1188

Stoletov K, Kato H, Zardouzian E et al (2010) Visualizing extravasation dynamics of metastatic tumor cells. J Cell Sci 123(Pt 13):2332–2341

Stott SL, Lee RJ, Nagrath S et al (2010) Isolation and characterization of circulating tumor cells from patients with localized and metastatic prostate cancer. Sci Transl Med 2(25):25ra23

Toss A, Mu Z, Fernandez S et al (2014) CTC enumeration and characterization: moving toward personalized medicine. Ann Transl Med 2(11):108

Tsai JH, Yang J (2013) Epithelial-mesenchymal plasticity in carcinoma metastasis. Genes Dev 27 (20):2192–2206

Tulley S, Zhao Q, Dong H et al (2016) Vita-assay method of enrichment and identification of circulating cancer cells/circulating tumor cells (CTCs). Methods Mol Biol 1406:107–119

Uen YH, Lu CY, Tsai HL et al (2008) Persistent presence of postoperative circulating tumor cells is a poor prognostic factor for patients with stage I-III colorectal cancer after curative resection. Ann Surg Oncol 15(8):2120–2128

Ulivi P (2016) Non-invasive methods to monitor mechanisms of resistance to tyrosine kinase inhibitors in non-small-cell lung cancer: where do we stand? Int J Mol Sci 17(7):1186

van Zijl F, Krupitza G, Mikulits W (2011) Initial steps of metastasis: cell invasion and endothelial transmigration. Mutat Res 728(1–2):23–34

Vona G, Sabile A, Louha M et al (2000) Isolation by size of epithelial tumor cells: a new method for the immunomorphological and molecular characterization of circulatingtumor cells. Am J Pathol 156(1):57–63

Wang H, Hara Y, Liu X et al (2015) Detection and enumeration of circulating tumor cells based on their invasive property. Oncotarget 6(29):27304–27311

Wong SC, Chan CM, Ma BB et al (2009) Clinical significance of cytokeratin 20-positive circulating tumor cells detected by a refined immunomagnetic enrichment assay in colorectal cancer patients. Clin Cancer Res 15(3):1005–1012

Yin CQ, Yuan CH, Qu Z et al (2016) Liquid biopsy of hepatocellular carcinoma: circulating tumor-derived biomarkers. Dis Markers 2016:1427849

Yu M, Stott S, Toner M et al (2011) Circulating tumor cells: approaches to isolation and characterization. J Cell Biol 192(3):373–382

Yu M, Bardia A, Wittner BS et al (2013) Circulating breast tumor cells exhibit dynamic changes in epithelial and mesenchymal composition. Science 339(6119):580–584

Zhang Z, Ramnath N, Nagrath S (2015) Current status of CTCs as liquid biopsy in lung cancer and future directions. Front Oncol 5:209

Chapter 8
Molecular Profiling and Significance of Circulating Tumor Cell Based Genetic Signatures

Nisha Kanwar and Susan J. Done

Abstract Cancer kills by metastasizing beyond the primary site. Early detection, surgical intervention and other treatments have improved the survival rates of patients with cancer, however, once metastasis occurs, responses to conventional therapies become significantly less effective, and this remains the leading cause of death. Circulating tumor cells (CTCs) are tumor cells that have preferentially disseminated from the primary tumor mass into the hematological system, and are *en route* to favorable distant sites where if they survive, can develop into metastases. They may be the earliest detectable cells with metastatic ability, and are gaining increasing attention because of their prognostic value in many types of cancers including breast, prostate, colon and lung. Recent technological advances have removed barriers that previously hindered the detection and isolation of these rare cells from blood, and have exponentially improved the genetic resolution at which we can characterize signatures that define CTCs. Some of the most significant observations from such examinations are described here. Firstly, aberrations that were thought to be unique to CTCs are detected at subclonal frequencies within primary tumors with measurable heterogeneity, indicating pre-existing genetic signatures for metastasis. Secondly, these subclonal events are enriched in CTCs

N. Kanwar
Department of Laboratory Medicine and Pathobiology, University of Toronto, Toronto, ON, Canada

The Campbell Family Institute for Breast Cancer Research at the Princess Margaret Cancer Centre, Toronto, ON, Canada
e-mail: nishak@uhnresearch.ca

S.J. Done (✉)
Department of Laboratory Medicine and Pathobiology, University of Toronto, Toronto, ON, Canada

Department of Medical Biophysics, University of Toronto, Toronto, ON, Canada

The Campbell Family Institute for Breast Cancer Research at the Princess Margaret Cancer Centre, Toronto, ON, Canada

Laboratory Medicine Program, University Health Network, Toronto, ON, Canada
e-mail: Susan.Done@uhn.ca

M.J.M. Magbanua, J.W. Park (eds.), *Isolation and Molecular Characterization of Circulating Tumor Cells*, Advances in Experimental Medicine and Biology 994,
DOI 10.1007/978-3-319-55947-6_8

and metastases, pointing towards the selection of a more 'fit' component of tumor cells with survival advantages. Lastly, this component of cancer cells may also be the chemoresistant portion that escapes systemic treatment, or acquires resistance during progression of the disease. The future of cancer management may include a standardized method of measuring intratumor heterogeneity of the primary as well as matched CTCs. This will help identify and target rare aberrations within primary tumors that make them more adept to disseminate, and also to monitor the development of treatment resistant subclones as cancer progresses.

Keywords Metastasis • CTC-signatures • Genetic profiling • Intratumor heterogeneity • Tumor subclones • Chemoresistance

8.1 Cancer Dissemination and Metastasis

There have been significant advances in early screening and targeted therapies to reduce deaths from cancer; however, metastasis remains the leading cause of patient mortality. In metastasis, a select few cells acquire the ability to invade tissues that surround the primary tumor, thus allowing them to break free and enter the circulation via intravasation of the blood or lymphatic systems. Once in circulation, this 'occult' process goes undetected, they travel to distant organs, and in some cases like 'seeds', displaying specific receptors that home them to their respective 'soil', they are able to survive, extravasate, reinitiate aberrant cell division, and propagate secondary tumors at new sites. A recent study designed a computer generated model for cell growth and dispersal, in a clinically relevant time frame, utilizing estimates for rates of cell division, death, and dispersal, and calculated that it would take 8 years for a lesion to grow from one cell to one billion cells in the absence of dispersal, but less than 2 years with dispersal (Waclaw et al. 2015). They were also able to show that a tumor's response to chemotherapy is dependent on dispersal, regardless of growth rate of the primary tumor. Furthermore, if accumulating mutations increased the dispersal probability before or during treatment, regrowth was also faster. Thus, it is a small component of the primary tumor that, often undetected, possesses the capacity for dispersal via dissemination with important implications for disease progression and survival.

Although tumor cells are shed in a range of 10s -1000s from very early on in tumorigenesis, they must survive in vessels against shear stress forces, anoikis, and unfavorable growth niches; and a majority of them will be in circulation for only a few days before undergoing apoptosis. It is this rare population of circulating cells with metastatic propensity that escape chemotherapy and radiation, making them an aggressive subset, that requires the attention of new targeted therapies to prevent their spread and stop the threat of metastasis. One of the hallmarks of curable cancer is early detection so that the tumor may be removed and treated locally by radiation before it spreads. If, however, cells are already in circulation at early time points, the approach needs to be a systemic one, where the cells in circulation must be targeted and eradicated before they receive the signals to propagate at new and distant sites.

There is evidence to show that the dissemination of tumor cells is an early event. The previous notion that larger tumors gave rise to metastases has been challenged by findings that suggest dissemination can even occur in the earliest invasive stages of cancer progression in both murine models and human breast cancer, and it occurs independently of tumor size (Hüsemann et al. 2008). Disseminated tumor cells have been found in niches such as the bone marrow and lymph nodes before the onset of overt metastasis (Pantel et al. 2008; Hüsemann et al. 2008; Woelfle et al. 2003). Furthermore, disseminated tumor cells were found in circulation in patients with small (less than 2 mm) tumors and also in patients with undetectable primary tumors (less than 7% of cases of breast cancer) (Weigelt et al. 2005; Schmidt-Kittler et al. 2003). These cells can remain dormant in niches such as the bone marrow or a future site of metastasis such as the lung, and upon induction by growth stimuli of the microenvironment, they can be reprogrammed to establish secondary tumors (Wikman et al. 2008). These observations provide evidence that the initial steps of metastasis occur early on within primary tumors and are programmed to allow dissemination via pre-determined routes to potentially pre-determined niches for either a dormant phase or an aggressive proliferative phase. This also raises an important caveat in the current methods to produce molecular signatures – rather than analyzing bulk tumors, efforts need to be made to analyze tumors at single cell resolution which would lead to the discovery of low level signatures present in those rare cells destined for dissemination, and help identify novel targets to prevent this metastatic transition altogether.

Rare cell isolation techniques have provided us with refined detection tools that enable us to find disseminated tumors cells in blood, bone marrow and other niche organs that sustain them. Tumor cells found in circulating blood are referred to as circulating tumor cells or CTCs, while tumor cells found in the bone marrow are referred to as disseminated tumor cells or DTCs. It is still unclear as to which niche houses the earliest population of tumor cells that have left the primary site, or what route they took to arrive there (hematogenous or lymphatic systems). Notably, although lymph node metastasis is an accurate prognostic indicator of distant metastases, there are about 20–30% of patients whose cancer metastasizes without involvement of the lymph nodes, indicating hematogenous spread of tumor cells to the metastatic sites (Pantel and Brakenhoff 2004). There is growing evidence that the secondary organ's microenvironment is a deciding factor in whether or not CTCs will extravasate there and survive. For example, transforming growth factor beta (TGFβ) expressed in the bone or lungs, TGFα in the liver, and CXCR4/7 chemokine receptors expressed on tumor cells, home to their ligands in the lung, liver and bone marrow, respectively, and thus influence the ability of metastatic cells to grow in the respective organs via the activation of various signaling pathways involved in migration, actin polymerization, proliferation and survival (Pantel et al. 2008; Chambers et al. 2002). Thus, it might not be an access point, but rather, pre-established signals from optimal secondary sites that decide the route circulating cells will take.

Cells in circulation are rare, with approximately 1 cell in 10^9 nucleated blood cells (Krishnamurthy et al. 2010). A major obstacle in characterizing CTCs is obtaining a sufficient number, void of contaminating white blood cells. The 'ideal' CTC marker would be one that is expressed exclusively in tumor cells, not in any subset of hematopoietic cells, and not repressed during the period of circulation when the cells are isolated. Currently it is impossible to differentiate between CTCs of prognostic value or metastatic potential from those that will remain dormant, undergo apoptosis, or be targeted by the immune system. CTCs are isolated based on the heterogeneous expression of known epithelial or hematopoietic markers (CK, EpCAM, CD45) or based on prior knowledge of the primary tumor or cancer type (HER2, EGFR, PSA, etc.). Enrichment is usually a pre-requisite to any isolation protocol, and improves the detection of cells by at least 10,000-fold. Several methods for enrichment of CTCs have been described – immunomagnetic bead separation, density centrifugation, size based exclusion, flow cytometric separation, and more recently microfluidic devices such as the CTC-chip and Herringbone chip (Pantel et al. 2008; Pantel and Brakenhoff 2004; Flores et al. 2010; Stott et al. 2010; Nagrath et al. 2007). In 2008, the FDA approved the CellSearch™ System for the isolation and enumeration of tumor cells from blood or bone marrow of metastatic breast cancer patients (Van der Auwera et al. 2010). Since then there have been numerous publications validating its sensitivity in isolation of these rare tumor cells (Giordano and Cristofanilli 2012; Andreopoulou et al. 2012; Lucci et al. 2012; Farace et al. 2011; Kraan et al. 2011). The system includes fixation and labeling of cells with markers for epithelial and white blood cells, followed by immunomagnetic separation of epithelial cells. An automated system then enumerates signals to provide an output of number of epithelial cells per mL of blood or bone marrow analyzed. The array of markers used to identify tumor cells is progressively increasing – HER2 was recently added to the breast cancer panel (Flores et al. 2010).

The CTC chip uses microfluidic principles for the capture of viable CTCs from small volumes of blood (Nagrath et al. 2007). Immuno-nanoparticles are replaced by 78,000 microposts over a surface of $970mm^2$, each coated with antibodies to EpCAM. There have been several improvements to microfluidic enrichment, such as the herringbone chip (angled microchannels create vortices during blood flow for enhanced capture of cells to channel walls), the iCHIP (size based sorting of cells followed by inertial force separation and sorting), and the DEPArray (CTCs are sorted into 'cages' based on dielectrophoresis on the basis of their electric charge) (Stott et al. 2010; Karabacak et al. 2014; Carpenter et al. 2014). There have also been developments such as the CellCollector and leukapheresis which involve *in vivo* capture of CTCs from devices attached directly to a patients peripheral arm vein, which allows for enrichment of higher numbers of cells (median of 7500 versus 10s–100s), from much larger volumes of blood (1.5 litres compared to 10 mL), within a smaller time frame for processing of the cells while they are still viable (30 minutes compared to a few hours or days) (Theil et al. 2016; Fischer et al. 2013). The caveat, however, in any enrichment method that involves labeling tumor cells, is the heterogeneity of breast cancers where there will be variability in expression of these markers depending on molecular subtype in the case of *EGFR* or differentiation in the case of *MGB2* (mammaglobin) or even epithelial-to-mesenchymal transition (EMT) in the case of *KRT19, EpCAM* and *TWIST*. With the rapid development of more standardized and sensitive methods to isolate CTCs, the clinical utility of these cells is likely to become more apparent.

8.2 Clinical Value of Tumor Cells in Circulation

The mere presence of CTCs and DTCs in patients with cancer is a negative prognostic indicator. There have been several studies that showed that the presence of DTCs in the bone marrow of patients with primary breast cancer has a negative prognostic impact. A multicenter retrospective study included 4703 patients with metastatic breast cancer across Europe and the U.S., and concluded that over a 10-year follow up period, patients with DTCs had significantly decreased overall and disease-free survival compared to patients who did not have DTCs in their bone marrow (Braun et al. 2005). Presence of DTCs was also correlated with higher tumor grade, presence of lymph node metastases as well as overt metastases, and a poorer prognosis, independent of tumor size (Braun et al. 2005). Since there is the issue of invasiveness and patient discomfort when it comes to obtaining repetitive bone marrow samples for the isolation of DTCs, as well as the difficulty in obtaining metastatic samples, CTCs measured in a blood sample provide an easy to collect and relatively non-invasive method of monitoring disease progression and its response to therapies in real-time, and provide prognostic information by probing for specific molecular markers. The prognostic relevance of CTCs in metastatic breast cancer has also been demonstrated by numerous groups, pioneered by a prospective study where 177 metastatic breast cancer patients were shown to have a reduced overall and disease free survival if they had 5 or more CTCs per 7.5 mL of blood (Cristofanilli et al. 2004). In a follow up study with the same group of patients, it was reported that the number of CTCs was a better indicator of disease progression than traditional techniques such as imaging with PET, CT or MRI scans (Cristofanilli et al. 2007; Bidard et al. 2010; Nelson 2010; Liu et al. 2009). Ignatiadis et al. were one of the first groups to show the prognostic importance of CTCs present in the blood of early breast cancer patients, and has been succeeded by larger cohorts such as the German SUCCESS trial of 1489 patients which recently showed that the presence of even 1 CTC had prognostic value in early breast cancer (Ignatiadis et al. 2008). Most recently, a meta analysis of 19 early stage breast cancer studies ($n = 2993$) and 22 metastatic breast cancer studies ($n = 3069$) also showed prognostic value for CTCs (Zhang et al. 2012). Both CTCs and DTCs were included in the tumor marker assessment for breast cancer by the American Society of Clinical Oncology in 2007 (TNM stage $cM_O(i+)$; no clinical presence of overt metastases but presence of individual tumor cells in the blood, bone marrow or lymph nodes) (Harris et al. 2007). The report was based on prospective randomized controlled trials, prospective therapeutic trials (level

1 studies) or meta-analyses testing the utility of a marker (level 2 studies). The clinical utility of CTCs and DTCs however, is yet to be established and requires further studies especially in early breast cancer, as well as in determining how enumeration or characterization of CTCs can affect treatment decisions.

8.3 Genetic Alterations Associated with CTCs and Cancer Metastasis

Two main models of metastasis have been proposed. The first is the linear progression model where a primary tumor's malignant genetic status is complete and decided first, and the disseminated tumor cells evolve from these founder cells (Klein 2009). The second is the parallel progression model, where tumor cells disseminate early on, and evolve into their own genetically malignant entities, independently of the primary tumor, at distant sites (Stoecklein and Klein 2010). Recent studies have shown that primary tumors may have a gene expression signature that is predictive of metastasis (Schmidt-Kittler et al. 2003; van de Vijver et al. 2002; Schardt et al. 2005). Furthermore, primary tumor expression signatures also define the route of metastatic spread – hematogenous or lymphatic. Woelfle et al. compared primary tumors with and without disseminated tumor cells (DTCs) in the bone marrow or lymph node metastases and found that distinct signatures were able to predict bone marrow versus lymphatic micrometastases, with minimal overlap of only nine genes (Woelfle et al. 2003). Genes involved in the disseminated tumor cell (DTC) positive primary tumor signature included JAK/STAT, and the HIF-1α pathways, implicated in tumor cell survival, invasion, and angiogenesis. HIF-1α also activates other genes such as lysyl oxidase which activates focal adhesion kinases to enhance invasion, and CXCR4 involved in homing and survival of cancer cells at secondary sites (Woelfle et al. 2003).

There has been a recent effort to characterize CTCs using gene expression and whole genome copy number or sequence profiling (Magbanua et al. 2012; Heitzer et al. 2013; Shipitsin et al. 2007; Powell et al. 2012). Whole genome amplification and single-cell genomic technologies have enabled the study of DNA and gene expression profiles of small focal areas of tumors and single CTCs. Results from these studies have shown that gene expression signatures of CTCs may be unique to their originating tissue type, as well are enriched for targetable pathways such as stem cell, EMT, TGFB1, and non-canonical Wnt signaling (Aktas et al. 2009; Kasimir-Bauer et al. 2012; Yu et al. 2012; Powell et al. 2012; Sieuwerts et al. 2008; Smirnov 2005). Furthermore, aberrations previously thought to be private to CTCs, were detected at low frequencies within the primary tumor itself, emphasizing the early programming of tumor cells to enter circulation (Heitzer et al. 2013; Gerlinger et al. 2012; Magbanua et al. 2012; Shah et al. 2009). Klein et al. showed through molecular characterization of primary tumors and their matched DTCs that once cells have left the primary tumor at early stages, they develop independently with a unique set of aberrations and are more heterogeneous compared to DTCs in patients with distant metastases at late stages (Klein et al. 2002). Furthermore, genomic aberrations that are characteristic of the breast primary tumors (16q-, 13q-, 17p- and 8q+) were absent from the genomic profiles of DTCs analyzed by array Comparative Genomic Hybridization (aCGH), although their malignant origin could be confirmed by microdeletions also found in primary tumors (16q22-, 8q11-) (Klein et al. 2002; Schardt et al. 2005). The prevailing pattern observed was that the DTCs were distinct from primary tumors, which were more like their lymph node metastases than the DTCs (Schmidt-Kittler et al. 2003; Mathiesen et al. 2012). Such discrepancies were also reported in CTCs when compared to primary tumors for markers such as ER, PgR, HER2 and EGFR mutations. These observations are in concordance with studies that showed discrepancies between molecular alterations of primary and metastasized secondary tumors. Flores et al. designed a study to establish the relationship between the HER2 status of primary tumors, CTCs, and metastatic lesions in 75 patients with breast cancer using fluorescence *in situ* hybridization (FISH) (Flores et al. 2010). Interestingly, patients with HER2 positive primaries had HER2 positive CTCs 98% of the time, compared to patients with HER2 negative primaries, where 33% of patients showed discordance with HER2 positive CTCs (Flores et al. 2010). The unexpected finding was that in these 33% of patients, 90% of the metastatic lesions matched the primary tumor (Flores et al. 2010). Other studies with similar endpoints have reported HER2 discrepancies of up to 40% between primary tumors and matched CTCs (Gradilone et al. 2011). This observation brings forward the phenomenon of aggressive characteristics being acquired transitionally to progress select cells through individual steps in metastasis such as invasion and intravasation, which are lost at later stages not requiring these functions. Logically it follows through, that a disseminated tumor cell that is in a transitional state between a primary and a metastatic tumor, should have a transitional genetic profile, subject to change as it encounters new environments and selective pressures. This also explains the difference in genomic profiles of DTCs isolated from lymph nodes versus bone marrow (Klein and Stoecklein 2009). Furthermore, it is very likely that a common set of genomic events exists to allow for the survival of cells in this state, for example, HER2 gain has been described as the most frequent region of gain in DTCs whether they disseminated via the blood or lymphatic routes, and it is not concordant with the primary tumors (Stoecklein and Klein 2010; Klein and Stoecklein 2009).

Smirnov et al. were able to perform global gene expression profiling of CTCs from prostate, colorectal and breast cancers and elegantly showed that these profiles were indeed tissue specific, although they also shared some commonality. They found that genes such as *KRT19* and *AGR2* were expressed in CTCs from all samples and not expressed in normal samples (Smirnov 2005). The tissue specific genes were *S100A14/16* and *CEACAM5* for breast and colorectal cancers, *KLK2/3, MSMB, DDC, AR, HPN* for prostate cancers; and *SCGB2A1/2* and *PIP* for breast cancers alone (Smirnov 2005). Most of these genes function in cell proliferation, migration and oncogenesis. The combination of this gene signature was able to classify tumor and normal correctly with 79.3% accuracy, which was comparable with the classification power of gene expression signatures obtained from primary tumors (Smirnov 2005).

It has been proposed that cells in circulation are a subset of tumor progenitor cells fitting the phenotype of aggressiveness, low proliferation and resistance to therapy. Lu et al. addressed the question of EMT and the inadequacy of most of the methods used to enrich for CTCs or DTCs using epithelial cell markers such as cytokeratin19 and EpCAM. In this study, CTCs were enriched based on invasive function rather than inconsistent expression of a marker. The collagen adhesion matrix selects for cells that are able to invade, remove and ingest matrix fragments by formation of invadopodia (Lu et al. 2010). They were able to conclude that the presence of invasive CTCs correlated to higher stage, lymph node positivity and poorer survival of patients with early breast cancer (Lu et al. 2010). Furthermore, if propagated in culture, the gene expression signature of these cells showed that they had properties of EMT stem cells expressing *TWIST1* and *CD44* (Lu et al. 2010). Fluorescence activated cell sorting (FACS) analysis showed that this was not a property held by all CTCs, as they could be separated into three distinct populations highlighting the heterogeneous nature of these cells – one showing epithelial lineage as EpCAM+, the other showing progenitor cell lineage as CD44+, and the third showing the intersection of cells expressing both markers. Other tumor specific markers expressed were TERT, MUC16, ER and PgR (Lu et al. 2010). Surprisingly HER2, VIM and other aggressiveness markers were not expressed in a specific population (Lu et al. 2010). Gradilone et al. have further propelled the idea of CTCs or DTCs having a stem-cell like phenotype, whereby they investigated the expression of ATP-binding cassette family genes – or the multidrug resistance related proteins (MRPs) (Gradilone et al. 2011). They reported a significant correlation between the stem cell marker *ALDH1* and the expression of a number of MRPs, in addition to the co-expression of HER2 and ERα in a discordant manner compared to primary tumors (Gradilone et al. 2011). These results taken together paint a clearer picture of aggressive disseminated cells gaining a proliferative, invasive and survival advantage with the divergence of their expression profiles.

From our own studies, we isolated CTCs from breast cancer patients based on depletion of the CD45+ fraction of whole blood (Kanwar et al. 2015). Thus, we minimized any enrichment bias of cells based on markers such as EpCAM or cytokeratins, only, which have been shown to be expressed quite heterogeneously in CTCs. We also ensured that the selected cells were completely void of contaminating white blood cells, even at low numbers, by detecting CTCs using the glucose oxidase enzyme which is absent in mammalian cells; and by isolating single CTCs by laser capture microdissection. Using high resolution copy number analysis, we identified a signature of recurrent copy number alterations on chromosome 19 in circulating tumor cells (CTCs) from breast cancer. These regions have not been previously reported to be associated with breast cancer metastasis, although they are altered in a small subset of breast cancer patients (3%) of the basal or ER negative subtypes.

The signature we identified consists of genes that regulate common CTC-like functions such as motility, invasion, resistance to anoikis, and intravasation. After compiling a list of minimum common regions of gain, or MCRs, we identified 90 out of 353 MCRs (25%) that were gained in 15–16 of 17 samples. These were gains on 1p36, 1q21, 7q11-22, 9q34, 11p15, 12q24, 16q22, 17q21-25, 20q, 22q, and across the entire chromosome 19. Notably, 49 out of the 90 MCRs were on chromosome 19. Chromosome 19 alterations have been implicated in many types of cancers (Yu et al. 2009; Beroukhim et al. 2010; Antoniou et al. 2010; Bayani et al. 2011). The MCRs that we identified contain several genes with possible roles in CTC-like functionality of tumor cells. Particularly, *LTBP4* (19q13.2) plays a role in activation of *TGFB1*, which has been previously implicated as a key EMT signaling pathway in CTCs and interacting cell populations (Yu et al. 2013; Powell et al. 2012; Shipitsin et al. 2007). *NUMBL* (19q13.2) has functions in metastasis and maintenance of tumor initiating cells, which could be present in the pool of disseminated cells. *JUND* (19p13.11) has been shown to activate aromatase promoters in breast tumor tissue that leads to higher estrogen signaling and breast cancer progression (Chen et al. 2011). It also has been shown to protect cells from p53 induced apoptosis, which is a property that some CTCs possess in order to survive in circulation and at distant sites before forming secondary tumors (Weitzman et al. 2000). *BSG* (19p13.3), also known as *EMMPRIN* or CD147 is a well-characterized gene that induces stromal cells to produce metalloproteinases which aid in the invasion process of tumor cells. Previously, Klein C. et al. showed in a study of single disseminated tumor cells in bone marrow from breast, prostate and lung cancer patients, that mRNA and protein levels of *BSG* were elevated in 82% of cells examined, and is thus an attractive candidate for a CTC specific marker (Klein et al. 2002). *ANGPTL4* (19p13.2) is another widely studied gene in breast, gastric, liver, colorectal, esophageal and prostate cancers with tumor and metastasis promoting functions such as angiogenesis, invasion, intravasation and anoikis resistance (Zhu et al. 2011; Tan et al. 2012; Zhang et al. 2013).

MicroRNAs are gaining much attention for their potential use as biomarkers for cancer progression and metastasis. We identified *MIR-516* and *MIR-371-373* on 19q13.42 amplified in CTC genomes, that belong to two clusters of microRNA families that are frequently co-amplified in embryonic stem cells and cancer (Bayani et al. 2011; Rippe et al. 2010; Laurent et al. 2008). It was recently shown that *MIR-516* was highly expressed in ER+, lymph node negative breast cancers and was associated with shorter time to distant metastasis (Foekens et al. 2008). *MIR-373* has been widely implicated in aggressive cancers. It was shown to be responsible for migratory and invasive phenotypes in breast cancer, *in vitro* and *in vivo*, via down-regulation of its target *CD44* (Huang et al. 2008). Another cluster of microRNAs that was gained contains *MIR-24, 27* and *23* and the *MIR-181* family (19p13.13). *MIR-24* has been implicated as a regulator of apoptosis by inhibiting *caspase9* and *apaf1*, which together form a complex known as the apoptosome that initiates apoptosis (Walker and Harland 2009). High expression of MIR-27 has also been linked to therapeutic resistance in leukemia, colon, esophageal, gastric, and ovarian cancers (Zhao et al. 2011; Feng et al. 2011; Zhang et al. 2010; Li et al. 2010). The MIR-181 family has been shown to allow cells to evade anoikis and grow as spheroids in an anchorage-independent manner, which is a distinct feature of cancer stem cells (Ji et al. 2009; Wang et al. 2009a). Two of the validated targets of mir-181 are *TIMP3*, inhibitor of metalloproteinase 2 and 9; and *ATM*, which when down-regulated results in resistance to DNA-damaging chemotherapy (Wang et al. 2009a). Taken together, these could synergistically allow invasion, survival and resistance to chemotherapy, thus propagating tumor cell dissemination and metastatic disease via CTCs.

Although some MCRs were less frequently amplified (4–13 patients), they contained important genes with clinical relevance when overexpressed in primary breast cancers, such as *MUC16*, *CCNE1*, and *KLK* genes. A recent study used a collagen adhesion matrix assay to enrich for CTCs with invasive functions from the blood of breast cancer patients. *MUC16* was among the significantly up-regulated genes including stem cell and EMT markers such as *CD44*, *EpCAM*, *TWIST1* and *TERT* (Lu et al. 2010). *CCNE1* is overexpressed in 25% of breast tumors and has been shown to be an independent prognostic factor in breast cancer, specifically for ER- tumors which show a higher incidence of carrying the 19q12 amplicon (Keyomarsi et al. 2002; Sieuwerts 2006; Natrajan et al. 2012). The 19q12 amplicon was also studied in ovarian cancer, and *CCNE1* was found to be overexpressed early on in the progression of ovarian cancer, and was associated with treatment resistance to platinum based drugs such as cisplatin, and poor overall survival of patients (Etemadmoghadam et al. 2010). Clinically, KLK3/PSA is an established serum biomarker for prostate and ovarian cancer detection, prognosis and monitoring. Kallikreins are involved in early tumor progression by protease-activated receptor (PAR) activation, and angiogenesis by extracellular matrix degradation, allowing both tumor cells and endothelial cells to migrate and reform to their respective invasive functions (Borgoño and Diamandis 2004). In breast cancer, a majority of kallikreins have been reported to be down-regulated, however, several roles have been identified for up-regulation of *KLK* genes. *KLK1* promotes extravasation of MDA-MB-231 tumor cells to lungs *in vivo* (Wolf et al. 2001). *KLK10* was found to be an independent predictive marker for response to tamoxifen treatment, where high levels correlated with poor response, shorter progression-free and survival overall (Yousef and Diamandis 2002; Luo et al. 2002).

We also queried the copy number profile of the *TGFB1* gene and identified 2 amplicons that were present in 12 and 13 patients. *TGFB1* is known to have dual functions as a tumor suppressor in early breast cancer, and is a potent promoter of EMT, invasion and metastasis in late stages. It has also been shown to be involved in mammary stem cell maintenance with higher expression in CD44+CD24- cells, it increases colonization of tumor cells in the lung via *ANGPTL4* in ER- breast cancer, thus increasing metastasis, and it can also suppress the activity of cytotoxic T cells and natural killer cells, thus allowing evasion of immune-surveillance (Barcellos-Hoff and Akhurst 2009). Biswas S et al. showed *in vivo*, that ionizing radiation or doxorubicin treatment in a mouse metastasis model led to an increase in circulating TGFB1, increased levels of CTCs, as well as higher incidence of lung metastasis (Biswas et al. 2007). Various other groups have also identified a relationship between CTCs and TGFB1, whereby high levels of TGFB1 were associated with tumor cell survival, intravasation and metastasis; and more specifically, Shim KS et al. showed that persisting CTCs and TGFB1 levels in blood 2 weeks post surgery in colorectal cancer was associated with earlier metastasis recurrence in the liver (Muraoka-Cook 2004; Muraoka et al. 2002; Shim et al. 1999). Shipitsin M et al. studied the heterogeneity of CD44+ stem cells in breast tumor tissues, and found that these cells had a TGFB response type of mRNA expression signature, which they termed the 'TGFB cassette' (Shipitsin et al. 2007). Patients expressing this 'cassette' had shorter distant metastasis free survival. They concluded that based on heterogeneous expression of this 'cassette' in CD44+ cells, different cells within the same tumor were likely to respond differently to TGFB signaling. It is possible that these responsive cells are programmed for paracrine CTC-like behavior.

In our study, genomes of CTCs clustered into two groups, a larger more homogeneous group and a smaller more heterogeneous group. The two groups were almost mutually exclusive, except for two MCRs in common, on chromosome 19p13 and 21q21, containing genes such as *ITGB2*, *TFF3*, *SERTAD3*, *LTBP4*, and *NUMBL* that are involved in metastasis and anti-apoptotic signaling during anoikis in migrating cells. Such functions are indicative of acquired behavior that would be common to all tumor cells that disseminate and enter circulation in the blood. Recently, Yu et al. showed that CTCs exist in a dynamic pool of epithelial-like and mesenchymal-like cells, the latter being associated with progressive disease (Yu et al. 2013). This mesenchymal component of CTCs was enriched for 45 genes, including *TFF1/3*, *ITGB4* and *LTBP4*. On the other hand, the dissimilarity between the two groups is suggestive of cancer cells transitioning through metastatic stages that may be reflected in their genomes. Cluster A had minimal alterations that may be sufficient for dissemination, such as amplification of *AKT2* (19q13), *SMAD2* (18q21), and *MIR-602* (9q34), however, this cluster also had many focal amplifications consisting of tumor suppressive genes including *PTEN*, *CADM2*, *EPHA5*, and *ESR2*. A previous study that performed gene expression profiling of CTCs observed overexpression of *PTEN* in 83% of the samples regardless of clustering (Powell et al. 2012). Similarly, Yu M. et al. and Miyomoto D.T. et al. recently showed that there were three distinct pools of CTCs in breast and prostate cancer, each responding differentially to chemotherapy. In breast cancer, CTCs were more homogeneously epithelial or mesenchymal, and a third mixed population, expressed markers from both groups (Yu et al. 2013). In prostate cancer, CTCs had gene expression signatures that were AR sensitive or resistant, and again, a third mixed population expressing genes from both signatures (Miyamoto et al. 2012). The eventual fate of a circulating cell could be modulated by the net pro and anti oncogenic or survival signals inherent to these cells, and also in the external microenvironment. It has been suggested that because of this balance, CTCs are in a state of dormancy, and they might contain a sub-population of tumor-initiating cells that are quiescent and resistant to chemotherapy (Wikman et al. 2008). For example, cells that express both EGFR and p38 are in a state of growth arrest or dormancy if the EGFR/p38 ratio is low, but will start proliferating at a secondary site if the EGFR/p38 ratio is high (Wikman et al. 2008). Our Cluster B had genomes with extensive alteration, particularly on chromosome 19, with genes such as ANGPTL4, BSG, MIR-23 and MIR373, that could define those CTCs that may be capable of evasion of anoikis, survival and a passage to dormant niches or metastatic sites. Furthermore, all CTCs within this cluster showed amplification of a 1.2 Mb region containing the ERBB2 gene. Genes within these amplicons potentially confer CTCs with intravasation ability, survival or chemo-resistant properties, and could be developed into CTC specific markers in blood. Although CTC genome profiles did not cluster according to the subtype of the primary tumors, MCRs on chromosome 19 were also associated with triple negative and HER+ tumors, which are more aggressive in nature, with higher incidence of CTCs (Nadal et al. 2012; Fehm et al. 2010). Additionally patients with distant metastases, as well as patients who presented at a younger age (<50 years) clustered close together suggesting an increase in homogeneity of CTC genomes in metastatic cancer compared to early breast cancer.

Considering the homogeneity of CTCs for certain genomic gains, specifically on chromosome 19, we determined how these regions were represented in primary breast tumors. Analysis of The Cancer Genome Atlas (TCGA) copy number data from 787 invasive breast carcinomas revealed a low frequency of 3–4% of samples with CTC-like MCRs of gain. The most common was not surprisingly, a minimal common region containing *CCNE1*, followed by others containing *KLK7-12*, C19MC and the *MIR-371-3* cluster. Upon examination of copy number data from our own laboratory, chromosome 19p12-q13.11 was gained in 38% primary invasive ductal carcinoma (IDC) samples and 10% of lymph node metastasis samples (Wang et al. 2009b). Additionally, there have been several papers that have illuminated a plausible role for gains on chromosome 19 in the more aggressive subtypes of breast cancer such as the basal versus luminal subtype, triple negative, and ER negative subtypes (Staaf et al. 2010, 2011; Natrajan et al. 2012; Horlings et al. 2010; Turner et al. 2010). Taken together, these results suggest that there indeed is an existing proportion of primary breast cancers with gains across chromosome 19, and possibly unidentified novel driver genes that appear to be more highly represented in the proportion of cells that are able to leave the primary site.

8.4 Intratumor Heterogeneity and Low Frequency CTC-Signatures

It is recognized that invasive breast cancers exhibit heterogeneity at the genomic level although the degree and extent has not been well documented (Campbell and Polyak 2007; Polyak 2007; Shipitsin et al. 2007). Over the last few years it has become clear that breast cancer is not a single disease. Inter-tumor heterogeneity exists between tumors on the morphological and molecular levels. On the molecular level there are four intrinsic subtypes based on gene expression signatures: luminal A, luminal B, HER2 and basal subtypes; each with unique tumorigenic features and responses to targeted therapies. More recently the Molecular

Taxonomy of Breast Cancer International Consortium (METABRIC) study integrated genomic copy number and gene expression data to conclude that breast cancer was much more heterogeneous, with ten subtypes showing distinct clinical outcomes (Curtis et al. 2012). Heterogeneity may also occur within the same patient in geographically separate areas of the same tumor (intratumor heterogeneity). Tumor heterogeneity develops along two axes: temporal (variability over time), and spatial (variability over location). Tumor cells are continuously cycling through cell growth and cell death, and exist as a heterogeneous mixture of subclones of varying fitness. They acquire new driver mutations that may give them a growth advantage over neighboring subclones. As the tumor mass expands, the composition of the tumor at different locations can be quite different (Waclaw et al. 2015). This spatial heterogeneity is also likely the reason why tumors fail to respond to treatments over time, or why they recur at the same site. Targetable aberrations in one part of the tumor are missed when they are not included in diagnostic sampling because of spatial heterogeneity. There is also an increasing degree of genetic diversity in lesions as cancer progresses, leading to temporal heterogeneity. In breast cancer this occurs over three transitions: *in situ* carcinoma to invasive breast cancer; evolution of the primary invasive cancer; and progression from primary to metastatic breast cancer via dissemination (Zardavas et al. 2015). Many studies have reported a shift in abundance of a major clone from ductal carcinoma *in situ* (DCIS) to IDC, as well as from primary to metastatic cancer (Rashid-Kolvear et al. 2007; Radford et al. 1995a, b; Heselmeyer-Haddad et al. 2012; Hernandez et al. 2012). Chemotherapy also induces a selection pressure on subclonal cell populations that influences tumor progression. Tumors after treatment are likely significantly different in composition and behavior compared to the original diagnostic sample. Therefore assessment of temporal heterogeneity before and after treatment can provide critical insight to predict therapeutic response and metastatic progression.

Most studies are based on the analysis of a single sample from whole tumors, and so look at dominant genomic changes present in larger portions of the tumor. It is important to address the broader question of clonal evolution and intratumor heterogeneity at the single cell level, especially when some clones are present at low frequencies within the tumor. Schmidt et al. showed that in multifocal prostate cancer, CTCs originated from distinct foci, even if they were as small as 0.2 cm, again suggesting that the blueprint for dissemination is probably in the primary tumor, detectable in single cells, if not on a bulk tumor basis. It may be that there is an increasing degree of genetic diversity in lesions as cancer progresses. There is evidence to support this theory from our own recent studies and from LOH (loss of heterozygosity) studies of ductal carcinoma *in situ* (Rashid-Kolvear et al. 2007; Radford et al. 1995a, b). With an increasing number of genetic perturbations, eventually the necessary genetic event may occur in a particular subclone or tumor initiating cell within the tumor that allows invasion to take place. It has been reported that significant heterogeneity can occur on a single nucleotide mutation level. Using next generation sequencing, 6 of 32 somatic mutations found in a metastasized tumor were also found in the primary tumor from 9 years earlier, and were detected at low frequencies (1–13%) (Navin et al. 2010). Gerlinger et al. carried out an extensive exome sequencing analysis of 9 spatially separate regions from a renal-cell carcinoma, along with matched metastatic sites (Gerlinger et al. 2012). They found that 63–69% of somatic mutations were present heterogeneously, including *mTOR* activating mutations which would result in mTOR inhibitor therapies producing different responses within these regions.

A study on intratumor heterogeneity in colorectal cancer using interphase FISH techniques showed that there are distinct chromosomal regions which are gained through aneuploidy that define a pro-metastatic type of cell (Sayagués et al. 2010). Interestingly, they also found that in a proportion of cases, a minor clone present in the primary tumor was the most highly represented clone in its metastases. Another study attempted to classify primary ductal breast carcinomas as "monogenomic" tumors with a more homogenous genome profile; or as "polygenomic" tumors with multiple subpopulations of genomic clones (Navin et al. 2010). They analyzed individual tumors as sectors using both aCGH and FISH techniques. Their results showed intra-tumor heterogeneity in a significant proportion of both tumor types, where polygenomic tumors had up to three major tumor subpopulations with clear clonal evolution. As the tumor grows, the composition of the center versus the tumor peripheries can be quite different. The center of the tumor is hypothesized to comprise driver mutations possibly seen in cells that initiated the tumor, or are involved in cell renewal (mutations involved in dormancy, drug resistance, survival and thus tumor recurrence). The outer periphery of the tumor conversely, is hypothesized to comprise of replicative cells which are dividing at rates proportional to the number of surrounding empty sites and nourishment from surrounding newly developed blood supplies (Waclaw et al. 2015). Driver mutations in these cells would be involved in invasion, intravasation and dissemination.

CTCs might be the earliest detectable cells with metastatic abilities. CTCs may not be representative of the whole tumor as a result of spatial and temporal heterogeneity. Chemo-resistant CTCs have been shown to be HER2 positive although they originated from HER2 negative primary tumors (Flores et al. 2010; Fehm et al. 2010). A proportion of these patients had metastatic tumors which were also HER2 positive. Such discrepancies were also found with ER, PgR and EGFR status suggesting vast heterogeneity and evolution of genetic markers in CTCs (Fehm et al. 2009, 2010). Single nucleotide sequencing of 50 nuclei in breast tumors revealed that no two cancer cells have the same genome (Wang et al. 2014). Multiple regions from single tumors must be sampled, as well as sampled over time via liquid biopsies, to address both spatial and temporal heterogeneity, and capture subclonal events that occur during tumor evolution. An accurate measure of heterogeneity (H) needs to be developed and standardized to determine the clinical value of H over site, stage and treatment response of a tumor. In the future, mathematical models or those based on ecological measures of evolution and heterogeneity within species could be introduced into the clinic to help guide treatment combinations and provide prognostic information. It would also be useful to determine the effect of other factors such as the microenvironment and how they contribute to tumor heterogeneity, as well as interactions between the tumor and stroma, hypoxia, tumor-infiltrating lymphocytes (TILs), metalloproteinases, and the vasculature. A better understanding of the degree and extent of cellular variation within individual breast cancers will lead to improvements in treatment approaches, and provide insight into mechanisms of relapse and how to block it. It is likely that, in the future, measurements of variability or heterogeneity will become a routine part of breast cancer care and lead to improved results for patients.

A few studies have compared heterogeneity between primary and matched metastatic tumors using aCGH and FISH or whole genome sequencing (WGS) and found that the degree and extent of heterogeneity between the two compartments may be directly related to the amount of time between diagnosis of the primary and occurrence of metastatic disease (Kuukasjärvi et al. 1997; Shah et al. 2012; Ding et al. 2010; Desmedt et al. 2008). While there are shared genetic alterations, they also observed *de novo* alterations in the metastatic lesions, as well as a trend for significant enrichment of the shared alterations in the metastases. Conversely, there was a subset of primary tumors that differed almost completely from their matched metastases, highlighting the importance of measuring temporal changes between compartments to better tailor treatments. Large scale studies that are starting to address heterogeneity are TRACERx (TRAcking non-small cell lung Cancer Evolution through therapy Rx) and DARWIN (Deciphering Anti-tumor Response With INtratumor heterogeneity), which will determine the relationship between factors such as immune response and clonal heterogeneity on clinical outcome, relapse and progression (Alizadeh et al. 2015).

It is becoming more and more apparent that aberrations that are prevalent in CTCs may reflect differences in CTC functionality compared to primary tumors. Single cell analysis of a larger cohort of primary tumors, critically those matched from CTC positive patients included in this study, might reveal the presence of these CTC-like gains at low frequencies, and shed more light on whether or not their presence is associated with tumor cell dissemination, metastasis, response to treatment and patient outcome. The underlying heterogeneity may be responsible for routes of dissemination of tumor cells and ultimately tumor behavior during disease progression. CTC-like alterations, even if present only focally within a primary tumor, could confer a more aggressive course of progression to metastasis. More importantly, by identifying markers that are specific to the more aggressive or chemo-resistant proportion of these cells, they could be targeted to block their spread to distant sites.

8.5 Functional Validation of CTC Signatures

The study of CTC signatures in a standard mouse model is a logical next step for functional validation, as it is more similar to the human mammalian system genetically, physiologically and anatomically. Recently, a group was successful in creating an experimental model for tumor heterogeneity in mice (Wagenblast et al. 2015). They infected a retroviral barcode library into mouse mammary carcinoma 4T1 cells and introduced the cell lines orthotopically into non-obese diabetic/severe combined immunodeficiency (NOD-SCID) mouse fat pads. Primary tumors, lymph nodes, blood, lungs, liver and brains were collected in order to quantify the barcode populations of subclones. They concluded that clone abundance of the primary tumors did not correlate with that of CTCs or metastases; lymph node metastases and distant metastases did not correlate; and CTCs and distant metastases were correlated. Furthermore, clones that were less represented in the primary tumors entered the bloodstream as CTCs and a few of these had the ability to colonize secondary sites.

Another group used the CTC-iChip to isolate CTCs from patient derived tumors in mice (Ting et al. 2014). They identified three gene expression signatures for CTCs: epithelial/classical, platelet derived and proliferative signatures. Epithelial and mesenchymal markers, *Aldh1a2* (stem cell marker) and extracellular matrix (ECM) markers (*Igfbp5*, *Klf4* and *Dcn*) were common across all three signatures. Interestingly, in contrast to primary tumors, where ECM gene products are secreted by surrounding stromal cells, and not by the epithelial cancer cells, they observed that rare cells at the epithelial-stromal interface of the xenografts express both keratins and ECM genes. This pattern of expression was also observed in matched CTCs from mice as well as humans, suggesting these were originating from the interface in primary tumors. ECM genes may be involved in the generation of CTCs from the primary tumors or to the survival of cancer cells deprived of stromal microenvironemental signals as they circulate in blood. ECM genes were also enriched in metastases versus primary tumors. Our own studies identified Decorin as strongly associated with presence of lymph node metastasis in a group of breast cancer patients. In a set of TMAs (n =990, 590 Stage 1 and 400 Stage 2) invasive breast cancers, decorin showed significant association with lymph node metastasis, higher nodal involvement and HER2 positivity (Cawthorn et al. 2012). Yu et al. used RNA sequencing to compare CTCs, primary and metastasis from mouse and human tumors, and found Wnt2 to be enriched in CTCs and metastases compared to primary tumors (Yu et al. 2012). Wnt2 increased metastasis *in vivo* without increasing the amount of CTCs, by increasing anchorage independent growth/ resistance to anoikis via FN1 an extracellular protein implicated in cell-matrix interactions and cell survival signals.

Several groups have shown *in vivo* that CTCs are indeed the seeds of metastasis, containing a population of metastasis initiating cells. In a xenograft assay of primary human luminal breast cancer, CTCs engrafted into the bone marrow of mice at the femoral medullary cavity were able to give rise to bone, lung and liver metastases (Baccelli et al. 2013). *In vitro* assays have also shown that cultured CTCs from patients are functional and will invade an extra cellular matrix (Lu et al. 2010). Single cell deep sequencing studies comparing CTCs, primary and metastatic tumors have shown that mutations that initially seemed specific to CTCs could be found in subclones of the primary tumor and metastases of the same patient, proving lineage from a common cell of origin (Dago et al. 2014; Heitzer et al. 2013; Lohr et al. 2014; Ni et al. 2013). CTCs tend to be more similar to their metastases compared to the primary tumor, partially due to the low abundance of these alterations in primary tumors. Furthermore, whole genomic profiles of CTCs do not change at different therapeutic timepoints in the way their mutational profiles have been shown to evolve, and indicates that specific chromosomal alterations occur early on, and are selectively maintained throughout the course of the disease.

8.6 Conclusions and Future Perspectives

Comparison of cancer samples from different sites or different time points within the same patient is beginning to shed more light on intratumor heterogeneity, clonal evolution and the resulting competition between different subclones post-treatment (Van Loo and Voet 2014). The study of spatially separate areas of the same tumors further adds to this complexity by showing morphological and genetic differences in tumor cells potentially undergoing differential selection at different locations within the tumor mass. Examination of a single or even a few biopsies may not paint an accurate picture of true underlying heterogeneity in tumors. Most current large-scale cancer genome-sequencing studies use DNA from millions of cells, containing intermixed sequences from different tumor clones and contaminating adjacent cells from the tumor microenvironment. Single cell sequencing, is now a standardized widely available tool with which we are able to access genetic information from CTCs and tumors at significant depths of resolution. Technologically, traditional Sanger sequencing can detect clones down to 10% frequency, versus mutation-specific PCR followed by targeted sequencing or mass spectrometry which detect subclonal events at 0.1% frequency (Hiley et al. 2014). Although these methods provide important information on the proportions and genomes of distinct cell populations within the tumor, detecting rare subclonal populations remains difficult. Visualizing genomic aberrations in single cells with FISH however, has the unparalleled advantage of measuring aberrations in multiple regions within individual cells from different areas of a tumor, compared to the pooled nature of next generation sequencing analyses. In the future we anticipate that targeted or full cancer genomes of cancer biopsies and CTCs will routinely be sequenced as part of the clinical evaluation and likely personalized treatments in the future. CTCs are particularly important in this regard as they represent easily obtained liquid biopsies allowing real-time monitoring of both metastatic potential and patient specific tailoring of treatments.

Metastatic tumor tissue contains genetic abnormalities sufficient and necessary to result in patient death. Furthermore, successive rounds of treatments alter the genetic landscape of tumors in a systemic manner resulting in resistance and the emergence of new mutations both in the primary and metastatic setting. A study that examined genomic imbalances involved in progression from DCIS to IDC found that there was clear clonal selection where a major clone in the IDC was one of several clones in the DCIS component (Heselmeyer-Haddad et al. 2012). Clinically they were able to conclude that there were high degrees of chromosomal instability already present in the pre-invasive DCIS lesions, and among these many clones, thus, it was likely that there was already a pre-existing clone required for metastasis. It has been observed that in a case with a HER2 amplification in the primary components of breast cancer, although the amplification was identified in a subclonal population of the patients metastatic tumor, there was no detectable expression of the mRNA and protein (Geyer et al. 2010). It is possible that *de novo* genetic or epigenetic alterations occurred in the metastatic tumor as HER2 was no longer functionally required for the growth/survival at the secondary site. This highlights the importance of comparative analyses of metastatic, primary tumors, and even pre-invasive lesions to identify key driver mutations that are selected during cancer dissemination, progression and chemoresistance. CTCs appear to be more similar to the metastases than primary tumors in single nucleotide polymorphism/insertion deletion DNA mutation (SNP/INDEL) composition (Ni et al. 2013). Genomic analyses, including our own, have shown that patients share a majority of gains and losses of CTC regions, showing the potential of diagnosis via CTCs. Dago et al. showed that in a single patient undergoing treatment, resistant clones emerge during treatment failure. Notably, after 9 weeks of treatment, the original CTC population was not completely eliminated and the drug resistant clone was detectable (Dago et al. 2014). In a whole exome sequencing study of CTCs, lymph node metastases and primary tumors of two patients, it was found that divergent evolution exists, a TP53 mutation was found in all primary foci, the metastasis and CTCs (Lohr et al. 2014). This study also showed that although 56% of mutations were shared between primary tumors and metastases, strikingly, 76% of the mutations were found in the CTCs. These observations exemplify that CTC sequencing might provide an a priori indication of phenotypic transition and guide the selection of therapeutic regimens. Important tumor related genes, including those involved in drug resistance and phenotypic transitions were frequently mutated in CTCs, such enrichment may represent a selective advantage of CTCs to escape targeted therapy.

There are many instances of low frequency clones found in primary tumors that are extremely relevant therapeutically. In some reported cases, patients who relapsed with MET-amplified disease (resistant to EGFR inhibitors) following treatment with an EGFR inhibitor, harbored the *MET* amplification in <1% of cells, which was clearly selected over the course of treatment. These patients would have benefited from a combined MET and EGFR inhibitor treatment. Similar reports have been made for KRAS mutations detected in cell free DNA as resistance developed to EGFR inhibitors in colorectal cancers and BRAF in melanoma resistant to RAF/MEK inhibition (Diaz et al. 2012; Wagle et al. 2014). In colorectal cancer, EGFR resistant tumors have been known to harbor *ERBB2* amplifications in 3% of cases, *FLT3* amplifications in 3% of cases, and *MEK1* alterations in as few as 1.5% of cases. In breast cancer, although the most frequently mutated genes are *TP53* and *PIK3CA* (>10%), there are numerous driver genes that are mutated in <3% of tumors and are associated with treatment resistance (Ng et al. 2015). This was a key finding in the METABRIC study that integrated copy number and gene expression data using next generation sequencing platforms for 2000 patients with primary breast cancer (Curtis et al. 2012). Although the molecular characterization of metastases will improve the currently available prognostic and predictive models, taking biopsies from metastases in patients is an invasive procedure that is frequently impossible due to the lack of accessible lesions. It is advantageous to analyze CTCs as they are the intact, functional cancer cells circulating in peripheral blood.

There appears to be a mismatch between cost and benefit of anti-cancer therapies. Between 2002 and 2012, there have been 71 drugs approved by the FDA with a median survival benefit of 2.1 months against a cost of $2.7 million per life saved (McGranahan and Swanton 2015). Subclonal mutations have huge economic and therapeutic value to cancer outcome, and there needs to be in shift in the way we collect, analyze and make prognostic decisions (Jamal-Hanjani et al. 2015). There is a clear benefit to detecting cancer as an early event, at this time the driver events have occurred in a group of cells that allowed them to have a selective growth advantage compared to surrounding cells in a defined area of tissue. Therefore, the group of tumor cells responds to targeted therapies against that tissue. If detected as a later event however, the tumor cells have had the opportunity to evolve as a collection of heterogeneous subclones, and thus the initial targetable clones may not be necessary for survival anymore, leaving targeting therapies ineffective. Combined therapies would be the preferred alternative at this point.

In conclusion, we know mortality from breast cancer is not due to primary tumors, but rather a failure to treat and control the growth of metastases. The world-renowned pediatric pathologist, Sidney Farber, stated in 1962 that, *"The greatest need we have today in the human cancer problem, except for a universal cure, is a method of detecting the presence of cancer before there are any clinical signs of symptoms"*. Five decades onwards, as we make leaps in describing the complex nature and evolution of cancer, we are now closer to finding and predicting the course of tumor progression, and treating patients before the onset of metastasis. Enumeration of CTCs, the earliest detectable cells with metastatic potential, has already provided important prognostic information on progression and overall survival. In the future, genomic analyses could provide more in depth information for personalized therapy.

References

Aktas B, Tewes M, Fehm T et al (2009) Stem cell and epithelial-mesenchymal transition markers are frequently overexpressed in circulating tumor cells of metastatic breast cancer patients. Breast Cancer Res BCR 11:R46

Alizadeh AA, Aranda V, Bardelli A et al (2015) Toward understanding and exploiting tumor heterogeneity. Nat Med 21:846–853

Andreopoulou E, Yang L-Y, Rangel KM et al (2012) Comparison of assay methods for detection of circulating tumor cells in metastatic breast cancer: AdnaGen AdnaTest BreastCancer Select/Detect™ versus Veridex CellSearch™ system. Int J Cancer 130:1590–1597

Antoniou AC, Wang X, Fredericksen ZS et al (2010) A locus on 19p13 modifies risk of breast cancer in BRCA1 mutation carriers and is associated with hormone receptor–negative breast cancer in the general population. Nat Genet 42:885–892

Baccelli I, Schneeweiss A, Riethdorf S et al (2013) Identification of a population of blood circulating tumor cells from breast cancer patients that initiates metastasis in a xenograft assay. Nat Biotechnol 31:539–544
Barcellos-Hoff M, Akhurst RJ (2009) Transforming growth factor-β in breast cancer: too much, too late. Breast Cancer Res 11:202
Bayani J, Marrano P, Graham C et al (2011) Genomic instability and copy-number heterogeneity of chromosome 19q, including the kallikrein locus, in ovarian carcinomas. Mol Oncol 5:48–60
Beroukhim R, Mermel CH, Porter D et al (2010) The landscape of somatic copy-number alteration across human cancers. Nature 463:899–905
Bidard F-C, Mathiot C, Delaloge S et al (2010) Single circulating tumor cell detection and overall survival in nonmetastatic breast cancer. Annal Oncol Off J Eur Soc Med Oncol/ESMO 21:729–733
Biswas S, Guix M, Rinehart C et al (2007) Inhibition of TGF-β with neutralizing antibodies prevents radiation-induced acceleration of metastatic cancer progression. J Clin Investig 117:1305–1313
Borgoño CA, Diamandis EP (2004) The emerging roles of human tissue kallikreins in cancer. Nat Rev Cancer 4:876–890
Braun S, Vogl FD, Naume B et al (2005) A pooled analysis of bone marrow micrometastasis in breast cancer. N Engl J Med 353:793–802
Campbell LL, Polyak K (2007) Breast tumor heterogeneity: cancer stem cells or clonal evolution? Cell Cycle (Georgetown, Tex) 6:2332–2338
Carpenter EL, Rader J, Ruden J et al (2014) Dielectrophoretic capture and fenetic analysis of single neuroblastoma tumor cells. Front Oncol 4:201
Cawthorn TR, Moreno JC, Dharsee M et al (2012) Proteomic analyses reveal high expression of decorin and endoplasmin (HSP90B1) are associated with breast cancer metastasis and decreased survival. PLoS One 7:e30992
Chambers AF, Groom AC, MacDonald IC (2002) Metastasis: dissemination and growth of cancer cells in metastatic sites. Nat Rev Cancer 2:563–572
Chen D, Reierstad S, Fang F et al (2011) JunD and JunB integrate prostaglandin E2 activation of breast cancer-associated proximal aromatase promoters. Mol Endocrinol 25:767–775
Cristofanilli M, Budd GT, Ellis MJ et al (2004) Circulating tumor cells, disease progression, and survival in metastatic breast cancer. N Engl J Med 351:781–791
Cristofanilli M, Broglio KR, Guarneri V et al (2007) Circulating tumor cells in metastatic breast cancer: biologic staging beyond tumor burden. Clin Breast Cancer 7:471–479
Curtis C, Shah SP, Chin S-F et al (2012) The genomic and transcriptomic architecture of 2,000 breast tumours reveals novel subgroups. Nature 486:346–352
Dago AE, Stepansky A, Carlsson A et al (2014) Rapid phenotypic and genomic change in response to therapeutic pressure in prostate cancer inferred by high content analysis of single circulating tumor cells. PLoS One 9:e101777
Desmedt C, Haibe-Kains B, Wirapati P et al (2008) Biological processes associated with breast cancer clinical outcome depend on the molecular subtypes. Clin Cancer Res 14:5158–5165
Diaz LA Jr, Williams RT, Wu J et al (2012) The molecular evolution of acquired resistance to targeted EGFR blockade in colorectal cancers. Nature 486:537–540
Ding L, Ellis MJ, Li S et al (2010) Genome remodelling in a basal-like breast cancer metastasis and xenograft. Nature 464:999–1005
Etemadmoghadam D, George J, Cowin PA et al (2010) Amplicon-dependent CCNE1 expression is critical for clonogenic survival after cisplatin treatment and is correlated with 20q11 gain in ovarian cancer. PLoS One 5:e15498
Farace F, Massard C, Vimond N et al (2011) A direct comparison of CellSearch and ISET for circulating tumour-cell detection in patients with metastatic carcinomas. Br J Cancer 105:847–853
Fehm T, Hoffmann O, Aktas B et al (2009) Detection and characterization of circulating tumor cells in blood of primary breast cancer patients by RT-PCR and comparison to status of bone marrow disseminated cells. Breast Cancer Res BCR 11:R59

Fehm T, Müller V, Aktas B et al (2010) HER2 status of circulating tumor cells in patients with metastatic breast cancer: a prospective, multicenter trial. Breast Cancer Res Treat 124:403–412
Feng D-D, Zhang H, Zhang P et al (2011) Down-regulated miR-331-5p and miR-27a are associated with chemotherapy resistance and relapse in leukaemia. J Cell Mol Med 15:2164–2175
Fischer JC, Niederacher D, Topp SA et al (2013) Diagnostic leukapheresis enables reliable detection of circulating tumor cells of nonmetastatic cancer patients. Proc Natl Acad Sci 110:16580–16585
Flores LM, Kindelberger DW, Ligon AH et al (2010) Improving the yield of circulating tumour cells facilitates molecular characterisation and recognition of discordant HER2 amplification in breast cancer. Br J Cancer 102:1495–1502
Foekens JA, Sieuwerts AM, Smid M et al (2008) Four miRNAs associated with aggressiveness of lymph node-negative, estrogen receptor-positive human breast cancer. Proc Natl Acad Sci USA 105:13021–13026
Gerlinger M, Rowan AJ, Horswell S et al (2012) Intratumor heterogeneity and branched evolution revealed by multiregion sequencing. N Engl J Med 366:883–892
Geyer FC, Weigelt B, Natrajan R et al (2010) Molecular analysis reveals a genetic basis for the phenotypic diversity of metaplastic breast carcinomas. J Pathol 220:562–573
Giordano A, Cristofanilli M (2012) CTCs in metastatic breast cancer. Recent Results Cancer Res 195:193–201
Gradilone A, Naso G, Raimondi C et al (2011) Circulating tumor cells (CTCs) in metastatic breast cancer (MBC): prognosis, drug resistance and phenotypic characterization. Annal Oncol Off J Eur Soc Med Oncol/ESMO 22:86–92
Harris L, Fritsche H, Mennel R et al (2007) American Society of Clinical Oncology 2007 update of recommendations for the use of tumor markers in breast cancer. J Clin Oncol Off J Am Soc Clin Oncol 25:5287–5312
Heitzer E, Auer M, Gasch C et al (2013) Complex tumor genomes inferred from single circulating tumor cells by array-CGH and next-generation sequencing. Cancer Res 73:2965–2975
Hernandez L, Wilkerson PM, Lambros MB et al (2012) Genomic and mutational profiling of ductal carcinomas in situ and matched adjacent invasive breast cancers reveals intra-tumour genetic heterogeneity and clonal selection. J Pathol 227:42–52
Heselmeyer-Haddad K, Berroa Garcia LY, Bradley A et al (2012) Single-cell genetic analysis of ductal carcinoma in situ and invasive breast cancer reveals enormous tumor heterogeneity yet conserved genomic imbalances and gain of MYC during progression. Am J Pathol 181:1807–1822
Hiley C, de Bruin EC, McGranahan N et al (2014) Deciphering intratumor heterogeneity and temporal acquisition of driver events to refine precision medicine. Genome Biol 15:453
Horlings HM, Lai C, Nuyten DSA et al (2010) Integration of DNA copy number alterations and prognostic gene expression signatures in breast cancer patients. Clin Cancer Res 16:651–663
Huang Q, Gumireddy K, Schrier M et al (2008) The microRNAs miR-373 and miR-520c promote tumour invasion and metastasis. Nat Cell Biol 10:202–210
Hüsemann Y, Geigl JB, Schubert F et al (2008) Systemic spread is an early step in breast cancer. Cancer Cell 13:58–68
Ignatiadis M, Kallergi G, Ntoulia M et al (2008) Prognostic value of the molecular detection of circulating tumor cells using a multimarker reverse transcription-PCR assay for cytokeratin 19, mammaglobin A, and HER2 in early breast cancer. Clin Cancer Res 14:2593–2600
Jamal-Hanjani M, Quezada SA, Larkin J et al (2015) Translational Implications of Tumor Heterogeneity. Clin Cancer Res 21:1258–1266
Ji J, Yamashita T, Budhu A et al (2009) Identification of microRNA-181 by genome-wide screening as a critical player in EpCAM-positive hepatic cancer stem cells. Hepatology (Baltimore, MD) 50:472–480
Kanwar N, Hu P, Bedard P et al (2015) Identification of genomic signatures in circulating tumor cells from breast cancer. Int J Cancer 137:332–344

Karabacak NM, Spuhler PS, Fachin F et al (2014) Microfluidic, marker-free isolation of circulating tumor cells from blood samples. Nat Protoc 9:694–710

Kasimir-Bauer S, Hoffmann O, Wallwiener D et al (2012) Expression of stem cell and epithelial-mesenchymal transition markers in primary breast cancer patients with circulating tumor cells. Breast Cancer Res BCR 14:R15

Keyomarsi K, Tucker SL, Buchholz TA et al (2002) Cyclin E and survival in patients with breast cancer. N Engl J Med 347:1566–1575

Klein CA (2009) Parallel progression of primary tumours and metastases. Nat Rev Cancer 9:302–312

Klein CA, Stoecklein NH (2009) Lessons from an aggressive cancer: evolutionary dynamics in esophageal carcinoma. Cancer Res 69:5285–5288

Klein CA, Blankenstein TJF, Schmidt-Kittler O et al (2002) Genetic heterogeneity of single disseminated tumour cells in minimal residual cancer. Lancet 360:683–689

Kraan J, Sleijfer S, Strijbos MH et al (2011) External quality assurance of circulating tumor cell enumeration using the CellSearch(®) system: a feasibility study. Cytometry B Clin Cytom 80:112–118

Krishnamurthy S, Cristofanilli M, Singh B et al (2010) Detection of minimal residual disease in blood and bone marrow in early stage breast cancer. Cancer 116:3330–3337

Kuukasjärvi T, Karhu R, Tanner M et al (1997) Genetic heterogeneity and clonal evolution underlying development of asynchronous metastasis in human breast cancer. Cancer Res 57:1597–1604

Laurent LC, Chen J, Ulitsky I et al (2008) Comprehensive microRNA profiling reveals a unique human embryonic stem cell signature dominated by a single seed sequence. Stem Cells 26:1506–1516

Li Z-M, Hu S, Xiao L et al (2010) Expression of microRNA 27a and its correlation with drug resistance in human ovarian cancer A2780/Taxol cells. Zhonghua Fu Chan Ke Za Zhi 45:372–375

Liu MC, Shields PG, Warren RD et al (2009) Circulating tumor cells: a useful predictor of treatment efficacy in metastatic breast cancer. J Clin Oncol 27:5153–5159

Lohr JG, Adalsteinsson VA, Cibulskis K et al (2014) Whole-exome sequencing of circulating tumor cells provides a window into metastatic prostate cancer. Nat Biotechnol 32:479–484

Lu J, Fan T, Zhao Q et al (2010) Isolation of circulating epithelial and tumor progenitor cells with an invasive phenotype from breast cancer patients. Int J Cancer 126:669–683

Lucci A, Hall CS, Lodhi AK et al (2012) Circulating tumour cells in non-metastatic breast cancer: a prospective study. Lancet Oncol 13:688–695

Luo L-Y, Diamandis EP, Look MP et al (2002) Higher expression of human kallikrein 10 in breast cancer tissue predicts tamoxifen resistance. Br J Cancer 86:1790–1796

Magbanua MJM, Sosa EV, Roy R et al (2012) Genomic profiling of isolated circulating tumor cells from metastatic breast cancer patients. Cancer Res 73:30–40

Mathiesen RR, Fjelldal R, Liestøl K et al (2012) High-resolution analyses of copy number changes in disseminated tumor cells of patients with breast cancer. Int J Cancer 131:E405–E415

McGranahan N, Swanton C (2015) Biological and therapeutic impact of intratumor heterogeneity in cancer evolution. Cancer Cell 27:15–26

Miyamoto DT, Lee RJ, Stott SL et al (2012) Androgen receptor signaling in circulating tumor cells as a marker of hormonally responsive prostate cancer. Cancer Discov 2:995–1003

Muraoka RS, Dumont N, Ritter CA et al (2002) Blockade of TGF-beta inhibits mammary tumor cell viability, migration, and metastases. J Clin Invest 109:1551–1559

Muraoka-Cook RS (2004) Conditional overexpression of active transforming growth factor 1 *in vivo* accelerates metastases of transgenic mammary tumors. Cancer Res 64:9002–9011

Nadal R, Fernandez A, Sanchez-Rovira P et al (2012) Biomarkers characterization of circulating tumour cells in breast cancer patients. Breast Cancer Res BCR 14:R71

Nagrath S, Sequist LV, Maheswaran S et al (2007) Isolation of rare circulating tumour cells in cancer patients by microchip technology. Nature 450:1235–1239

Natrajan R, Mackay A, Wilkerson PM et al (2012) Functional characterization of the 19q12 amplicon in grade III breast cancers. Breast Cancer Res 14:R53
Navin N, Krasnitz A, Rodgers L et al (2010) Inferring tumor progression from genomic heterogeneity. Genome Res 20:68–80
Nelson NJ (2010) Circulating tumor cells: will they be clinically useful? J Natl Cancer Inst 102:146–148
Ng CK, Martelotto LG, Gauthier A et al (2015) Intra-tumor genetic heterogeneity and alternative driver genetic alterations in breast cancers with heterogeneous HER2 gene amplification. Genome Biol 16:107
Ni X, Zhuo M, Su Z et al (2013) Reproducible copy number variation patterns among single circulating tumor cells of lung cancer patients. Proc Natl Acad Sci 110:21083–21088
Pantel K, Brakenhoff RH (2004) Dissecting the metastatic cascade. Nat Rev Cancer 4:448–456
Pantel K, Brakenhoff RH, Brandt B (2008) Detection, clinical relevance and specific biological properties of disseminating tumour cells. Nat Rev Cancer 8:329–340
Polyak K (2007) Breast cancer: origins and evolution. J Clin Invest 117:3155–3163
Powell AA, Talasaz AH, Zhang H et al (2012) Single cell profiling of circulating tumor cells: transcriptional heterogeneity and diversity from breast cancer cell lines. PLoS One 7:e33788
Radford DM, Fair KL, Phillips NJ et al (1995a) Allelotyping of ductal carcinoma in situ of the breast: deletion of loci on 8p, 13q, 16q, 17p and 17q. Cancer Res 55:3399–3405
Radford DM, Phillips NJ, Fair KL et al (1995b) Allelic loss and the progression of breast cancer. Cancer Res 55:5180–5183
Rashid-Kolvear F, Pintilie M, Done SJ (2007) Telomere length on chromosome 17q shortens more than global telomere length in the development of breast cancer. Neoplasia (New York, NY) 9:265–270
Rippe V, Dittberner L, Lorenz VN et al (2010) The two stem cell microRNA gene clusters C19MC and miR-371-3 are activated by specific chromosomal rearrangements in a subgroup of thyroid adenomas. PLoS One 5:e9485
Sayagués JM, Abad MM, Melchor HB et al (2010) Intratumoural cytogenetic heterogeneity of sporadic colorectal carcinomas suggests several pathways to liver metastasis. J Pathol 221:308–319
Schardt JA, Meyer M, Hartmann CH et al (2005) Genomic analysis of single cytokeratin-positive cells from bone marrow reveals early mutational events in breast cancer. Cancer Cell 8:227–239
Schmidt-Kittler O, Ragg T, Daskalakis A et al (2003) From latent disseminated cells to overt metastasis: genetic analysis of systemic breast cancer progression. Proc Natl Acad Sci U S A 100:7737–7742
Shah SP, Morin RD, Khattra J et al (2009) Mutational evolution in a lobular breast tumour profiled at single nucleotide resolution. Nature 461:809–813
Shah SP, Roth A, Goya R et al (2012) The clonal and mutational evolution spectrum of primary triple-negative breast cancers. Nature 486:395–399
Shim KS, Kim KH, Han WS et al (1999) Elevated serum levels of transforming growth factor-beta1 in patients with colorectal carcinoma: its association with tumor progression and its significant decrease after curative surgical resection. Cancer 85:554–561
Shipitsin M, Campbell LL, Argani P et al (2007) Molecular definition of breast tumor heterogeneity. Cancer Cell 11:259–273
Sieuwerts AM (2006) Which cyclin E prevails as prognostic marker for breast cancer? Results from a retrospective study involving 635 lymph node-negative breast cancer patients. Clin Cancer Res 12:3319–3328
Sieuwerts AM, Kraan J, Bolt-de Vries J et al (2008) Molecular characterization of circulating tumor cells in large quantities of contaminating leukocytes by a multiplex real-time PCR. Breast Cancer Res Treat 118:455–468
Smirnov DA (2005) Global gene expression profiling of circulating tumor cells. Cancer Res 65:4993–4997

Staaf J, Jönsson G, Ringnér M et al (2010) High-resolution genomic and expression analyses of copy number alterations in HER2-amplified breast cancer. Breast Cancer Res BCR 12:R25

Staaf J, Jönsson G, Ringnér M et al (2011) Landscape of somatic allelic imbalances and copy number alterations in HER2-amplified breast cancer. Breast Cancer Res BCR 13:R129

Stoecklein NH, Klein CA (2010) Genetic disparity between primary tumours, disseminated tumour cells, and manifest metastasis. Int J Cancer 126:589–598

Stott SL, Hsu C-H, Tsukrov DI et al (2010) Isolation of circulating tumor cells using a microvortex-generating herringbone-chip. Proc Natl Acad Sci U S A 107:18392–18397

Tan MJ, Teo Z, Sng MK et al (2012) Emerging roles of angiopoietin-like 4 in human cancer. Mol Cancer Res MCR 10:677–688

Theil G, Fischer K, Weber E et al (2016) The use of a new cell collector to isolate circulating tumor cells from the blood of patients with different stages of prostate cancer and clinical outcomes – a proof-of-concept study. PLoS One 11:e0158354

Ting DT, Wittner BS, Ligorio M et al (2014) Single-Cell RNA Sequencing Identifies Extracellular Matrix Gene Expression by Pancreatic Circulating Tumor Cells. Cell Rep 8:1905–1918

Turner N, Lambros MB, Horlings HM et al (2010) Integrative molecular profiling of triple negative breast cancers identifies amplicon drivers and potential therapeutic targets. Oncogene 29:2013–2023

van de Vijver MJ, He YD, van't Veer LJ et al (2002) A gene-expression signature as a predictor of survival in breast cancer. N Engl J Med 347:1999–2009

Van der Auwera I, Peeters D, Benoy IH et al (2010) Circulating tumour cell detection: a direct comparison between the CellSearch System, the AdnaTest and CK-19/mammaglobin RT-PCR in patients with metastatic breast cancer. Br J Cancer 102:276–284

Van Loo P, Voet T (2014) Single cell analysis of cancer genomes. Curr Opin Genet Dev 24:82–91

Waclaw B, Bozic I, Pittman ME et al (2015) A spatial model predicts that dispersal and cell turnover limit intratumour heterogeneity. Nature 525:261–264

Wagenblast E, Soto M, Gutiérrez-Ángel S et al (2015) A model of breast cancer heterogeneity reveals vascular mimicry as a driver of metastasis. Nature 520:358–362

Wagle N, Van Allen EM, Treacy DJ et al (2014) MAP kinase pathway alterations in BRAF-mutant melanoma patients with acquired resistance to combined RAF/MEK inhibition. Cancer Discov 4:61–68

Walker JC, Harland RM (2009) microRNA-24a is required to repress apoptosis in the developing neural retina. Genes Dev 23:1046–1051

Wang B, Hsu S-H, Majumder S et al (2009a) TGFβ-mediated upregulation of hepatic miR-181b promotes hepatocarcinogenesis by targeting TIMP3. Oncogene 29:1787–1797

Wang C, Iakovlev VV, Wong V et al (2009b) Genomic alterations in primary breast cancers compared with their sentinel and more distal lymph node metastases: an aCGH study. Genes Chromosomes Cancer 48:1091–1101

Wang Y, Waters J, Leung ML et al (2014) Clonal evolution in breast cancer revealed by single nucleus genome sequencing. Nature 512:155–160

Weigelt B, Peterse JL, van't Veer LJ (2005) Breast cancer metastasis: markers and models. Nat Rev Cancer 5:591–602

Weitzman JB, Fiette L, Matsuo K et al (2000) JunD protects cells from p53-dependent senescence and apoptosis. Mol Cell 6:1109–1119

Wikman H, Vessella R, Pantel K (2008) Cancer micrometastasis and tumour dormancy. APMIS 116:754–770

Woelfle U, Cloos J, Sauter G et al (2003) Molecular signature associated with bone marrow micrometastasis in human breast cancer. Cancer Res 63:5679–5684

Wolf W, Michael Evans D, Chao L et al (2001) A synthetic tissue kallikrein inhibitor supresses cancer cell invasiveness. Am J Pathol 5:1797–1805

Yousef GM, Diamandis EP (2002) Expanded human tissue kallikrein family – a novel panel of cancer biomarkers. Tumour Biol J Int Soc Oncodev Biol Med 23:185–192

Yu W, Kanaan Y, Bae YK et al (2009) Chromosomal changes in aggressive breast cancers with basal-like features. Cancer Genet Cytogenet 193:29–37

Yu M, Ting DT, Stott SL et al (2012) RNA sequencing of pancreatic circulating tumour cells implicates WNT signalling in metastasis. Nature 487:510–513

Yu M, Bardia A, Wittner BS et al (2013) Circulating breast tumor cells exhibit dynamic changes in epithelial and mesenchymal composition. Science 339:580–584

Zardavas D, Irrthum A, Swanton C et al (2015) Clinical management of breast cancer heterogeneity. Nat Rev Clin Oncol 12:381–394

Zhang H, Li M, Han Y et al (2010) Down-regulation of miR-27a might reverse multidrug resistance of esophageal squamous cell carcinoma. Dig Dis Sci 55:2545–2551

Zhang L, Riethdorf S, Wu G et al (2012) Meta-analysis of the prognostic value of circulating tumor cells in breast cancer. Clin Cancer Res 18:5701–5710

Zhang H, Wei S, Ning S et al (2013) Evaluation of TGFβ, XPO4, elF5A2 and ANGPTL4 as biomarkers in HCC. Exp Ther Med 5:119–127

Zhao X, Yang L, Hu J (2011) Down-regulation of miR-27a might inhibit proliferation and drug resistance of gastric cancer cells. J Exp Clin Cancer Res 30:55

Zhu P, Tan Ming J, Huang R-L et al (2011) Angiopoietin-like 4 protein elevates the prosurvival intracellular $O_2-:H_2O_2$ ratio and confers anoikis resistance to tumors. Cancer Cell 19:401–415

Chapter 9
Detection of Gene Rearrangements in Circulating Tumor Cells: Examples of *ALK*-, *ROS1*-, *RET*-Rearrangements in Non-Small-Cell Lung Cancer and *ERG*-Rearrangements in Prostate Cancer

Cyril Catelain, Emma Pailler, Marianne Oulhen, Vincent Faugeroux, Anne-Laure Pommier, and Françoise Farace

Abstract Circulating tumor cells (CTCs) hold promise as biomarkers to aid in patient treatment stratification and disease monitoring. Because the number of cells is a critical parameter for exploiting CTCs for predictive biomarker's detection, we developed a FISH (fluorescent *in situ* hybridization) method for CTCs enriched on filters (filter-adapted FISH [FA-FISH]) that was optimized for high cell recovery. To increase the feasibility and reliability of the analyses, we combined fluorescent staining and FA-FISH and developed a semi-automated microscopy method for optimal FISH signal identification in filtration-enriched CTCs. Here we present

---

Cyril Catelain and Emma Pailler are contributed equally to the manuscript.

C. Catelain • M. Oulhen • A.-L. Pommier
Gustave Roussy, Université Paris-Saclay, "Circulating Tumor Cells" Translational Platform, AMMICA CNRS UMS3655 – INSERM US23, 114 rue Édouard Vaillant, F-94805 Villejuif, France

INSERM, U981 "Identification of Molecular Predictors and New Targets for Cancer Treatment", 114 rue Édouard Vaillant, F-94805 Villejuif, France
e-mail: cyril.catelain@gustaveroussy.fr; marianne.oulhen@gustaveroussy.fr; anne-laure.pommier@gustaveroussy.fr

E. Pailler • V. Faugeroux • F. Farace (✉)
Gustave Roussy, Université Paris-Saclay, "Circulating Tumor Cells" Translational Platform, AMMICA CNRS UMS3655 – INSERM US23, 114 rue Édouard Vaillant, F-94805 Villejuif, France

INSERM, U981 "Identification of Molecular Predictors and New Targets for Cancer Treatment", 114 rue Édouard Vaillant, F-94805 Villejuif, France

Univ Paris Sud, Université Paris-Saclay, 114 rue Édouard Vaillant, F-94270 Le Kremlin-Bicetre, France
e-mail: emma.pailler@gustaveroussy.fr; vincent.faugeroux@gustaveroussy.fr; francoise.farace@gustaveroussy.fr

M.J.M. Magbanua, J.W. Park (eds.), *Isolation and Molecular Characterization of Circulating Tumor Cells*, Advances in Experimental Medicine and Biology 994,
DOI 10.1007/978-3-319-55947-6_9

these methods and their use for the detection and characterization of *ALK*-, *ROS1*-, *RET*-rearrangement in CTCs from non-small-cell lung cancer and *ERG*-rearrangements in CTCs from prostate cancer patients.

Keywords Circulating tumor cells • Filtration-enrichment • Fluorescent staining • FA-FISH • Predictive biomarkers

9.1 Introduction

Chemotherapy remains an important mode of treatment for many cancers but is slowly being supplemented by a new generation of targeted therapies directed against specific molecular alterations in cancer cells which has proven to be more effective with markedly fewer side effects. In current practice, biomarkers predicting response to therapy could be assessed either in the primitive tumor tissue taken at diagnosis or in tumor biopsy samples (metastasis) collected during the course of the disease. Primitive tumor tissue can be difficult to obtain in patients with certain tumor types such as non-small-cell lung cancer (NSCLC). Subjecting patients to biopsies could be invasive, in some cases challenging, and associated with risk. Even in case such as prostate cancer (PCa) where the primary tissue is available, the samples may not be representative of a patient's metastatic disease which may arise many years after diagnosis. Therefore, a key challenge today is to overcome the hurdle of tumor tissue and single-biopsy sample availability.

NSCLC is the most frequent type of lung cancer and the most common cause of death from cancer (Jemal et al. 2011). Treatment paradigms for NSCLC have considerably evolved toward a stratification of patients in molecularly selected subsets who can be effectively treated by therapies targeting mutant driver oncogenes. Small-molecule tyrosine kinase inhibitors (TKI) targeting single driver oncogenic pathways essential for tumor cell survival have demonstrated high objective response rates in molecularly defined NSCLC patients harboring *epidermal growth factor receptor* (*EGFR*) gene mutations or *anaplastic lymphoma kinase* (*ALK*) fusion genes (Shames and Wistuba 2014; Oxnard et al. 2013; Sequist et al. 2007; Shaw et al. 2013). The list of NSCLC driver oncogenes includes three fusion genes namely *ALK*, *c-ros oncogene 1* (*ROS1*) and *ret proto-oncogene* (*RET*) (Soda et al. 2007; Kohno et al. 2012; Rikova et al. 2007). The most prevalent *ALK*-rearrangement consists in a fusion gene between the *ALK* gene and *echinoderm microtubule associated protein-like 4* (*EML4*) which has been identified in 4% of unselected patients with NSCLC (Chiarle et al. 2008; Pao and Girard 2011), while a range of different *ALK*-gene fusions can occur (Hallberg and Palmer 2016). *ALK* is the only gene rearrangement diagnosed in routine using either fluorescence *in situ* hybridization (FISH) or more recently immunochemistry (Kerr and Lopez-Rios 2016). *ALK*-rearranged patients can benefit from ALK inhibitor therapies such as crizotinib, alectinib or ceritinib (Solomon and Soria 2016). In 2011, crizotinib received US Food & Drug Association (FDA) approval as the first ALK-inhibitor for advanced *ALK*-rearranged NSCLC patients after demonstration of impressive clinical results. To ensure identification of *ALK*-rearranged patients most likely to benefit, the FDA approved crizotinib concurrently with a companion diagnostic test, the Vysis *ALK* Break Apart FISH Probe Kit. *ROS1* fusion genes have been identified in ~1% of NSCLC (Bergethon et al. 2012; Gainor and Shaw 2013). Rearrangement leads to fusion of the *ROS1*-gene on chromosome 6 with a number of different genetic partners, a process that can drive cellular transformation and constitutive ROS1 kinase activity (Davies and Doebele 2013). Patients with *ROS1*-rearranged NSCLC can also benefit from crizotinib therapy. *RET-rearrangement* gene was found in lung adenocarcinoma patients for the first time in 2012 by four independent groups (Kohno et al. 2012; Ju et al. 2012; Lipson et al. 2012; Takeuchi et al. 2012). Approximately 1% of lung adenocarcinomas were reported to harbor a novel gene fusion involving the *RET* tyrosine kinase gene partnered with either *kinesin family member 5B* (*KIF5B*) or *coiled-coil domain containing 6* (*CCDC6*). Because surgery is frequently not a component of treatment in NSCLC, the diagnosis of molecular biomarkers is usually done in small tumor biopsies or fine needle aspirates which are challenging as mentioned above. Furthermore, the diagnosis of biomarkers is often hindered by the limited tumor tissue quantities available.

PCa is the commonest cancer in men accounting for 10% for all cancer-related death. Androgen-deprivation therapy is a standard of care treatment for PCa and efficiently controls the growth of androgen-dependent tumors. Unfortunately, the majority of these cancers ultimately become refractory to hormone deprivation and emerges as castration resistant (Tannock et al. 2004). The treatment of metastatic castration-resistant prostate cancer (mCRPC) patients has dramatically changed in the last 5 years thank to the development of active drugs such as the chemotherapy agent cabazitaxel, the androgen receptor (AR) pathway inhibitors abiraterone acetate and enzalutamide, and the immunotherapy sipuleucel-T (Kantoff et al. 2010; Ryan et al. 2013; Scher et al. 2012). However, not all patients benefit from all these agents and predictive biomarkers are needed to assess clinical response and guide treatment. The fusion between the androgen-regulated *transmembrane protease serine 2* (*TMPRSS2*) gene promoter and *v-ets avian erythroblastosis virus E26 oncogene homolog* (*ERG*) genes, *AR* amplification and alterations in PI3K/AKT/mTOR pathway are used to classify mCRPC patients into molecular subgroups. Although these biomarkers currently have no direct relevance for a therapeutic decision, it is expected that future treatments entering the clinic in mCRPC will be rationally delivered in molecularly selected patient populations, according to the presence of these biomarkers. The molecular characterization of cancer samples is hampered by the availability of metastatic tumor tissue in mCRPC patients. Metastasis biopsy is challenging to perform in daily practice, as the metastatic disease is often located to the bone.

Finding more effective means to identify predictive biomarkers which could aid in treatment decision or patient stratification is a major clinical issue in NSCLC and mCRPC patients. Peripheral blood represents an easily accessible and non-invasive source of spreading tumor cells. Circulating tumor cells (CTCs) which migrate from primitive tumor or metastatic sites are the main route of metastatic dissemination and may contain clones with tumorigenic potential (Baccelli et al. 2013). In contrast to tumor biopsies, CTCs offer an attractive option to identify molecular biomarkers, which could be easily repeated during treatment providing longitudinal information on the selected biomarker. Moreover CTCs may be released from various metastatic sites and have been reported to reflect the tumor heterogeneity (Heitzer et al. 2013; Massard et al. 2016). In order to identify and characterize biomarkers in CTCs from NSCLC and mCRPC patients, our approach was first to develop a FISH method called FA-FISH to directly detect gene rearrangements in filtration-enriched CTCs. Secondly, to increase the feasibility and reliability of this method, we combined fluorescent staining and FISH and developed a semi-automated microscopy method optimized for FISH signals detection in filtration-enriched CTCs. Using these methods, we examined *ALK*-, *ROS1*- and *RET*-rearrangements in CTCs from NSCLC patients, as well as *ERG*-rearrangements in mCRPC patients. Here, we report our experience in the detection and characterizations of CTCs harboring these gene rearrangements.

9.2 Development of the FA-FISH Method and the Semi-automated Analysis of CTCs Captured on Filters

9.2.1 The FA-FISH (Filter Adapted - Fluorescent In Situ *Hybridization) Method*

In 2011 we reported a study showing higher CTC recovery in metastatic NSCLC and PCa patients using ISET (isolation by size of epithelial tumor cells) filtration technique (Farace et al. 2011). As the number of CTCs is a critical parameter to identify molecular biomarkers, we decided to develop FISH for CTCs enriched on filters (FA-FISH) (Pailler et al. 2013). A 1-mL sample of blood will typically contain five to ten million leukocytes, five billion erythrocytes, and a very small number of rare circulating cells, including CTCs. The filtration techniques are based on the observation that tumor cells of most types of solid cancers are most often larger than blood cells (leukocytes and erythrocytes). The ISET system uses filters designed to allow the elimination of all erythrocytes and most leukocytes from the sample. ISET filters are composed of ten spots. After filtration, one ISET spot typically retain leucocytes (ranging from 6000 to 20,000, mostly granulocytes) and fifty non-hematopoietic cells among which are found CTCs. Each spot (corresponding to filtration of 1 mL of blood) could be precisely cut out for independent analyzes.

The FA-FISH method required several technical optimizations compared to the FISH method established for tissue or cell slides. The first step was to determinate the optimal incubation time required for the enzymatic digestion of the cell membrane. Two rounds of fixation of the cells present on the filter have been added in order to preserve the cell integrity. Because the filter membrane inevitably retains fluorescent background signals, we diminished this background by optimizing the temperature of hybridization for each probe and discarding non-specific staining with stringent washes. This direct FA-FISH method was used to detect *ALK*-rearrangement in ISET-enriched CTCs from *ALK*-rearranged patients showing high specificity and sensibility (Pailler et al. 2013).

9.2.2 Semi-automated Microscopy of Combined Fluorescent Staining and FA-FISH in Filtration-Enriched CTCs

Manual FISH analyses of filtration-enriched CTCs are time-consuming due to the high numbers of white blood cells DAPI$^+$/CD45$^+$ retained on the filters, laborious and operator-dependent. Scanner software is commonly able to analyze around 100 cells per tumor sample by FISH. Using standard scanning conditions it was therefore not conceivable to scan all the FISH signals present in the cells (6000–20,000, as mentioned above) retained on a 1 mL ISET spot. To decrease the numbers of cells to scan, we limited the FISH analysis to DAPI$^+$/CD45$^-$ cells: this option provided the additional advantage of excluding DAPI$^+$/CD45$^+$ subpopulations which could occasionally harbor unspecific break apart FISH signals when apoptotic or damaged.

While offering important advantages such as sensitivity of CTC capture and flexibility for CTC characterization, filtration systems such as ISET have drawbacks. One problem is the difficulty to design a filter membrane which sits entirely flat, regardless of the material used: virtually all filter membranes developed today are not microscopically flat. Another is that pores inevitably retain white blood cell debris and fluorescence signals which disturb microscopy analysis, thus cells placed on pores are frequently difficult to analyze. These two problems make the automation of microscopy challenging to implement.

Given these difficulties, we established a multi-step process for optimal FISH signal identification in filtration-enriched CTCs where filters were (i) treated by fluorescent staining, (ii) scanned on the Ariol system and analyzed automatically to locate DAPI$^+$/CD45$^-$ cells, (iii) treated by FA-FISH, (iv) scanned in the small regions containing the DAPI$^+$/CD45$^-$ cells with specific parameters (z-stacking, step i.e. distance between two z-stacks, exposure time), (v) and analyzed for detection, interpretation and validation of FISH signals within DAPI$^+$/CD45$^-$ cells (Pailler et al. 2016).

Another advantage of this semi-automated microscopy method is the possibility to combine successive assays on the same filter. Automation allows precise location of cells on filters, thus relocating cell data and images from successive experiments performed on the same filter. The combination of assays increases the amount of available information, contributing to a better characterization of CTCs and reliability of the results. Therefore, data issued from successive experiments may be gathered, further improving and refining CTC characterization.

9.3 Detection *ALK*-Rearranged CTCs in NSCLC Patients

After establishing the direct FA-FISH method, we have examined the presence of *ALK*-rearrangement in CTCs of 18 *ALK*-rearranged and 14 *ALK*-negative patients (Pailler et al. 2013). In this report, we showed that the specificity and the sensibility were of 100% at a cutoff value of four *ALK*-rearranged CTCs per 1 mL blood (median, nine CTCs per 1 mL; range, four to 34 CTCs per 1 mL). No or only one *ALK*-rearranged CTC (median, one per 1 mL; range, zero to one per 1 mL) was detected in *ALK*-negative patients. The concordance between CTCs and tumors were 99.9%. *ALK*-rearrangement patterns were determined in CTCs and compared to those present in tumor biopsies. While heterogeneous patterns (split of the red and green and isolated red signals) were present in tumor biopsies, *ALK*-rearranged CTCs harbored a unique FISH pattern which was associated with either a single copy or a gain of native *ALK* copies consisting in the split of red and green signals (Fig. 9.1a). This unique rearrangement (3′5′) was consistently observed in all patient CTCs regardless of the frequency of cells harboring this rearrangement within the tumor specimen, including patients in whom this pattern was not detected in the tumor biopsy. These data suggested that CTCs bearing this unique *ALK*-rearrangement may have acquired invasive and migratory properties that are lacking in tumor cells with other *ALK*-rearrangement patterns. Therefore we tested epithelium-mesenchymal transition (EMT) markers in *ALK*-rearranged CTCs and found that these cells were negative for cytokeratins and E-cadherin and express exclusively mesenchymal markers (vimentin, N-cadherin). When tumor biopsy specimens were analyzed for the epithelial and mesenchymal marker expression, we observed important inter- and intra-tumor heterogeneity for these markers. Interestingly, ALK protein expression correlated with a low or absence of epithelial marker expression and higher levels of vimentin expression.

Thus, *ALK*-rearranged CTCs expressed a mesenchymal phenotype contrasting with heterogeneous epithelial and mesenchymal marker expressions in tumors. Overall, our results suggested that CTCs with this unique *ALK*-rearrangement expressing a mesenchymal phenotype may result from the selection of tumor cells that display migratory and higher potential invasive properties. These CTCs may possibly contain highly metastatic cells, such as cancer stem cells or tumor-initiating cells. Although a single tumor biopsy sample might not be representative of the entire tumor, these results suggested that *ALK*-rearranged CTCs might originate from various metastatic sites. By reflecting the metastatic disease process, CTCs may be more informative of biomarker status than a single biopsy taken at a given time.

Moreover, we detected qualitative and quantitative variations of CTCs bearing abnormal *ALK*-FISH patterns in five patients treated with crizotinib. This result showed that CTCs could possibly help to monitor the impact of *ALK*-inhibitor treatments and guide therapeutic decision during treatment course in *ALK*-rearranged patients.

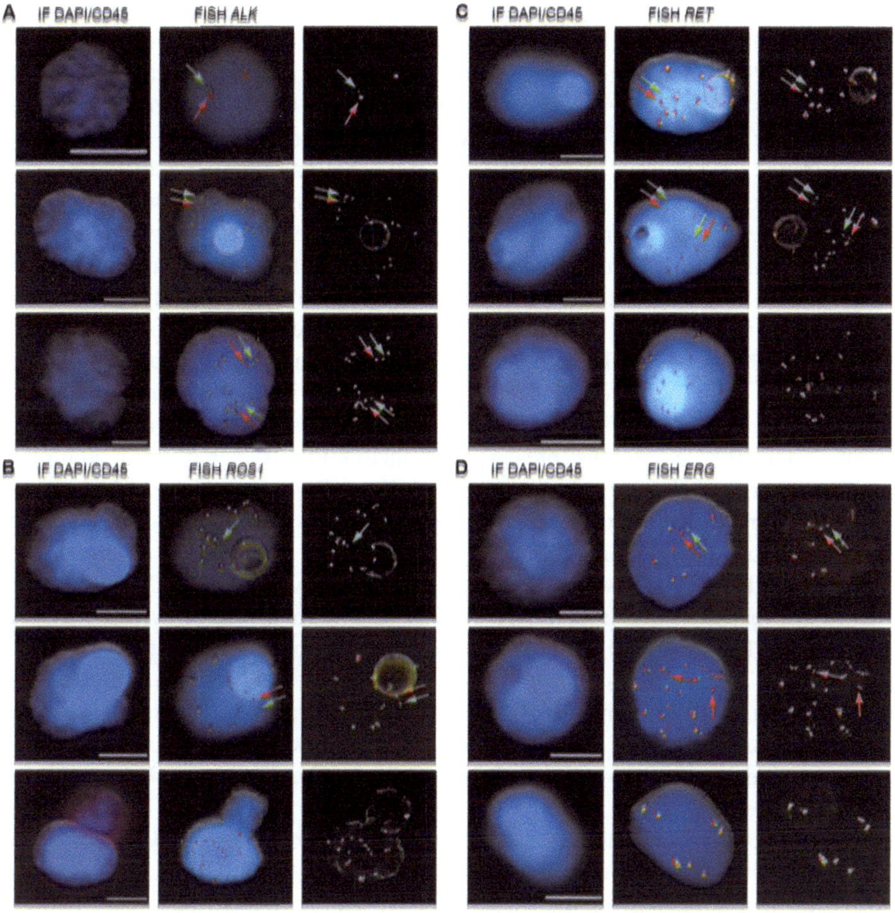

Fig. 9.1 Examples of gene rearrangement detection in filtration-enriched CTCs from NSCLC and mPCa patients by combined fluorescent staining and fluorescent *in situ* hybridization (FISH). (**a**) Example of *ALK*-rearrangement detection in NSCLC patients with an *ALK*-rearranged tumor. (**b**) Example of *ROS1*-rearrangement detection in NSCLC patients with a *ROS1*-rearranged tumor. (**c**) Example of *RET*-rearrangement detection in NSCLC patients with a *RET*-rearranged tumor. (**d**) Example of *ERG*-rearrangement detection in mPCa patients with an *ERG*-rearranged tumor. Gene rearrangements are shown by *green* and *red*. Scale: *white bars* = 10 μm (Reprinted with permission from Pailler et al. 2016)

9.4 Detection *ROS1*- and *RET*-Rearranged CTCs in NSCLC Patients

Using combined fluorescent staining, and FA-FISH and the semi-automated microscopy method, we evaluated whether *ROS1*-rearrangements could be detected in CTCs from *ROS1*-rearranged NSCLC patients (Pailler et al. 2015). Four *ROS1*-rearranged patients treated by the *ROS1*-inhibitor were examined and CTCs sampled at two time points (before and during the crizotinib treatment). *ROS1*-rearrangement was in parallel examined in CTCs from four *ROS1*-negative NSCLC patients. In *ROS1*-rearranged patients, median number of *ROS1*-rearranged CTCs at baseline was 34.5 per 3 mL blood (range, 24–55). In *ROS1*-negative patients, median background hybridization of *ROS1*-rearranged CTCs was 7.5 per 3 mL blood (range, 7–11). The two types of *ROS1* FISH patterns (split of the red and green, isolated green signals) were identified in CTCs (Fig. 9.1b) while only one type was detected in the tumor biopsies. *ROS1*-gene alterations observed in CTCs at baseline from *ROS1*-rearranged patients were compared with those present in tumor biopsies and CTCs during crizotinib treatment. Tumor heterogeneity, assessed by *ROS1* copy number, was significantly higher in baseline CTCs compared with paired tumor biopsies in the three patients experiencing partial response or stable disease. We also observed that the copy number in *ROS1*-rearranged CTCs increased significantly in the two patients who progressed during crizotinib treatment. To further assess the presence of aneuploid CTCs harboring abnormal *ROS1* pattern and their chromosomal instability (CIN) status, we developed two tests: 1/ the measurement of the DNA content by Hoechst 33342 quantification and 2/ a multi-FISH chromosomal method carried out with the AneuVysion Multicolor DNA Probe Kit (Abbott Molecular, Inc.). Results showed that CTCs from *ROS1*-rearranged patients had high DNA content and high levels of aneuploidy and numerical CIN. Thus, this study provided the first proof-of-concept that CTCs can be used for noninvasive and sensitive detection of *ROS1*-rearrangement in NSCLC patients. Furthermore, CTCs from *ROS1*-rearranged patients showed considerable heterogeneity of *ROS1*-gene abnormalities and elevated numerical CIN, a potential mechanism to escape *ROS1*-inhibitor therapy in *ROS1*-rearranged NSCLC tumors.

More recently, we used the same approach to examine whether *RET*-rearrangements could be detected in CTCs from five NSCLC patients harboring this gene rearrangement in the tumor biopsy. Multiple abnormal FISH patterns including the *RET*-gene rearrangement were observed in CTCs from *RET*-rearranged patients (Fig. 9.1c) (Pailler et al. 2016). Similarly to the results from *ROS1*-rearranged patients, these data indicated a considerable degree of heterogeneity of *RET*-gene abnormalities in CTCs from these patients.

9.5 Detection *ERG*-Rearranged CTCs in mCRPC Patients

Recently, our group reported the results of the prospective PETRUS study of biomarker assessment in paired primary prostatic tumors, metastatic biopsies and CTCs from a cohort of 54 mCRPC (Massard et al. 2016). *ERG*-rearrangement was examined in ISET-enriched CTCs using fluorescent staining combined to FA-FISH and the semi-automated microscopy method. Using a negative cohort of ten breast cancer patients, we evaluated the hybridization background of *ERG* probes and found a median value of *ERG*-rearranged cells of 0 cell per 3 mL blood (range 0–6/

3 mL). The median value of *ERG*-rearranged CTCs was 16 per 3 mL (range, 3–57 per 3 mL) in the eight patients exhibiting *ERG*-rearrangement in the metastatic biopsy. The median value of *ERG*-rearranged CTCs was 3 per 3 mL (range, 0–6 per 3 mL) in the nine patients without *ERG*-rearrangement in the metastatic biopsy. At a threshold of seven *ERG*-rearranged CTCs per 3 mL blood, *ERG*-rearrangements were detected in CTCs of seven out of the eight patients exhibiting *ERG*-rearrangements in the metastatic biopsy while all mCRPC patients negative for *ERG*-rearrangements in the biopsy were negative in CTCs. The concordance between CTCs and tumors was of 88%. In contrast to tumor samples, multiple *ERG*-rearrangement patterns were detected in ISET-enriched CTCs indicating an higher heterogeneity of CTCs (Fig. 9.1d). These multiple rearrangement patterns observed in *ERG*-rearranged CTCs were associated with gain of native *ERG* copies far more prevalent than in the tumor samples including metastatic sites.

9.6 Conclusion

Although technically challenging, we have established an experimental process and a semi-automated microscopy method allowing to detect gene rearrangements such as *ALK*, *ROS1*, *RET* and *ERG* in filtration-enriched CTCs from NSCLC and mPCa patients respectively. By increasing the feasibility and reliability of filtration-enriched CTC assays, this automation method may be helpful to progress towards their standardization and validation. These results are still proofs-of-concept that required to be validated in collaborative efforts with others groups to progress towards to the clinic. These studies also provided information on the biological characteristics of CTCs such as the EMT status of *ALK*-rearranged CTCs and the elevated numerical CIN of *ROS1*-rearranged CTCs. Overall, our results may provide new insights on the role of CTCs in the metastatic progression of these tumors and the mechanism by which tumor cells can escape sensitivity to kinase inhibitor therapy.

Competing Interests The authors declare that they have no competing interests.

Funding CC is supported by the Agence Nationale pour la Recherche (ANR-CE17-0006-01). EP is supported by the LabEx LERMIT (grant no ANR-10-LABX-0033-LERMIT) and the Fondation pour la Recherche Médicale (grant no FDT20150532072). VF is supported by the Fondation pour la Recherche Médicale (grants no FDT20160435543). The authors are grateful for the research support of the Fondation de France (grant no 201300038317), the Fondation ARC pour la Recherche sur le Cancer (grant no 20131200417), Innovative Medicines Initiative 11th Call CANCER ID (IMI-JU-11-2013, 115749), Institut National du Cancer (PRT-K14-032) and Agence Nationale de la Recherche (ANR-CE17-0006-01).

Author's Contributions Manuscript drafted by FF and CC. All authors have read and approved the final version of the manuscript.

References

Baccelli I, Schneeweiss A, Riethdorf S et al (2013) Identification of a population of blood circulating tumor cells from breast cancer patients that initiates metastasis in a xenograft assay. Nat Biotechnol 31(6):539–544

Bergethon K, Shaw AT, Ou SH et al (2012) ROS1 rearrangements define a unique molecular class of lung cancers. J Clin Oncol 30(8):863–870

Chiarle R, Voena C, Ambrogio C et al (2008) The anaplastic lymphoma kinase in the pathogenesis of cancer. Nat Rev Cancer 8(1):11–23

Davies KD, Doebele RC (2013) Molecular pathways: ROS1 fusion proteins in cancer. Clin Cancer Res 19(15):4040–4045

Farace F, Massard C, Vimond N et al (2011) A direct comparison of CellSearch and ISET for circulating tumour-cell detection in patients with metastatic carcinomas. Br J Cancer 105 (6):847–853

Gainor JF, Shaw AT (2013) Novel targets in non-small cell lung cancer: ROS1 and RET fusions. Oncologist 18(7):865–875

Hallberg B, Palmer RH (2016) The role of the ALK receptor in cancer biology. Ann Oncol 27 (Suppl 3):iii4–iii15

Heitzer E, Auer M, Gasch C et al (2013) Complex tumor genomes inferred from single circulating tumor cells by array-CGH and next-generation sequencing. Cancer Res 73(10):2965–2975

Jemal A, Bray F, Center MM et al (2011) Global cancer statistics. CA Cancer J Clin 61(2):69–90

Ju YS, Lee WC, Shin JY et al (2012) A transforming KIF5B and RET gene fusion in lung adenocarcinoma revealed from whole-genome and transcriptome sequencing. Genome Res 22(3):436–445

Kantoff PW, Higano CS, Shore ND et al (2010) Sipuleucel-T immunotherapy for castration-resistant prostate cancer. N Engl J Med 363(5):411–422

Kerr KM, Lopez-Rios F (2016) Precision medicine in NSCLC and pathology: how does ALK fit in the pathway? Ann Oncol 27(Suppl 3):iii16–iii24

Kohno T, Ichikawa H, Totoki Y et al (2012) KIF5B-RET fusions in lung adenocarcinoma. Nat Med 18(3):375–377

Lipson D, Capelletti M, Yelensky R et al (2012) Identification of new ALK and RET gene fusions from colorectal and lung cancer biopsies. Nat Med 18(3):382–384

Massard C, Oulhen M, Le Moulec S et al (2016) Phenotypic and genetic heterogeneity of tumor tissue and circulating tumor cells in patients with metastatic castrationresistant prostate cancer: a report from the PETRUS prospective study. Oncotarget 7(34):55069–55082

Oxnard GR, Binder A, Janne PA (2013) New targetable oncogenes in non-small-cell lung cancer. J Clin Oncol 31(8):1097–1104

Pailler E, Adam J, Barthelemy A et al (2013) Detection of circulating tumor cells harboring a unique ALK rearrangement in ALK-positive non-small-cell lung cancer. J Clin Oncol 31 (18):2273–2281

Pailler E, Auger N, Lindsay CR et al (2015) High level of chromosomal instability in circulating tumor cells of ROS1-rearranged non-small-cell lung cancer. Ann Oncol 26(7):1408–1415

Pailler E, Oulhen M, Billiot F et al (2016) Method for semi-automated microscopy of filtration-enriched circulating tumor cells. BMC Cancer 16:477

Pao W, Girard N (2011) New driver mutations in non-small-cell lung cancer. Lancet Oncol 12 (2):175–180

Rikova K, Guo A, Zeng Q et al (2007) Global survey of phosphotyrosine signaling identifies oncogenic kinases in lung cancer. Cell 131(6):1190–1203

Ryan CJ, Smith MR, de Bono JS et al (2013) Abiraterone in metastatic prostate cancer without previous chemotherapy. N Engl J Med 368(2):138–148

Scher HI, Fizazi K, Saad F et al (2012) Increased survival with enzalutamide in prostate cancer after chemotherapy. N Engl J Med 367(13):1187–1197

Sequist LV, Bell DW, Lynch TJ et al (2007) Molecular predictors of response to epidermal growth factor receptor antagonists in non-small-cell lung cancer. J Clin Oncol 25(5):587–595
Shames DS, Wistuba II (2014) The evolving genomic classification of lung cancer. J Pathol 232 (2):121–133
Shaw AT, Kim DW, Nakagawa K et al (2013) Crizotinib versus chemotherapy in advanced ALK-positive lung cancer. N Engl J Med 368(25):2385–2394
Soda M, Choi YL, Enomoto M et al (2007) Identification of the transforming EML4-ALK fusion gene in non-small-cell lung cancer. Nature 448(7153):561–566
Solomon B, Soria JC (2016) The continuum of care for ALK-positive NSCLC: from diagnosis to new treatment options = an overview. Ann Oncol 27(Suppl 3):iii1–iii3
Takeuchi K, Soda M, Togashi Y et al (2012) RET, ROS1 and ALK fusions in lung cancer. Nat Med 18(3):378–381
Tannock IF, de Wit R, Berry WR et al (2004) Docetaxel plus prednisone or mitoxantrone plus prednisone for advanced prostate cancer. N Engl J Med 351(15):1502–1512

Chapter 10
Enrichment, Isolation and Molecular Characterization of EpCAM-Negative Circulating Tumor Cells

Rita Lampignano, Helen Schneck, Martin Neumann, Tanja Fehm, and Hans Neubauer

Abstract The presence of EpCAM-positive circulating tumor cells (CTCs) in the peripheral blood is associated with poor clinical outcomes in breast, colorectal and prostate cancer, as well as the prognosis of other tumor types. In addition, recent studies have suggested that the presence of CTCs undergoing epithelial-to-mesenchymal transition and, as such, may exhibit reduced or no expression of epithelial proteins e.g. EpCAM, might be related to disease progression in metastatic breast cancer (MBC) patients. Analyzing the neoplastic nature of this EpCAM-low/negative (EpCAM-neg) subpopulation remains an open issue as the current standard detection methods for CTCs are not efficient at identifying this subpopulation of cells. The possible association of EpCAM-neg CTCs with EpCAM-positive (EpCAM-pos) CTCs and role in the clinicopathological features and prognosis of MBC patients has still to be demonstrated. Several technologies have been developed and are currently being tested for the identification and the downstream analyses of EpCAM-pos CTCs. These technologies can be adapted and implemented into workflows to isolate and investigate EpCAM-neg cells to understand their biology and clinical relevance. This chapter will endeavour to explain the rationale behind the identification and analyses of all CTC subgroups, as well as to review the current strategies employed to enrich, isolate and characterize EpCAM-negative CTCs. Finally, the latest findings in the field will briefly be discussed with regard to their clinical relevance.

Keywords Single cell isolation • Molecular analysis • EPCAM-negative

---

R. Lampignano • H. Schneck • M. Neumann • T. Fehm
Department of Obstetrics and Gynecology, University Hospital and Medical Faculty of the Heinrich-Heine University Duesseldorf, Duesseldorf, Germany

H. Neubauer (✉)
Forschungslabore der Frauenklinik des, Universitätsklinikums Düsseldorf, Life Science Center, Merowingerplatz 1A, 40225 Düsseldorf, Germany
e-mail: Hans.Neubauer@med.uni-duesseldorf.de

M.J.M. Magbanua, J.W. Park (eds.), *Isolation and Molecular Characterization of Circulating Tumor Cells*, Advances in Experimental Medicine and Biology 994,
DOI 10.1007/978-3-319-55947-6_10

10.1 Circulating Tumor Cells – Optimal Candidates as "Liquid Biopsy"

Circulating tumor cells (CTCs) are cancer cells that can be found in the blood circulation after they have descended from primary tumours, their recurrences or from metastatic lesions (Joosse et al. 2015). Due to the lack of unique characteristics for these carcinoma cells, epithelial markers like the epithelial cell adhesion molecule (EpCAM) were chosen to identify and enrich CTCs in the peripheral blood, an environment which is normally negative for epithelial cells. The presence of EpCAM-positive CTCs in the peripheral blood is clearly associated with poor clinical outcomes in breast (Cristofanilli et al. 2004), colorectal (Cohen et al. 2008) and prostate cancer (de Bono et al. 2008), but has also been linked to prognosis in other tumor entities (Krebs et al. 2011; Hiltermann et al. 2012).

In opposite to tumor biopsies, CTCs can be obtained in a low invasive, fast and easy fashion, making them ideal candidates to serve as 'liquid biopsy'. The big hope is that current treatment regimen can be optimized based on the CTCs' geno- or phenotype in order to provide a benefit for the patients suffering from cancer (Pantel and Alix-Panabières 2010). To realize this, CTC analysis has to go beyond pure CTC enumeration to detailed single CTC enrichment and molecular characterization, finally aiming to understand the CTCs' biology as well as uncovering mechanisms involved in therapy resistance and systemic cancer progression. This demand to comprehensively investigate the CTCs' molecular and functional properties is complicated by the low frequency of CTCs in the peripheral blood, their genotypic and phenotypic heterogeneity and their variable capacities to metastasize (Pantel and Alix-Panabières 2010). Because of these challenges, an important step towards CTC characterization consists in the development of highly sensitive and specific enrichment and analysis strategies, which – in the optimal situation – do not discriminate between CTC subpopulations. Up to now, most established methods to detect CTCs are based on their expression of EpCAM. However, since some cancers were reported to express EpCAM at variable levels, the question was raised if we are only looking at the tip of the iceberg (Rao et al. 2005; Konigsberg et al. 2011; Mostert et al. 2011; Barradas and Terstappen 2013).

10.2 Not All Tumor Derived Cells in the Blood Are EpCAM-Positive

The epithelial cell adhesion molecule (EpCAM), a glycosylated transmembrane protein, was identified more than 35 years ago as one of the first tumour-associated antigens (Herlyn et al. 1979). Besides its function in homotypic cell adhesion, EpCAM represents a cell surface receptor which is involved in cellular processes such as proliferation, migration and differentiation (Maetzel et al. 2009). This protein is strongly expressed in epithelia and in most carcinomas, while being absent on cells in the peripheral blood (Balzar et al. 1999; Patriarca et al. 2012). For this reason, it became the prime antigen to identify and isolate CTCs and was implemented as antigen of choice into the FDA-approved CellSearch® assay (Janssen Diagnostics), which represents the 'gold standard' in the automatic CTC enrichment and detection (Terstappen et al. 1998; Cristofanilli et al. 2004).

However, solely relying on EpCAM expression for CTC enrichment has been recognized to have critical limitations as data indicate that EpCAM is heterogeneously or even not expressed on some cancers, cancer subtypes and CTCs (Rao et al. 2005; Konigsberg et al. 2011; Mostert et al. 2011). In support of this, it was reported that CellSearch® is unable to detect CTCs in about 36% of metastatic breast cancer patients (Mego et al. 2011), and similar data are also published for lung cancer as well (Bozzetti et al. 2015; de Wit et al. 2015; Chudziak et al. 2016). In addition, CellSearch® fails to efficiently detect EpCAM-low/negative breast cancer cell lines. These are primarily related to the basal-like subtype exhibiting a more aggressive mesenchymal phenotype (Sarrió et al. 2008; Sieuwerts et al. 2009; Punnoose et al. 2010).

These findings and recent reports – which demonstrate that EpCAM-negative CTC subpopulations can be observed apart from breast and lung cancer in several other tumor entities including prostate (Xu et al. 2015), esophageal (Driemel et al. 2014) and colorectal (Yokobori et al. 2013) cancer – underscore that EpCAM is indeed not applicable as a universally valid antigen to detect the whole CTC population (Lustberg et al. 2014; Schneck et al. 2015).

10.3 Modulation of EpCAM Expression

Several molecular mechanisms have been proposed to contribute to EpCAM modulation. These include downregulation by exposure to tumor necrosis-factor-α (TNF-α; (Gires et al. 2001) and to other cytokines (Flieger et al. 2001) as well as the loss of EpCAM expression upon hypermethylation of its gene promoter (Spizzo et al. 2007; Tai et al. 2007). Another explanation for a reduced EpCAM–positivity of CTCs can be deduced from the mechanism of its activation (Gires and Stoecklein 2014): its extracellular domain is cleaved by regulated intramembranous proteolysis and is released into the intercellular space (Maetzel et al. 2009).

The most important modulator of EpCAM expression, however, might be the process of epithelial-to-mesenchymal transition (EMT; Gires and Stoecklein 2014). During EMT, epithelial cells undergo phenotypic changes. They lose epithelial characteristics such as the expression of EpCAM, E-Cadherin, and keratins and gain mesenchymal traits such as the expression of vimentin. Eventually, cells lose their adhesive properties and gain motile and invasive features (Thiery 2002; Joosse et al. 2015). In agreement with the EMT-model, Yu et al. found a significant number of CTCs in metastatic breast cancer, which exhibit a partial or complete EMT phenotype and which are associated with disease progression (Yu et al. 2013). This observation could be confirmed by other groups who observed that EpCAM-negative breast cancer cells express high amounts of EMT-related genes (Gorges et al. 2012).

EMT is assumed to not only contribute to tumor invasion. It may also directly contribute to therapy resistance as well as to the escape from cell death by conferring stem cell capabilities (Thiery 2009). Therefore, it may be worthy testing whether proteins associated to staminality and EMT might be combined with EpCAM-based enrichment to detect and isolate the entire CTC content in patient's peripheral blood.

But still, although highly aggressive and invasive properties have recently been reported for EpCAM-negative CTCs (Gorges et al. 2012; Yu et al. 2013), the impact of EMT-like cancer cells, concerning metastatic tumor spread, still has to be investigated and metastasis-initiating cell fractions need to be identified.

10.4 Enrichment of EpCAM-Negative CTCs

For the detection and isolation of EpCAM-negative CTCs the same general considerations have to be taken into account that are valid for EpCAM-positive CTCs: both are rare events within the peripheral blood requiring highly sensitive and specific enrichment methods to precisely capture cells down to a frequency of 1 in 10^7–10^8 white blood cells (WBCs)/ml. Consequently, these assays should enable to enrich a maximum number of true positive events while the identification of false positive events – by e.g. non-specific labelling or false negative results, or by no or low expression of an antigen – should be kept to a minimum (Allan and Keeney 2010). Apart from sensitivity and specificity, CTC enrichment further demands for purity, reproducibility and reliability (Gabriel et al. 2016). Purity of EpCAM-positive CTCs is normally verified by staining the cells for nuclear DNA, positive immune labeling for cytokeratins and negativity for the leukocyte common antigen CD45. In addition to these characteristics, putative EpCAM-negative CTCs should be confirmed by testing them for the absence of EpCAM expression (Fig. 10.1).

To overcome the above described major intrinsic limitations of the EpCAM-based CTC isolation methodologies, in recent years several investigators have developed enrichment approaches which can be divided in a) label-dependent methods that target antigens presented by CTCs which are distinct from EpCAM (Mostert et al. 2011; Albuquerque et al. 2012; Mostert et al. 2012; Schneck et al. 2015) and b) label-independent techniques that enrich for CTCs based on their different physical cell properties such as size, deformability and density (Alix-Panabières and Pantel 2013; Joosse et al. 2015; Fig. 10.2). All of these alternative techniques are still at an experimental stage and due to lacking clinical validation they have not been approved for diagnostic purposes yet (Parkinson et al. 2012).

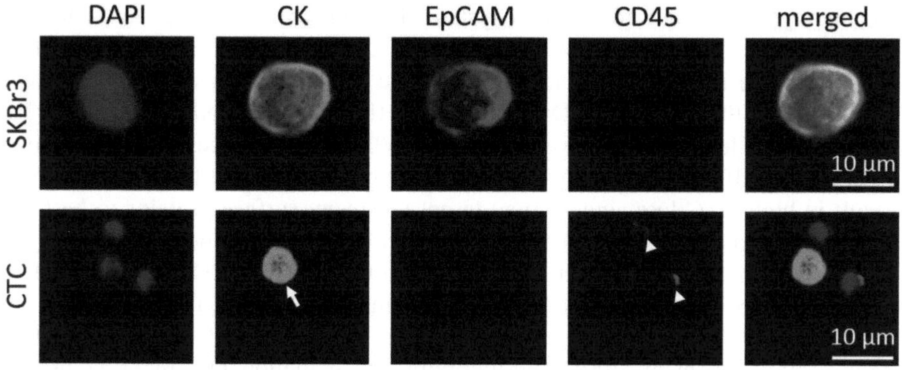

Fig. 10.1 Verification of EpCAM-negative cells
Images below depict a SKBR3 breast cancer cell (*upper row*) and a potential EpCAM-negative CTC (*lower row*) taken with immunofluorescence microspcopy. The EpCAM-negative epithelial cell (*lower row, arrow*) displays an intact nucleus (DAPI), expression of cytokeratins (CK) and negativity for EpCAM and CD45. *Arrow heads* indicate co-enriched leukocytes which are negative for CK and EpCAM but positive for CD45. The representative SKBR3 breast cancer cell is depicted as positive control for expression of CK and EpCAM. In the merge all fluorescence signals are overlayed

10.4.1 Label-Dependent Separation Technologies

Label-dependent strategies mostly rely on antibodies that target epithelial-specific and/or tumour-associated antigens. They are commonly applied to distinguish CTCs from cells of hematopoietic origin such as leukocytes. Label-dependent enrichment is primarily employed using immunomagnetic separation technologies (Esmaeilsabzali et al. 2013). Therein, antibodies are bound to matrixes such as magnetic (micro) beads (0.5–5 μm) or nanoparticles (50–250 nm) that can be provided pre-coupled or compiled according to the users' specific needs (Schneck et al. 2015). After a brief incubation of the blood sample with such antibody-coated particles, captured cells are separated from non-labeled cells by exposing them to a magnetic field (Esmaeilsabzali et al. 2013). In general, such immuno-affinity assays either allow for negative (indirect capturing) or positive (direct capturing) selection of the cells of interest.

10.4.2 Negative (Indirect Capturing) Selection of Cells

Since numerous blood-borne cells may share similar properties with mesenchymal or stem-like CTCs, leukocytes (WBCs) and erythrocytes are often depleted in order to avoid compromising the purity of enriched CTC fractions (Yang et al. 2009; Liu 2011). This can be achieved, for example, by immunodepletion using CD45 antibody-coupled Dynabeads™ (Thermo Fisher, USA) or RosetteSep™ (StemCell

Technologies, Canada). In the latter system bispecific antibodies lead to the formation of multicellular rosettes by crosslinking leukocytes and erythrocytes (Liu 2011; Lu 2015). The issue is to find the right balance between purity of CTCs and their loss since on the one hand CD45-based depletion was reported to reach 99.98% efficacy – still leaving up to several thousand WBCs/mL of processed blood sample (Liu 2011; Bulfoni et al. 2016). On the other hand, using an antibody cocktail may result in high CTC loss since it may target too many surface proteins to be truly non-specific to the CTC population. In support of this, immunodepletion with the RosetteSep™ CTC enrichment cocktail, which targets CD2, CD16, CD19, CD38, CD45, CD66b, glycophorin A (GYPA), and either CD36 or CD56 depending on tumor origin, was reported to result in a rather low recovery of epithelial cell line cells (~60%; He et al. 2008). Furthermore, the depletion rate reported by the manufacturer for this cocktail exhibits considerable variation, ranging from 3.2 to 4.7 log depletion.

Of course the advantage of leukocyte depletion is that it allows the isolation of cells that do not fulfill all the above-mentioned criteria accepted for CTC validation, such as round nuclei in cells expressing cytokeratin and lacking CD45. This is extremely important when aiming to isolate EMT-positive CTCs that do not show any immunoreactivity for EpCAM, cytokeratin and CD45. A disadvantage may be – and this still has to be demonstrated - that CTCs clustered with hematopoietic cells may be co-depleted by negative selection. However, CTCs with a mesenchymal phenotype can be recovered after immunodepletion (Lapin et al. 2016).

10.4.3 Positive (Direct Capturing) Selection of the Cells

Because of the limitations of EpCAM-based isolation methods and their potential challenges described above, many research groups are targeting alternative cell surface antigens using single antibodies or antibody cocktails to enrich for EpCAM-negative CTCs (Mikolajczyk et al. 2011; Lustberg et al. 2014; Pribluda et al. 2015; Schneck et al. 2015). Amongst others, these antigens include HER2 (human epidermal growth factor receptor 2), MUC1 (mucin 1), EGFR (epidermal growth factor receptor), osteoblast (OB-) and neural (N-) cadherin, the CUB domain-containing protein 1 (CDCP1, CD318), and PSMA (prostate-specific membrane antigen) which were employed for the enrichment of, inter alia, breast, colorectal, prostate, lung, and gastric cancer cells (Mikolajczyk et al. 2011; Kirby et al. 2012; Yu et al. 2013; Bitting et al. 2013; Galletti et al. 2014; Gabriel et al. 2016). CTC numbers in breast cancer samples were also proposed to be increased using a combination of anti-EpCAM enrichment with antibodies specific for the Thomsen-Friedenreich antigen (CD176; Schindlbeck et al. 2008), the melanoma cell adhesion molecule (MCAM, or cell surface glycoprotein MUC18 [CD146]; Mostert et al. 2011) or the integrin alpha 6 (CD49f; Mostert et al. 2012). Additionally, EpCAM-depleted breast cancer samples can be enriched for EpCAM-low/negative and CK-positive events using antibodies against the receptor for hyaluronic acid (HA) CD44, CD49f, CD146, cell surface CK8, ADAM8 (a disintegrine and metalloproteinase 8), c-Met/HGFR (hepatocyte growth factor receptor) and Trop2/TACSTD2 (tumour-associated calcium signal transducer 2), or magnetic beads coated with the extracellular matrix components such as HA (Schneck et al. 2015). By applying the latter antibodies immobilized to Dynabeads™ and Adembeads™, EpCAM-low/negative cells could be detected in 69% (20/29) of blood samples obtained from patients with metastatic breast cancer, while enrichment with Trop2, CD49f and CK8 attained 80% (76/95) of all identified potential CTCs (Schneck et al. 2015). However, exploiting non tumour-specifc antigens for capturing (e.g. CD44, CD49f, CD146) it has to be taken into consideration that additional validation steps on protein or genomic level are indispensable for proving that captured cells indeed originate from cancer. One possibility is single-cell aCGH (array-based comparative genomic hybridization), by which genomic aberrations can be determined and the malignant nature of suchlike isolated EpCAM-low/negative cells can be validated (Schneck et al. 2015).

Aside from bead-based approaches to isolate EpCAM-negative CTCs, alternative antibodies may also be attached to nanostructured surfaces (Wang et al. 2011; Lin et al. 2014), immunomagnetic microchannels (Hoshino et al. 2011) and other microfluidic chips (CTC−/Herringbone-Chip; (Stott et al. 2010), or even to medical wires approaches (CellCollector™, GILUPI; Saucedo-Zeni et al. 2012) which are so far used to isolate EpCAM-positive CTCs but whose versatility, in terms of detecting a broader CTC spectrum, may be extended in this way.

One issue of positive CTC selection and isolation may be that binding of cell surface markers with antibodies might induce cell signaling leading to phenotypic changes, e.g. EpCAM is involved in cellular signaling processes such as proliferation, migration and differentiation (Maetzel et al. 2009), as stated above. This may especially be disadvantageous when isolating viable CTCs for subsequent transcriptome analysis or for *in vitro* or *in vivo* functional assays.

Taken together, EpCAM-negative cells can already be isolated with antibodies specific for cell surface proteins but the biology and clinical relevance of these cells still has to be investigated.

10.4.4 Label-Free Separation Technologies

Label-free separation approaches exploit the different biophysical properties of CTCs and WBCs, such as their density, size, and deformability. Their obvious advantage is the potential to isolate heterogeneous and intact CTCs, regardless of their surface marker expression level, at high throughput and low cost.

10.4.4.1 Density-Based Gradient Centrifugation

Density-based gradient centrifugation has been traditionally used to fractionate blood into its cellular constituents. Since CTCs have a similar cells density as the mononuclear blood cells (Seal 1959) this technology is used to enrich for CTCs independently on their marker expression (Seal 1959; Weitz et al. 1998; Rosenberg et al. 2002). The scene is currently dominated by the standard method of Ficoll-Paque™ and by the novel OncoQuick™. The latter was specifically designed for CTC isolation and combines an altered density gradient separation medium with a porous barrier and a modified centrifugation protocol (Rosenberg et al. 2002). The barrier prevents contaminations of the interphase which is built up during centrifugation and contains both the mononuclear cells and the tumor cells. The performances of both assays have been compared in a study by Rosenberg et al. (2002) which intended to achieve a more effective enrichment of CTCs. In the experiments using blood samples spiked with cells of the colorectal carcinoma cell line HT-29, an increased tumor cell recovery rate was observed with the OncoQuick™ protocol. In fact, by significantly lowering the amount of the mononuclear cells in the enriched fraction, a faster and a more reliable CTC detection by immunocytochemistry or RT-PCR was accomplished. Pösel et al. (2012) suggested that a possible explanation for the higher cell loss observed with the Ficoll-Paque™ protocol could be the increased cytotoxicity of the separation medium.

The OncoQuick™ assay was successfully applied to enrich CTCs in blood samples from 30% of 37 gastrointestinal cancer patients (Rosenberg et al. 2002) and from 40% of 63 women with advanced breast cancer (Müller et al. 2005). In comparison to the CellSearch® instrument, CTCs were found in 23% of blood samples obtained from 61 patients' blood samples processed by OncoQuick™ protocol, as opposed to 54% obtained by immunomagnetic enrichment (Balic et al. 2005). Although the patients included into this study suffered from different metastasized cancers (breast, colon, rectal, gastric, ovarian, prostate, liver, esophagus, lung, testes, pancreas, kidney and two carcinoma of unknown primary) and provided CTCs with heterogeneous EpCAM expression levels and biophysical properties, the data show a high cell loss in tumor cell recovery by density-gradient centrifugation which may be due to the heterogenous densities of CTCs.

10.4.4.2 Size and Deformability: Filtration Systems

Some research groups described CTCs as being larger (Seal 1964; Allard et al. 2004; Cho et al. 2012; Coumans et al. 2013; Sollier et al. 2013) and stiffer (Marrinucci et al. 2007; Hou et al. 2008; Leong et al. 2010; Marrinucci et al. 2012; Shaw Bagnall et al. 2015) than hematopoietic cells, whence many enrichment technologies have been established to achieve high recovery rates by exploiting these physical differences. Among them, there are several assays using filter membranes (Seal 1964; Romsdahl et al. 1965; Vona et al. 2000; Zheng et al.

2007; 2011 Ntouroupi et al. 2008; Lin et al. 2010; Chung et al. 2011; Desitter et al. 2011; Adams et al. 2011; Kahn et al. 2004). Track-etched membranes are currently applied to capture tumor cells from whole blood using the "isolation by size of tumor cells" approach (ISET®, (Vona et al. 2000). The ISET® method consists of 10–12 wells containing a polycarbonate track-etched membrane which is perforated with 8 µm-diameter pores. By applying this filtration system, which is capable to process up to 1 ml of fixed blood, multiple clinical studies report successful recoveries of CTCs from liver cancer, melanoma, lung and prostate cancer (Vona et al. 2004; De Giorgi et al. 2010; Lecharpentier et al. 2011; Krebs et al. 2012; Chen et al. 2013), as well as higher CTC positity in comparison with the CellSearch® system in the following types of cancer: lung (50% *vs.* 39%, Hofman et al. 2011; 100% *vs.* 45%, Farace et al. 2011; 80% *vs.* 23%, Krebs et al. 2012; 100% *vs.* 33%, Pailler et al. 2013), prostate (100% *vs.* 90%, Farace et al. 2011), breast (85% *vs.* 75%, Farace et al. 2011), pancreas (93% *vs.* 43%, Khoja et al. 2012) and liver (100% *vs.* 32%, Morris et al. 2014). This discrepancy suggests that filtration may isolate additional CTC subpopulations which are not captured with an EpCAM-based strategy.

Certainly, the critical question is which one is the ideal filter in terms of pore size and numbers, filter material and thickness to discriminate between CTCs and WBCs. To address this question the most common filtration assays have been compared in a comprehensive study by Coumans et al. (2013) where the best recovery rates for different tumor cell lines spiked into whole blood were achieved with filters made out of a stiff, flat material, which does not interact with blood cells. Besides, the membranes should be 10 µm thick and should contain approx. 100,000 regularly spaced pores with a diameter of 5 µm. Using these parameters the recovery rates for cells of tumor cell lines Colo-320 and SW-480 which are of comparable diameter to CTCs (10.8–12.9 µm *vs* 10.7–13.1 µm for patients′ CTCs), were in average 20% and 70% respectively, and were comparable to those of the tested hemotopoietic cell lines HL-60 and K-562 (Coumans et al. 2013).

Microfiltration has recently been used to detect EpCAM-negative CTC in blood samples previously depleted of EpCAM-positive cells (CellSearch®). By successively combining both the technologies, CTC positivity rate in metastatic lung cancer patients could be increased from 15% EpCAM-positive only up to 41% EpCAM-positive/negative (de Wit et al. 2015).

Despite the speed and the high efficiency of filtration methods in capturing CTCs, some aspects still need to be improved: the harvesting rates and purity of CTCs, membrane clogging, which varies from sample to sample, and the difficulty to detach cells retained by the membranes in order to allow their downstream analysis. In addition, co-isolation of WBCs is very likely to occur, since the size of some WBCs overlaps with that of CTCs and this may therefore lead to the detection of false positive events by immunocytochemistry, as leukocytes were reported to slightly stain for cytokeratins as well as for EpCAM (Tibbe et al. 2007). Moreover, microfiltration will not enrich for small CTCs, although their clinical relevance is currently still controversial, since their small dimension could be either a sign of dormancy – associated with an increased metastatic potential – or a sign of cell death, as high percentages of EpCAM-positive tumor cells have been observed to be apoptotic (Marrinucci et al. 2012).

Another novel promising technology to isolate CTCs in a label-free fashion similar to the filtration is the Parsortix™ system. It consists in a three-dimensional microfiltration technique which captures CTCs while the blood sample is flowing through a disposable cassette containing a stair-like separation unit. The smallest step may be either 10 μm or 6.5 μm high, and has to be passed through by the cells. Since CTCs are larger and stiffer than WBCs they cannot slip through this gap and get stuck in it. Finally the captured cells can be released into a collection tube by reversing the flow direction.

By processing up to 10 ml of blood samples spiked with cells derived from primary tumours, different groups report recovery rates with Parsortix™ ranging from 30% up to 70% (Xu et al. 2015; Chudziak et al. 2016; Hvichia et al. 2016) with a leukocyte background between 1000 and 2000 cells in average. In comparison to the CellSearch® similar recovery rates were observed (PC3 cells: 43% Parsortix™ vs 40% CellSearch®, Xu et al. 2015; HT29 cell: 78% Parsortix™ vs 83% CellSearch®, Chudziak et al. 2016). In contrast, lower recovery rates were achieved with Parsortix™ in comparison to IsoFlux™ (PC3 cells: 40% vs. 90%, Xu et al. 2015). Interestingly, in samples of prostate, lung, breast and colon cancer the Parsortix™ harvested more CTCs than the CellSearch® (Xu et al. 2015; Chudziak et al. 2016; Hvichia et al. 2016) and similar amounts to the IsoFlux™ in prostate cancer (Xu et al. 2015), suggesting a high proportion of EpCAM-negative CTCs.

Parsortix™ was also shown to be compatible with the blood preservative tubes CellSave® (Chudziak et al. 2016; Hvichia et al. 2016), Streck Cell-Free RNA and Streck CytoCheck (Chudziak et al. 2016) making this system quite versatile and providing the possibility to process stored blood samples. Furthermore, tumor cells used in spiking experiments as well as CTCs recovered by Parsortix™ preserve their viability for further functional characterizations (Xu et al. 2015; Hvichia et al. 2016).

10.4.4.3 Size and Deformability: Microfluidic Systems

In the last decade, several size and deformability-based microfluidic platforms have been established to separate CTCs from the hematopoietic blood components.

Tan et al. (2009) developed a microdevice which contains crescent-shaped isolation arrays consisting of pillars with fixed 5 μm gaps width where cells in the blood can be fractionated and CTCs are captured. By applying this technology, they reported capturing and purity rates for breast and colon cancer cells of more than 80%. In addition the viability of the captured cells was ensured.

By exploiting shear gradient lift forces, another high-throughput microfluidic approach has been designed by Di Carlo and co-workers (Hur et al. 2011; Mach et al. 2011; Sollier et al. 2013). In this Vortex Chip blood samples are pumped through microchannels which contain square-shaped enlargements in regular distances. When CTCs in the laminar flow reach the square-shaped enlargements, due to their bigger size they are driven by the shear gradient lift force towards the centre, where they start to circulate. Whereas, smaller hematopoietic cells pass through the squares in the collection phase and are hence separated from tumor cells. The microvortices containing CTCs are stable until the flow rate is changed and the cells are subsequently flushed out of the device. This system was reported to process up to 10 ml of blood spiked with 500 cancer cells within 3 min, achieving a cell recovery of about 20%, purity rates of approx. 40% and a cell viability of about 90% (Hur et al. 2011; Mach et al. 2011). With an optimized version of the vortex chip, 7.5 ml of blood were processed in 20 min, achieving successful enrichment of CTCs from 4/4 breast and 8/8 lung cancer samples, with more than 5 cells recovered in 9/12 samples and a 57–94% purity rate (Sollier et al. 2013).

Hou et al. (2013) also exploited the inertial lift forces to develop another device for continuous CTC separation. The ClearCell® FX device consists of a spiral microchannel with a trapezoidal cross-section. Therein CTCs larger than 11 μm are concentrated along the short inner channel whereas WBCs flow along the outer channel. By applying this device to blood samples spiked with cells derived from tumor cell lines, more than 85% recovery rate was achieved. In a clinical validation experiment the ClearCell® FX was able to capture CTCs in 20/20 lung cancer samples with a recovery of 5–88 CTCs/ml at a flow rate of 3 ml/h. In some samples CTC microemboli as large as 50–100 μm were successfully captured as well, which may enable the analysis of CTC clusters.

Subsequently, Khoo et al. (2014) presented an improved multiplexed spiral version which is able to process 7.5 ml of blood in less than 5 min. They report a CTC positivity rate of 56/56 clinical samples with a recovery rate of 12–1275 CTCs/ml in breast cancer and 10–1535 CTCs/ml in lung cancer samples.

As described for filtration approaches, microfluidic methods do not discriminate between EpCAM-positive and EpCAM-negative CTCs. It can therefore be assumed that their application will increase CTC positivity rate and the numbers of isolated intact and heterogeneous CTCs. This has been confirmed in a study using the multi-orifice flow fractionation (p-MOFF) system, in which 4 of 24 metastatic breast cancer patients (16.6%) had only EpCAM-positive CTCs but about 1/3 of the patients had EpCAM-negative CTCs and about 50% of patients had both EpCAM-negative and EpCAM-positive CTCs suggesting that EpCAM-negative CTCs constitute the larger percentage of overall CTCs, even among patients who have both EpCAM-negative and EpCAM-positive CTCs (Hyun et al. 2016).

In summary, considering the advantages of CTC capture by microfluidic devices – such as excellent purity, high recovery rates, low leukocyte contamination, sample storage, low processing times, cells viability and possible downstream analysis – there are high chances that in the near future improved microfluidic systems will dominate the scene of CTC enrichment strategies.

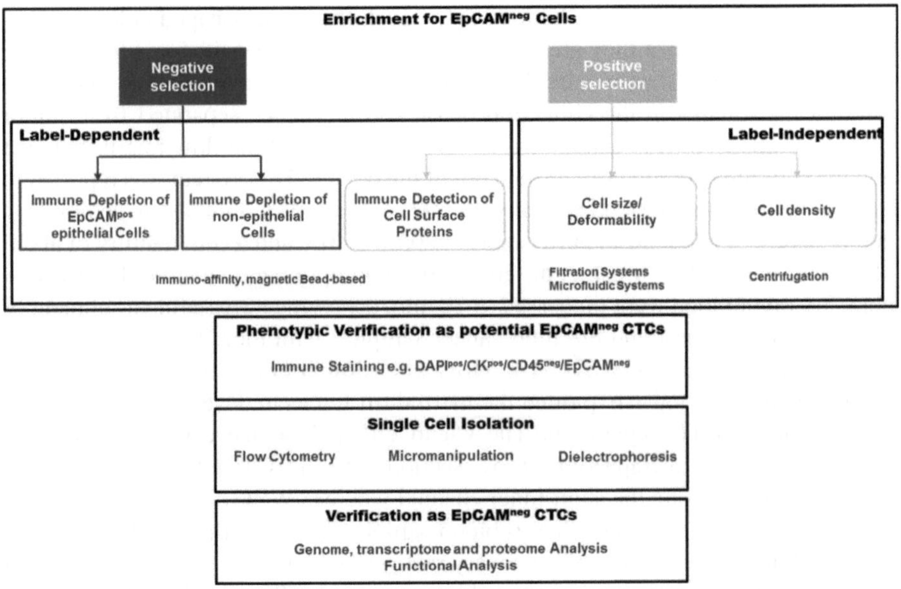

Fig. 10.2 Enrichment, isolation and molecular characterization of EpCAM^{neg} CTCs

10.5 Isolation of EpCAM^{neg} CTCs

Enrichment of CTCs using different devices and technologies will always face the problem of a background of unwanted co-captured WBCs, which are complicating further downstream analysis of the tumour cells. The big hurdle to overcome is to isolate pure CTC populations or even single CTCs with high efficiency. Several techniques are applied for single CTC isolation which have in common that they isolate the cells from cell suspensions by manipulating very small drops of liquid (flow cytometry or micromanipulation) or by directing a single cell (dielectrophoresis). Additionally, all of them require one of the CTC pre-enrichment steps described above. This is putting a big emphasis on the establishment of detailed workflows combining compatible enrichment and isolation technologies (Neumann et al. 2016). In addition highly trained staff is needed for such technologies.

10.5.1 Fluorescence Activated Cell Sorting (FACS)

Flow cytometry is often a standard equipment in many medical facilities and therefore available for the detection and isolation of CTCs. The advantages of flow cytometry are its fast sample processing and readout, providing measurements about cell numbers, their sizes and the expression of biomarkers. Sorting of CTCs has been combined with prior CTC detection by the CellSearch® system which is advantageously providing CTCs which are already labeled with fluorescence-conjugated antibodies. But still the fluorochromes used in CellSearch® have to be tested for the respective flow cytometry system (Neves et al. 2014).

One disadvantage of flow cytometry compared to e.g. micromanipulation is that it does not provide visual quality control of the isolated CTCs. The morphology of the CTC can already provide information about its integrity and the quality of its genomic DNA for molecular characterization (Polzer et al. 2014). Besides, CTCs are isolated in a relatively large volume of buffer, which may also complicate downstream analysis. However, if enough CTCs are expected within a sample, flow cytometry provides the capacity for automated high-throughput single CTC isolation (Neves et al. 2014).

10.5.2 Dielectrophoresis (DEP)

The isolation of single CTCs using dielectrophoresis exploits the differences in dielectric properties of cancer cells compared to normal blood cells. Currently, there are various technologies which utilize DEP in different manners. One of them, the DEPArray™ system (Silicon Biosystems, Italy), was built to isolate CTCs after they have been detected in the CellSearch® system (Fabbri et al. 2013). The content of a CellSearch® cartridge is loaded into a DEPArray™ single-use microfluidic bullet, which consists of an array of individual controllable electrodes and embedded sensors (Fabbri et al. 2013; Bolognesi et al. 2016). Next, dielectrophoretic cages are build up surrounding a single cell to postion it on the array. Fluorescent images are generated and the individuall cell of interest is moved to the outlet of the cartridge and it is finally released into a tube. This fully automated isolation process takes place within 3 h. One drawback of the DEPArray™ system is that a relatively high volume of the original sample is lost in the tubing system leading to potential cell losses. Besides, the device is best suitable for fixed cell suspensions (Fabbri et al. 2013; Bulfoni et al. 2016). An important advantage of the DEPArray™ system is that it enables visual quality control of the isolated CTCs (Polzer et al. 2014).

10.5.3 Micromanipulation

Micromanipulation can be performed manually by using pipettes or manually-controlled micromanipulators. In order to optimize cell picking in terms of speed and accuracy, semi-automated solutions combining inverse fluorescence microscopes and semiautomated-controlled capillary holders, have been developed, such as the CellCelector™ system (ALS Automated Lab Solutions GmbH, Germany). In general, glass capillaries can be utilized in horizontal or vertical orientation, whereby the latter layout – realized by the CellCelector™ - enables a flexible deposition of CTCs on various formats e.g. culture plates, PCR tubes or glass slides making it a very versatile technology. Advantages of the micromanipulation comprise cell imaging (as discussed above) and less shear forces compared to flow cytometry. Beside that, the correlation between the CTC count in the CellSearch® and the CTCs detected within the CellCelector™ is almost 100% providing a suitable combination of CTC detection and single cell isolation (Neumann et al. 2016). In addition, the risk of aspirating unwanted material is below ≤9% for cell densities of 25–50 cells/100 mm^2 (own observations).

One drawback of both the DEPArray™ and micromanipulation is the amount of time needed to pick a certain number of cells. Single cell identification and isolation using CellCelector™ from one CellSearch® cartridge can be performed by an experienced operator within 1–2.5 h – depending on the CTC numbers – with cell identification being the most time-consuming part. Therefore, it is advisable to define when micromanipulation or FACS sorting may be used in order to avoid isolating cells of minor quality due to extensive isolation times, which may interfere with molecular characterization.

10.6 Molecular Characterization of EpCAM-Negative CTCs

Beyond tumor cell capture and isolation, molecular characterization – e.g. mesenchymal, proliferative and stem cell-like features of EpCAM-positive and EpCAM-negative CTCs is required to gain more insights into their biology, which might pave the way for precision medicine and personalized therapy in the future. Like EpCAM-positive CTCs, EpCAM-negative cells can be characterized using either nucleic acid-based (DNA/RNA), protein-based or function-based approaches which are reviewed elsewhere (Magbanua and Park 2014; Lianidou et al. 2013).

Molecular characterization of CTCs is a growing field which is currently highly active. However, as already stated for the establishment of workflows, the compatibility of different applications has to be tested in order to answer the question if the analysis of both EpCAM-positive and EpCAM-negative CTCs is of academic or of clinical relevance (Polzer et al. 2014; Schneck et al. 2015).

10.7 Clinical Relevance of EpCAM^{neg} CTCs

While the clinical relevance of EpCAM-positive CTCs detected by the CellSearch® is indisputable (Bidard 2014), patients with undetectable CTCs generally have a more favorable outcome. However, some of these supposedly CTC-negative patients might also face worse prognoses, potentially due to the presence of

EpCAM-negative CTCs in their blood (Lustberg et al. 2014). This assumption is now beginning to be evaluated. Already in 2011, Mego et al. (2011) have provided the first evidence that EpCAM-negative CTCs might be of clinical relevance. In their retrospective study comprising a large cohort of metastatic breast cancer patients, the lack of EpCAM-positive CTC was positively correlated with brain metastasis. Following, an EpCAM-negative cell subpopulation was isolated and further characterized by generating breast cancer patient derived CTC lines and investigating biomarkers accounting for this pronounced metastatic competency (Zhang et al. 2013). Thereupon, a 'brain metastasis selected marker' (BMSM) signature was defined for CTCs being negative for EpCAM, but expressing ALDH1 (aldehyde dehydrogenase 1), HER2, EGFR, HPSE (heparanase) and Notch1, entailing high invasiveness and increased brain metastatic propensities when being xenografted into nude mice (Zhang et al. 2013). Vishnoi et al. (2015) further proposed that stem-like EpCAM-negative CTCs with a combinatorial expression of uPAR (urokinase-type plasminogen activator receptor) and integrin β1 are important for developing brain metastases, either as alternative or additive to the BMSM profile. Both markers are linked to breast cancer dormancy. Consequently, they posited that analyzing these EpCAM-negative CTC subsets provides a clinically useful tool with respect to brain involvement in metastatic breast cancer, thereby representing a step forward towards early detection and treatment strategies (Vishnoi et al. 2015). In a study of Lustberg et al. (2014) encompassing patients of different breast cancer subtypes, CK-positive circulating cells were characterised. Cells that met CTC-criteria (EpCAM-positive, CK-positive, CD45-negative) as well as other CK-positive 'atypical' circulating cell populations (EpCAM-positive, CD45-positive; EpCAM-negative, CD45-positive; EpCAM-negative, CD45-negative) could be identified using flow cytometry and immune-histochemistry. Patients presenting high levels of EpCAM-negative and CD45-negative cells ($\geq$100 events/ml) were associated with a significantly decreased overall survival (OS; $p = 0.0292$), whereas no correlation with progression-free survival (PFS) could be observed (Lustberg et al. 2014). Additionally, the authors proposed that circulating events being negative for EpCAM, but double positive for CK and CD45, might represent tumor-associated macrophages which may adversely affect patients' outcome as well (Lustberg et al. 2014).

On the other hand clinical utility of EpCAM−negative CTCs has also been questioned. A pilot study including lung cancer patients also aimed to determine whether the identified EpCAM-negative CTCs are of clinical significance (de Wit et al. 2015). Therein, blood samples were first processed by CellSearch® to subsequently enrich and enumerate the remaining EpCAM-depleted blood fractions for EpCAM-negative events by a combined filtration and staining approach. As opposed to the aforementioned study with breast cancer patients, the presence of EpCAM-negative CTCs was no independent prognosticator for OS ($p = 0.308$, cutoff of $\geq$1 CTC; de Wit et al. 2015). However, in their study the EpCAM − negative CTCs were detected using pan-cytokeratin antibodies, and thus pure mesenchymal CTCs in the EpCAM − negative cell fraction may have been missed. Apart from this, the tumor origin of identified CTCs was not confirmed. Mesenchymal CTCs may constitute large portions of the total CTC fraction (Yu et al. 2013), and transient phenotypes that are partly epithelial and partly mesenchymal may also exist (Yu et al. 2013; Poruk 2016). In contrast to the findings of de Wit et al., several studies have demonstrated that mesenchymal and transient CTC phenotypes are associated with inferior prognosis regardless of EpCAM expression (Aktas 2009; Mego 2012; Yokobori et al. 2013; Ueo 2015), thus emphasizing the neccessity of EpCAM-independent CTC enrichment.

Very recently, Bulfoni et al. (2016) conducted a prospective observational case study enrolling 56 patients with metastatic breast cancer to correlate the presence of different CD45-negative cell populations with clinical data. Blood samples were analyzed by using the DEPArray™ technology and staining of the sorted cells for epithelial (including EpCAM) and mesenchymal marker cocktails. Based on the marker expression, all cells lacking CD45 were classified into four groups: epithelial (E) and epithelial/mesenchymal (EM) CTCs, mesenchymal (MES) cells, and cells that were negative for all applied markers (NEG). Overall, a higher number of NEG cells was associated with the triple-negative breast cancer subtype – highly proliferating primary tumor – and with the presence of brain metastases (Bulfoni et al. 2016), whereby the latter seem to be in line with the data proposed by Zhang et al. (2013) demonstrating that CTCs with a brain metastatic potential do not express EpCAM and supporting the importance of going beyond the pure enumeration of CTC expressing this antigen. Conversely, bone metastases were strongly associated with the absolute and relative abundance of CTC expressing epithelial antigens, which is consistent with the observed association of bone metastases with a CTC number $\geq$5 cells/7.5 ml of peripheral blood, as estimated by the CellSearch® (Cristofanilli et al. 2004). Regarding association with prognosis, CTCs expressing both epithelial and mesenchymal markers significantly correlated with decreased PFS ($p = 0.016$) and OS ($p = 0.022/0.0016$), while the presence of MES cells was associated with a more favorable OS (Bulfoni et al. 2016).

Taken together, many experimental settings and clinical investigations have described the presence of non-epithelial/EpCAM-negative and undetectable CTCs in the blood of cancer patients, with only a few addressing the question whether these cells are of clinical relevance. Nevertheless, all of the herein mentioned studies acknowledge that CTC research with respect to the characterization of EpCAM-negative cell subsets and biomarkers enabling their identification is worthwhile and might be crucial to decipher a holistic view of mechanisms in metastasis (Bulfoni et al. 2016).

One important consequence may be concluded from current studies on EpCAM-negative CTCs: if CTCs in EMT predict the OS of the metastatic disease – as e.g. reported by Bulfoni et al. – this would suggest the existence of a subset of tumours whose prognosis is not significantly modified by currently available therapies. A similar conclusion has been reached by the clinical study SWOG S0500 (Smerage et al. 2014), where early switching to an alternate cytotoxic therapy in patients with persistently increased EpCAM-positive CTC after

21 days of first-line chemotherapy, was not effective in prolonging the OS. Those authors suggested that it would be more profitable for this subpopulation of patients to be recruited into prospective trials of novel therapies and to take advantage of molecular analyses of metastasis, CTC, or circulating cell-free DNA to guide treatment choices (Smerage et al. 2014). Based on the results reviewed above, one may also have to include EpCAM-negative CTCs into this panel – keeping in mind that this is still based on small sample numbers.

10.8 Conclusion and Open Questions

Although the identification of CTCs gained a strong impetus after the milestone publication by Cristofanilli et al. in 2004, the field of molecular analysis of single CTCs is still in its infancy. For EpCAM-positive CTCs it has been shown for several cancer entities that their presence in the peripheral blood is clearly associated with poor clinical outcome. Their predictive value or their relevance for therapy monitoring is still unknown. For EpCAM-negative CTCs the situation is even less conclusive, leaving many open questions regarding their biology and clinical importance. Recent models suggest that the detection of CTCs in epithelial-to-mesenchymal transition might be related to disease progression in metastatic breast cancer patients. However, current detection methods are not efficient in identifying this subpopulation of cells. The neoplastic nature of these cell populations is still an open issue.

Currently, technologies are tested for the identification and downstream analysis of EpCAM-positive CTCs. These can also be implemented into workflows to investigate EpCAM-negative cells in order to understand their biology. One interesting question may address their clonal relatedness to EpCAM-positive CTCs. Do both CTC subpopulations originate from the same founder cell? Do they share equal sensitivity to treatment or are there differences in their resistance mechanisms? Do both CTC subtypes have the same capacity to metastasize and to persist in suitable microenvironments? Recent evidence suggests that CTC clusters possess increased metastatic potential compared to single CTCs, and that cancer patients with detectable CTC clusters have a shorter survival (Aceto 2014; Chang 2016). CTC clusters also reportedly express mesenchymal markers indicative of EMT (Yu et al. 2013). Perhaps EpCAM-negative CTCs have a different potential to form homo- or heterotypic cell clusters.

There are already many technologies on the market, which allow isolation and molecular characterization of EpCAM-negative CTCs. The important step will be to define the best combinations to answer these open questions.

References

Aceto N (2014) Circulating tumor cell clusters are oligoclonal precursors of breast cancer metastasis. Cell 158:1110–1122

Adams D, Makarova O, Zhu P et al (2011) Abstract 2369: isolation of circulating tumor cells by size exclusion using lithography fabricated precision microfilters. Cancer Res 71 (8 Suppl):2369–2369

Aktas B (2009) Stem cell and epithelial-mesenchymal transition markers are frequently overexpressed in circulating tumor cells of metastatic breast cancer patients. Breast Cancer Res 11:R46

Albuquerque A, Kaul S, Breier G et al (2012) Multimarker analysis of circulating tumor cells in peripheral blood of metastatic breast cancer patients: a step forward in personalized medicine. Breast Care 7:7–12

Alix-Panabières C, Pantel K (2013) Technologies for detection of circulating tumor cells: facts and vision. Lab Chip 14(1):57–62

Allan AL, Keeney M (2010) Circulating tumor cell analysis: technical and statistical considerations for application to the clinic. J Oncol 2010:426218

Allard WJ, Matera J, Miller MC et al (2004) Tumor cells circulate in the peripheral blood of all major carcinomas but not in healthy subjects or patients with nonmalignant diseases. Clin Cancer Res 10(20):6897–6904

Balic M, Dandachi N, Hofmann G et al (2005) Comparison of two methods for enumerating circulating tumor cells in carcinoma patients. Cytometry B Clin Cytom 68B(1):25–30

Balzar M, Winter MJ, de Boer CJ, Litvinov SV (1999) The biology of the 17-1A antigen (Ep-CAM). J Mol Med Berl Ger 77(10):699–712

Barradas AMC, Terstappen LWMM (2013) Towards the biological understanding of CTC: capture technologies, definitions and potential to create metastasis. Cancers 5(4):1619–1642

Bidard FC (2014) Clinical validity of circulating tumour cells in patients with metastatic breast cancer: a pooled analysis of individual patient data. Lancet Oncol 15:406–414

Bitting RL, Boominathan R, Rao C et al (2013) Development of a method to isolate circulating tumor cells using mesenchymal-based capture. Methods San Diego Calif 64(2):129–136

Bolognesi C, Forcato C, Buson G et al (2016) Digital sorting of pure cell populations enables unambiguous genetic analysis of heterogeneous formalin-Fixed paraffin-embedded tumors by next generation sequencing. Sci Rep 6:20944

Bozzetti C, Quaini F, Squadrilli A et al (2015) Isolation and characterization of circulating tumor cells in squamous cell carcinoma of the lung using a non-EpCAM-based capture method. PLoS One 10:e0142891

Bulfoni M, Gerratana L, Del Ben F et al (2016) In patients with metastatic breast cancer the identification of circulating tumor cells in epithelial-to-mesenchymal transition is associated with a poor prognosis. Breast Cancer Res 18:1–15

Chang MC (2016) Clinical significance of circulating tumor microemboli as a prognostic marker in patients with pancreatic ductal adenocarcinoma. Clin Chem 62(3):505–513

Chen C-L, Mahalingam D, Osmulski P et al (2013) Single-cell analysis of circulating tumor cells identifies cumulative expression patterns of EMT-related genes in metastatic prostate cancer. Prostate 73(8):813–826

Cho EH, Wendel M, Luttgen M et al (2012) Characterization of circulating tumor cell aggregates identified in patients with epithelial tumors. Phys Biol 9(1):16001

Chudziak J, Burt DJ, Mohan S et al (2016) Clinical evaluation of a novel microfluidic device for epitope-independent enrichment of circulating tumour cells in patients with small cell lung cancer. Analyst 141(2):669–678

Chung Y-K, Reboud J, Lee KC et al (2011) An electrical biosensor for the detection of circulating tumor cells. Biosens Bioelectron 26(5):2520–2526

Cohen SJ, Punt CJ, Iannotti N et al (2008) Relationship of circulating tumour cells to tumour response, progression-free survival, and overall survival in patients with metastatic colorectal cancer. J Clin Oncol 26(19):3213–3221
Coumans FAW, van Dalum G, Beck M et al (2013) Filter Characteristics Influencing Circulating Tumor Cell Enrichment from Whole Blood. PLoS One 8(4):e61770
Cristofanilli M, Budd GT, Ellis MJ et al (2004) Circulating tumor cells, disease progression, and survival in metastatic breast cancer. N Engl J Med 351:781–791
de Bono JS, Scher HI, Montgomery RB et al (2008) Circulating tumour cells predict survival benefit from treatment in metastatic castration-resistant prostate cancer. Clin Cancer Res Off J Am Assoc Cancer Res 14(19):6302–6309
De Giorgi V, Pinzani P, Salvianti F et al (2010) Application of a filtration- and isolation-by-size technique for the detection of circulating tumor cells in cutaneous melanoma. J Invest Dermatol 130(10):2440–2447
de Wit S, Dalum G van, Lenferink ATM et al (2015) The detection of EpCAM+ and EpCAM– circulating tumour cells. Sci Rep 5:12270.
Desitter I, Guerrouahen BS, Benali-Furet N et al (2011) A new device for rapid isolation by size and characterization of rare circulating tumor cells. Anticancer Res 31(2):427–441
Driemel C, Kremling H, Schumacher S et al (2014) Context-dependent adaption of EpCAM expression in early systemic esophageal cancer. Oncogene 33(41):4904–4915
Esmaeilsabzali H, Beischlag TV, Cox ME et al (2013) Detection and isolation of circulating tumor cells: principles and methods. Biotechnol Adv 31(7):1063–1084
Fabbri F, Carloni S, Zoli W et al (2013) Detection and recovery of circulating colon cancer cells using a dielectrophoresis-based device: KRAS mutation status in pure CTCs. Cancer Lett 335 (1):225–231
Farace F, Massard C, Vimond N et al (2011) A direct comparison of Cell Search and ISET for circulating tumour-cell detection in patients with metastatic carcinomas. Br J Cancer 105 (6):847–853
Flieger D, Hoff AS, Sauerbruch T et al (2001) Influence of cytokines, monoclonal antibodies and chemotherapeutic drugs on epithelial cell adhesion molecule (EpCAM) and Lewis Y antigen expression. Clin Exp Immunol 123(1):9–14
Gabriel MT, Calleja LR, Chalopin A et al (2016) Circulating tumor cells: a review of non–EpCAM-based approaches for cell enrichment and isolation. Clin Chem 62(4):571–581
Galletti G, Sung MS, Vahdat LT et al (2014) Isolation of breast cancer and gastric cancer circulating tumor cells by use of an anti HER2-based microfluidic device. Lab Chip 14 (1):147–156
Gires O, Kieu C, Fix P et al (2001) Tumor necrosis factor alpha negatively regulates the expression of the carcinoma-associated antigen epithelial cell adhesion molecule. Cancer 92(3):620–628
Gires O, Stoecklein NH (2014) Dynamic EpCAM expression on circulating and disseminating tumour cells: causes and consequences. Cell Mol Life Sci 71(22):4393–4402
Gorges TM, Tinhofer I, Drosch M et al (2012) Circulating tumour cells escape from EpCAM-based detection due to epithelial-to-mesenchymal transition. BMC Cancer 12:178
He W, Kularatne SA, Kalli KR et al (2008) Quantitation of circulating tumor cells in blood samples from ovarian and prostate cancer patients using tumor-specific fluorescent ligands. Int J Cancer 123(8):1968–1973
Herlyn D, Herlyn M, Steplewski Z et al (1979) Monoclonal antibodies in cell-mediated cytotoxicity against human melanoma and colorectal carcinoma. Eur J Immunol 9(8):657–659
Hiltermann TJN, Pore MM, van den Berg A et al (2012) Circulating tumour cells in small-cell lung cancer: a predictive and prognostic factor. Ann Oncol 23(11):2937–2942
Hofman V, Ilie MI, Long E et al (2011) Detection of circulating tumor cells as a prognostic factor in patients undergoing radical surgery for non-small-cell lung carcinoma: comparison of the efficacy of the CellSearch Assay™ and the isolation by size of epithelial tumor cell method. Int J Cancer 129(7):1651–1660
Hoshino K, Huang Y-Y, Lane N et al (2011) Microchip-based immunomagnetic detection of circulating tumor cell. Lab Chip 11(20):3449–3457

Hou HW, Li QS, Lee GYH et al (2008) Deformability study of breast cancer cells using microfluidics. Biomed Microdevices 11(3):557–564
Hou HW, Warkiani ME, Khoo BL et al (2013) Isolation and retrieval of circulating tumor cells using centrifugal forces. Sci Rep 3:1259
Hur SC, Mach AJ, Di Carlo D (2011) High-throughput size-based rare cell enrichment using microscale vortices. Biomicrofluidics 5(2):022206
Hvichia GE, Parveen Z, Wagner C et al (2016) A novel microfluidic platform for size and deformability based separation and the subsequent molecular characterization of viable circulating tumor cells. Int J Cancer 138(12):2894–2904
Hyun K-A, Koo G-B, Han H et al (2016) Epithelial-to-mesenchymal transition leads to loss of EpCAM and different physical properties in circulating tumor cells from metastatic breast cancer. Oncotarget 7(17):24677–24687
Joosse SA, Gorges TM, Pantel K (2015) Biology, detection, and clinical implications of circulating tumor cells. EMBO Mol Med 7(1):1–11
Kahn HJ, Presta A, Yang L-Y et al (2004) Enumeration of circulating tumor cells in the blood of breast cancer patients after filtration enrichment: correlation with disease stage. Breast Cancer Res Treat 86(3):237–247
Khoja L, Backen A, Sloane R et al (2012) A pilot study to explore circulating tumour cells in pancreatic cancer as a novel biomarker. Br J Cancer 106(3):508–516
Khoo BL, Warkiani ME, Tan DS-W et al (2014) Clinical validation of an ultra high-throughput spiral microfluidics for the detection and enrichment of viable circulating tumor cells. PLoS One 9(7):e99409
Kirby BJ, Jodari M, Loftus MS et al (2012) Functional characterization of circulating tumor cells with a prostate-cancer-specific microfluidic device. PLoS One 7(4):e35976
Konigsberg R, Obermayr E, Bises G et al (2011) Detection of EpCAM positive and negative circulating tumor cells in metastatic breast cancer patients. Acta Oncol 50(5):700–710
Krebs MG, Sloane R, Priest L et al (2011) Evaluation and prognostic significance of circulating tumor cells in patients with non–small-cell lung cancer. J Clin Oncol 29(12):1556–1563
Krebs MG, Hou J-M, Sloane R et al (2012) Analysis of circulating tumor cells in patients with non-small cell lung cancer using epithelial marker-dependent and -independent approaches. J Thorac Oncol 7(2):306–315
Lapin M, Tjensvoll K, Oltedal S et al (2016) MINDEC-an enhanced negative depletion strategy for circulating tumour cell enrichment. Sci Rep 6:28929
Lecharpentier A, Vielh P, Perez-Moreno P et al (2011) Detection of circulating tumour cells with a hybrid (epithelial/mesenchymal) phenotype in patients with metastatic non-small cell lung cancer. Br J Cancer 105(9):1338–1341
Leong FY, Li Q, Lim CT, Chiam K-H (2010) Modeling cell entry into a micro-channel. Biomech Model Mechanobiol 10(5):755–766
Lianidou ES, Mavroudis D, Georgoulias V (2013) Clinical challenges in the molecular characterization of circulating tumour cells in breast cancer. Br J Cancer 108:2426–2432
Lin HK, Zheng S, Williams AJ et al (2010) Portable filter-based microdevice for detection and characterization of circulating tumor cells. Am Assoc Cancer Res 16(20):5011–5018
Lin M, Chen J-F, Lu Y-T et al (2014) Nanostructure embedded microchips for detection, isolation, and characterization of circulating tumor cells. Acc Chem Res 47(10):2941–2950
Liu Z (2011) Negative enrichment by immunomagnetic nanobeads for unbiased characterization of circulating tumor cells from peripheral blood of cancer patients. J Transl Med 9:70–70
Lu Y (2015) Isolation and characterization of living circulating tumor cells in patients by immunomagnetic negative enrichment coupled with flow cytometry. Cancer 121 (17):3036–3045
Lustberg MB, Balasubramanian P, Miller B et al (2014) Heterogeneous atypical cell populations are present in blood of metastatic breast cancer patients. Breast Cancer Res 16(2):R23
Mach AJ, Kim JH, Arshi A et al (2011) Automated cellular sample preparation using a Centrifuge-on-a-Chip. Lab Chip 11(17):2827–2834

Maetzel D, Denzel S, Mack B et al (2009) Nuclear signalling by tumour-associated antigen EpCAM. Nat Cell Biol 11(2):162–171

Magbanua MJM, Park JW (2014) Advances in genomic characterization of circulating tumour cells. Cancer Metastasis Rev 33(2–3):757–769

Marrinucci D, Bethel K, Bruce RH et al (2007) Case study of the morphologic variation of circulating tumor cells. Hum Pathol 38(3):514–519

Marrinucci D, Bethel K, Kolatkar A et al (2012) Fluid biopsy in patients with metastatic prostate, pancreatic and breast cancers. Phys Biol 9(1):16003

Mego M (2012) Prognostic value of EMT-circulating tumor cells in metastatic breast cancer patients undergoing high-dose chemotherapy with autologous hematopoietic stem cell transplantation. J Cancer 3:369–380

Mego M, De Giorgi U, Dawood S et al (2011) Characterization of metastatic breast cancer patients with nondetectable circulating tumor cells. Int J Cancer 129(2):417–423

Mikolajczyk SD, Millar LS, Tsinberg P et al (2011) Detection of EpCAM-negative and cytokeratin-negative circulating tumor cells in peripheral blood. J Oncol 2011:252361

Morris KL, Tugwood JD, Khoja L et al (2014) Circulating biomarkers in hepatocellular carcinoma. Cancer Chemother Pharmacol 74(2):323–332

Mostert B, Kraan J, Bolt-de Vries J et al (2011) Detection of circulating tumor cells in breast cancer may improve through enrichment with anti-CD146. Breast Cancer Res Treat 127 (1):33–41

Mostert B, Kraan J, Sieuwerts AM et al (2012) CD49f-based selection of circulating tumor cells (CTCs) improves detection across breast cancer subtypes. Cancer Lett 319(1):49–55

Müller V, Stahmann N, Riethdorf S et al (2005) Circulating tumor cells in breast cancer: correlation to bone marrow micrometastases, heterogeneous response to systemic therapy and low proliferative activity. Am Assoc Cancer Res 11(10):3678–3685

Neumann MHD, Schneck H, Decker Y et al (2016) Isolation and characterization of circulating tumor cells using a novel workflow combining the CellSearch® system and the CellCelector™. Biotechnol Prog.

Neves RPL, Raba K, Schmidt O et al (2014) Genomic high-resolution profiling of single CKpos/CD45neg flow-sorting purified circulating tumor cells from patients with metastatic breast cancer. Clin Chem 60(10):1290–1297

Ntouroupi TG, Ashraf SQ, McGregor SB et al (2008) Detection of circulating tumour cells in peripheral blood with an automated scanning fluorescence microscope. Br J Cancer 99 (5):789–795

Pailler E, Adam J, Barthélémy A et al (2013) Detection of circulating tumor cells harboring a unique ALK rearrangement in ALK-positive non–small-cell lung cancer. J Clin Oncol 31 (18):2273–2281

Pantel K, Alix-Panabières C (2010) Circulating tumour cells in cancer patients: challenges and perspectives. Trends Mol Med 16(9):398–406

Parkinson DR, Dracopoli N, Petty BG et al (2012) Considerations in the development of circulating tumor cell technology for clinical use. J Transl Med 10:138

Patriarca C, Macchi RM, Marschner AK et al (2012) Epithelial cell adhesion molecule expression (CD326) in cancer: a short review. Cancer Treat Rev 38(1):68–75

Polzer B, Medoro G, Pasch S et al (2014) Molecular profiling of single circulating tumor cells with diagnostic intention. EMBO Mol Med 6(11):1371–1386

Poruk KE (2016) Circulating tumor cell phenotype predicts recurrence and survival in pancreatic adenocarcinoma. Ann Surg 264(6):1073–1081

Pösel C, Möller K, Fröhlich W et al (2012) Density gradient centrifugation compromises bone marrow mononuclear cell yield. PLoS One 7(12):e50293

Pribluda A, de la Cruz CC, Jackson EL (2015) Intratumoral heterogeneity: from diversity comes resistance. Am Assoc Cancer Res 21(13):2916–2923

Punnoose EA, Atwal SK, Spoerke JM et al (2010) Molecular biomarker analyses using circulating tumor cells. PLoS One 5(9):e12517

Rao CG, Chianese D, Doyle GV et al (2005) Expression of epithelial cell adhesion molecule in carcinoma cells present in blood and primary and metastatic tumors. Int J Oncol 27(1):49–57
Romsdahl MM, Valaitis J, McGrath RG et al (1965) Circulating tumor cells in patients with carcinoma: method and recent studies. JAMA 193(13):1087–1090
Rosenberg R, Gertler R, Friederichs J et al (2002) Comparison of two density gradient centrifugation systems for the enrichment of disseminated tumor cells in blood. Cytometry 49 (4):150–158
Sarrió D, Rodriguez-Pinilla SM, Hardisson D et al (2008) Epithelial-mesenchymal transition in breast cancer relates to the basal-like phenotype. Cancer Res 68(4):989–997
Saucedo-Zeni N, Mewes S, Niestroj R et al (2012) A novel method for the in vivo isolation of circulating tumor cells from peripheral blood of cancer patients using a functionalized and structured medical wire. Int J Oncol 41(4):1241–1250
Schindlbeck C, Stellwagen J, Jeschke U et al (2008) Immunomagnetic enrichment of disseminated tumor cells in bone marrow and blood of breast cancer patients by the Thomsen-Friedenreich-Antigen. Clin Exp Metastasis 25(3):233–240
Schneck H, Gierke B, Uppenkamp F et al (2015) EpCAM-independent enrichment of circulating tumor cells in metastatic breast cancer. PLoS One 10(12):e0144535
Seal SH (1959) Silicone flotation: a simple quantitative method for the isolation of free-floating cancer cells from the blood. Cancer 12(3):590–595
Seal SH (1964) A sieve for the isolation of cancer cells and other large cells from the blood. Cancer 17(5):637–642
Shaw Bagnall J, Byun S, Begum S et al (2015) Deformability of tumor cells versus blood cells. Sci Rep 5:18542
Sieuwerts AM, Kraan J, Bolt J et al (2009) Anti-epithelial cell adhesion molecule antibodies and the detection of circulating normal-like breast tumor cells. J Natl Cancer Inst 101(1):61–66
Smerage JB, Barlow WE, Hortobagyi GN et al (2014) Circulating tumor cells and response to chemotherapy in metastatic breast cancer: SWOG S0500. J Clin Oncol 32(31):3483–3489
Sollier E, Go DE, Che J et al (2013) Size-selective collection of circulating tumor cells using Vortex technology. Lab Chip 14(1):63–77
Spizzo G, Gastl G, Obrist P et al (2007) Methylation status of the Ep-CAM promoter region in human breast cancer cell lines and breast cancer tissue. Cancer Lett 246(1–2):253–261
Stott SL, Hsu C-H, Tsukrov DI et al (2010) Isolation of circulating tumor cells using a microvortex-generating herringbone-chip. Proc Natl Acad Sci U S A 107(43):18392–18397
Tai K-Y, Shiah S-G, Shieh Y-S et al (2007) DNA methylation and histone modification regulate silencing of epithelial cell adhesion molecule for tumor invasion and progression. Oncogene 26 (27):3989–3997
Tan SJ, Yobas L, Lee GYH et al (2009) Microdevice for the isolation and enumeration of cancer cells from blood. Biomed Microdevices 11(4):883–892
Terstappen LW, Rao C, Gross S et al (1998) Flow cytometry–principles and feasibility in transfusion medicine. Enumeration of epithelial derived tumor cells in peripheral blood. Vox Sang 74(Suppl 2):269–274
Thiery JP (2002) Epithelial–mesenchymal transitions in tumour progression. Nat Rev Cancer 2 (6):442–454
Thiery JP (2009) Epithelial-mesenchymal transitions in cancer onset and progression. Bull Acad Natl Med 193 (9):1969–1978 discussion 1978–9
Tibbe AGJ, Miller MC, Terstappen LWMM (2007) Statistical considerations for enumeration of circulating tumor cells. Cytometry A 71A(3):154–162
Ueo H (2015) Circulating tumour cell-derived plastin3 is a novel marker for predicting long-term prognosis in patients with breast cancer. Br J Cancer 112:1519–1526
Vishnoi M, Peddibhotla S, Yin W et al (2015) The isolation and characterization of CTC subsets related to breast cancer dormancy. Sci Rep 5:17533
Vona G, Sabile A, Louha M et al (2000) Isolation by size of epithelial tumor cells. Am J Pathol 156 (1):57–63

Vona G, Estepa L, Béroud C et al (2004) Impact of cytomorphological detection of circulating tumor cells in patients with liver cancer. Hepatology 39(3):792–797

Wang S, Liu K, Liu J et al (2011) Highly efficient capture of circulating tumor cells by using nanostructured silicon substrates with integrated chaotic micromixers. Angew Chem Int Ed 50 (13):3084–3088

Weitz J, Kienle P, Lacroix J et al (1998) Dissemination of tumor cells in patients undergoing surgery for colorectal cancer. Am Assoc Cancer Res 4(2):343–348

Xu L, Mao X, Imrali A et al (2015) Optimization and evaluation of a novel size based circulating tumor cell isolation system. PLoS One 10(9):e0138032

Yang L, Lang JC, Balasubramanian P et al (2009) Optimization of an enrichment process for circulating tumor cells from the blood of head and neck cancer patients through depletion of normal cells. Biotechnol Bioeng 102(2):521–534

Yokobori T, Linuma H, Shimamura T et al (2013) Plastin3 is a novel marker for circulating tumor cells undergoing the epithelial-mesenchymal transition and is associated with colorectal cancer prognosis. Cancer Res 73:2059–2069

Yu M, Bardia A, Wittner BS et al (2013) Circulating breast tumor cells exhibit dynamic changes in epithelial and mesenchymal composition. Science 339(6119):580–584

Zhang L, Ridgway LD, Wetzel MD et al (2013) The identification and characterization of breast cancer CTCs competent for brain metastasis. Sci Transl Med 5(180):180ra48

Zheng S, Lin H, Liu J-Q et al (2007) Membrane microfilter device for selective capture, electrolysis and genomic analysis of human circulating tumor cells. J Chromatogr A 1162(2):154–161

Zheng S, Lin HK, Lu B et al (2011) 3D microfilter device for viable circulating tumor cell (CTC) enrichment from blood. Bimed Microdevices 13(1)

Chapter 11
Expression of Epithelial Mesenchymal Transition and Cancer Stem Cell Markers in Circulating Tumor Cells

Stefan Werner, Arnulf Stenzl, Klaus Pantel, and Tilman Todenhöfer

Abstract The characterization of circulating tumor cells (CTC) has the potential not only to provide important insights into molecular alterations of advanced tumor disease but also to facilitate risk prediction. Epithelial mesenchymal transition (EMT) has been discovered as important process for the development of metastases and the dissemination of tumor cells into the blood stream. In different tumor types, CTC with a mesenchymal phenotype have been reported that have presumably underwent EMT. Moreover, CTC with stem-cell like characteristics have been postulated as important drivers of tumor progression. Different platforms have been introduced to allow CTC enrichment independent of expression of epithelial antigens, as these may be downregulated in EMT- or stem-cell-like CTC. Both for CTCs with EMT- or stem-cell features different markers have been proposed. However, there is still a lack of evidence on the association of these markers with functional features and characteristics for stem cells and cells undergoing EMT.

Keywords Epithelial mesenchymal transition (EMT) • Cancer stem cell • Circulating tumor cells

11.1 Role of Epithelial Mesenchymal Transition in Solid Tumors and CTC

Epithelial mesenchymal transition has been demonstrated to be an important process in the progression of solid cancers in preclinical models (De Craene and Berx 2013). The detachment of tumor cells from their primary site and the invasion

S. Werner • K. Pantel
Department of Tumor Biology, University Medical Center Hamburg-Eppendorf, Hamburg, Germany

A. Stenzl • T. Todenhöfer (✉)
Department of Urology, Eberhard-Karls-University, Teubingen, Germany
e-mail: Tilman.Todenhoefer@med.uni-tuebingen.de

M.J.M. Magbanua, J.W. Park (eds.), *Isolation and Molecular Characterization of Circulating Tumor Cells*, Advances in Experimental Medicine and Biology 994,
DOI 10.1007/978-3-319-55947-6_11

of blood vessels requires a phenotypic change of tumor cells including an increased mobility and changes in the cytoskeleton (Thiery 2002). These changes enable tumor cells to invade the walls of small vessels and to enter the blood stream. This process represents a first and important step of tumor cell dissemination and formation of metastases (Alix-Panabieres and Pantel 2014a; Schilling et al. 2012). Once entered into the blood stream, tumor cells are able to invade distant organs such as the bone marrow (Mohme et al. 2016; Todenhofer et al. 2015). After entering these distant sites, the cells switch into a dormant state ("tumor cell dormancy") and can form the bases for later metastases or can form metastases directly (Uhr and Pantel 2011). The exact molecular mechanisms for dormancy and development of metastases have not been fully elucidated yet and are under intense investigation. The therapeutic modulation of these processes has a significant potential to inhibit tumor cell progression.

Several factors have been shown to significantly promote the process of EMT in solid tumor cells. These factors include physical and mechanical stress including Hypoxia and radiation (Zhang et al. 2013). Tumor cells in hypoxic conditions upregulate Hypoxia-inducible factor 1 alpha (HIF 1alpha) (Ye et al. 2016). HIF1a is a transcription factor stimulating the expression of various genes including genes involved in EMT including N-Cadherin and Vimentin. The upregulation of EMT by Hypoxia is assumed to contribute to resistance mechanisms of tumor cells (Marie-Egyptienne et al. 2013). Interestingly, mechanical stress to tumor cells such as the performance of core needle biopsy has been also demonstrated to upregulate markers of EMT and thereby contribute to the process of tumor cell dissemination (Mathenge et al. 2014).

The role of EMT in CTC is widely unknown. To date, no clear evidence is present showing that all CTC undergo a state of EMT during the invasion of blood vessels or during their circulation through the blood stream. So far, no preclinical model could conclusively prove that EMT is inevitable for solid tumor cells to become a CTC. Moreover, the clinical relevance of epithelial transition characteristics of CTC is unclear, although recent evidence suggests that the presence of CTC with mesenchymal characteristics is associated with aggressive disease (Krawczyk et al. 2014).

The process of EMT is closely related to the concept of tumor stem cells (Barriere et al. 2014). Cancer stem cells are a subpopulation of solid tumors having the potential of self-renewal and proliferation. These cells are assumed to represent the main promoter of tumor growth (Pardal et al. 2003). Targeting these cells has become an important goal in treatment concepts for cancer (Yoshida and Saya 2016). The concept, that only cells with stem cell like characteristics have the potential for renewal and replication implicates, that only this subpopulation of CTC is able to form distant metastases (Kreso and Dick 2014). Therefore, the identification of CTC with stem-cell like characteristics is assumed to be highly relevant when interpreting the clinical significance of CTC (Yang et al. 2015). The exact characteristics of these stem-cell like CTC have not been fully discovered yet. The understanding of the exact molecular features of these cells is an essential step for the development of platforms that allow the enrichment and molecular analysis of these cells. To assess the main characteristics of tumor stem cells, CTC platforms allowing in-vitro assays and culture of CTC are required. To date, most CTC platforms do not allow further culture of CTC limiting the evaluation of the main features of stem cells, replication and self-renewal (Alix-Panabieres et al. 2016; Pantel and Alix-Panabieres 2016).

11.2 Platforms for EpCAM Independent Enrichment and Analysis of CTCs with EMT Features

Several techniques have been applied to achieve an enrichment and characterization of CTC. A significant proportion of CTC platforms use antibodies coupled to immunomagnetic beads or nanoparticles in order to enrich CTC based on the expression of cancer-specific antigens (Alix-Panabieres and Pantel 2014b; Hegemann et al. 2016; Schilling et al. 2012). One of the mainly used antigens is EpCAM, which has been shown to be absent on benign blood cells and expressed by epithelial tumor cells. However, it has been shown by several groups that a subpopulation of CTC, especially CTC that have undergone EMT, have reduced or no EpCAM expression, which leads to a failure of EpCAM based enrichment platforms (Alix-Panabieres and Pantel 2014b; Hyun et al. 2016). On the other hand, it has been shown that EpCAM positive cells can also be present in the circulation of patients with benign colon disease questioning the specificity of EpCAM as a marker of tumor cells (Pantel et al. 2012). Therefore, intense research has been going on aiming to develop platforms that can enrich CTC independent of their EpCAM expression. These techniques use physical and biological properties of CTC in order to enrich them. The two main goals that should be achieved by a system with a good performance are a high recovery rate of CTC and a high purity. The high recovery rate is necessary to prevent false negative results and the loss of cells with high biological and prognostic relevance. Unfortunately, there is still a lack of data giving us an idea which characteristics these cells leading to formation of metastasis and disease progression have and how they can be distinguished from CTC that will make no harm. To evaluate the performance of any CTC platform, data on recovery rates is urgently needed. The most commonly performed approach for determining recovery rates of CTC is the spiking of defined numbers of tumor cell lines into the peripheral blood with subsequent quantification (given that the approach allows quantification) (Todenhofer et al. 2016a; Weissenstein et al. 2012). The problem with using cell lines is that they often do not perfectly represent the biology and heterogeneity of tumors (Park et al. 2014). On the other hand, studies claiming a high sensitivity of a platform due to higher numbers of CTC compared to another platform observed in patients' samples has to be considered with caution, as the real number of CTC cannot be determined currently (Andreopoulou et al. 2012; Van der Auwera et al. 2010). This is a current limitation of all CTC systems. A high purity is required in order to reduce the necessity of downstream analyses for the identification of CTC within the enriched population. Such downstream analyses inevitably reduce the recovery rate and may limit the options for characterization of biologic properties of CTC (such as culturing of CTC, in-vitro drug testing or single cell RNA analysis) (Alix-Panabieres et al. 2016). An example: A microfluidic platform that performs enrichment of CTC based on deformability and size of cells provides a 100% recovery but purity of only 5–10% (due to contaminating leukocytes in the outflow channel with a ratio of 10 leukocytes per CTC). In order to exactly identify the CTC, further analysis is required. One option for further analysis could be immunocytochemical staining of the cells for CTC specific markers. However, most of the markers currently use for immunocytochemical detection of CTC have an epithelial origin (such as cytokeratins). These markers can be downregulated in cells undergoing EMT (Barriere et al. 2014). Data on non-epithelial CTC specific marker is sparse. Moreover, the advantage of a marker-independent enrichment strategy compared to a marker-based enrichment goes partially lost when applying a marker-based approach as a second step. A second downside of immunocytochemical analysis of cells is, that fixation usually affects viability of cells. Viability is crucial for in-vitro analysis, drug testing and other functional analysis, which have a high relevance for improving the understanding of the biology of CTCs (Alix-Panabieres et al. 2016). Therefore, a high purity is crucial to prevent further analyses, loss of cells and long blood processing times. Non-optimal purity or recovery is an issue with all currently used CTC platform, either EpCAM dependent or independent ones. Table 11.1 provides an overview on EpCAM independent technologies for CTC enrichment including their advantages and disadvantages.

Antigen-dependent enrichment techniques allowing a specific enrichment of CTC with mesenchymal phenotype have not been broadly implemented yet. Mesenchymal markers such as N-Cadherin and vimentin are frequently expressed on PBMCs. Therefore, these markers are not suitable for antigen-dependent enrichment of CTC. One potential approach allowing an enrichment of malignant EMT-like CTCs is the negative selection of CD45-positive leukocytes. This negative selection is also integrated in the CellSearch platform (in addition to the positive selection of EpCAM). However, recent studies have shown that platforms solely based on depletion of CD45-positive cells still lead to enrichment of a high number of CD45 negative PBMC. The contamination with benign cells significantly affects the performance of downstream applications aiming to identify CTC within the enriched cell population.

To date, there is no broadly used and established marker for specific enrichment of CTC with mesenchymal phenotype. Several approaches have been introduced, but none of them has been conclusively proven to enable a specific enrichment of cancer cells.

In order to identify cells with mesenchymal features, the selection of appropriate markers is of utmost importance. Several approaches are possible. First, the parallel assessment of epithelial and mesenchymal markers has been demonstrated to be feasible. However, this requires that the CTC still shows expression of epithelial markers and hasn't switched completely to a mesenchymal phenotype. The

Table 11.1 EpCAM independent techniques for enrichment and detection of circulating tumor cells (CTC)

Platform	Enrichment of CTC	Detection of CTC	Advantage	Disadvantage	References
Density gradient centrifugation (e.g.Percoll, Ficoll-Hypaque)	Centrifugation of whole blood leading to cell distribution according to density	Multiple downstream applications possible, including immunocytochemistry (e.g. for CK)	Easy application, low costs	Significant contamination of PBMC layer with benign PBMCs, low purity migration of CTC to plasma fraction	Nastaly et al. (2014), Zhu et al. (2016a) and Konigsberg et al. (2011)
Microfluidic enrichment based on physical features of cells (e.g. Parsotix system)	Microfluidic enrichment of large cells with decreased deformability	Multiple downstream applications feasible, including mRNA sequencing, immunocytochemistry	Short processing time, enrichment with no significant impact on viability	Contamination with leukocytes, Identification of CTC based on CK staining (fixation required), recovery rate dependent on CTC type	Hvichia et al. (2016), Todenhofer et al. (2016c) and Gorges et al. (2016)
Filter-based enrichment of CTC based on physical features (e.g. ScreenCell)	Size dependent enrichment of CTC	Multiple downstream applications feasible, including mRNA sequencing, immunocytochemistry	Easy application low costs	Limited data on cell recovery, loss of small CTC, clogging	Freidin et al. (2014) and Mascalchi et al. (2016)
Dielectrophoresis-based enrichment of CTC (ApoStream, DEPArray)	Different dielectric polarization charges due to differences in morphology and conductivity of CTC	Multiple downstream applications feasible, including mRNA sequencing, immunocytochemistry	High recovery rate, high viability after enrichment	Low sample volumes required, change of conductivity during procedure,	Gupta et al. (2012)
Immunomagnetic based depletion of leukocytes (e.g. EasySep, Dynabeads, MagSweeper)	Removal of erythrocytes and immunomagnetic depletion of white blood cells (CD45)	Multiple downstream applications feasible, including mRNA sequencing, immunocytochemistry	Independent of CTC phenotype, high viability		Powell et al. (2012)

epithelial marker that has been used most commonly in this context is cytokeratin (Kallergi et al. 2011). However, repression of cytokeratins is a phenomenon frequently described in the context of EMT (Lamouille et al. 2014). Therefore, a parallel assessment of cytokeratins and mesenchymal markers is likely to detect only intermediate state CTC and not CTC that have switched completely to a mesenchymal phenotype. However, the sole detection of mesenchymal markers bears the risk to identify benign cells expressing mesenchymal markers. Leukocytes have been shown to express mesenchymal markers such as vimentin (Wu et al. 2015). A further potential approach is to perform a negative selection for leukocyte markers in combination with the detection of mesenchymal markers (Dinney et al. 2014; Wu et al. 2015). In the context of CTC with an EMT-like phenotype, the following markers have been discussed and used most frequently.

11.2.1 Vimentin

Vimentin is a major cytoskeleton component of mesenchymal cells and a major determinant for cell motility. It regulates cellular integrity, stabilizes cytoskeleton interactions and mediates resistance to mechanical stress. The expression of vimentin in tumor cells has been connected to the development of metastases by various preclinical and translational studies (Hu et al. 2004; Zelenko et al. 2016). The role of vimentin in CTC has been addressed by various studies. In breast cancer, CTC with expression of vimentin have been found more frequently in patients with advanced disease compared to early cancer. Moreover, co-expression with other EMT markers such as TWIST has been described (Kallergi et al. 2011). The expression of vimentin in CTC has been also described as poor prognostic parameter in various cancers including prostate cancer, pancreatic cancer (Lindsay et al. 2016; Poruk et al. 2016). One of the main limitations of vimentin is, that intracellular expression of vimentin is not only present in tumor cells but also in benign blood cells (Gorges et al. 2016). Therefore, the identification of cell surface vimentin, which is mainly expressed on tumor cells, has drawn significant attention (Mitra et al. 2015b; Satelli et al. 2014). The identification of cell surface vimentin provided the basis for the development of assays designed to capture CTC from patients with sarcoma. Moreover, the expression of cell surface vimentin has been shown in other solid tumor types to correlate with therapy response and outcome (Satelli et al. 2015a; Satelli et al. 2015b).

11.2.2 TWIST1

TWIST1 is a basic helix-loop-helix transcription factor that is involved in cell lineage determination and differentiation. Mutations have been linked to development of the Sezary syndrome (Howard et al. 1997). Moreover, TWIST1 has been described as significant contributor to the process of EMT and the development of metastases (Zhu et al. 2016b). TWIST1 inhibits the expression of E-Cadherin, a marker with significant relevance for an epithelial phenotype (Vesuna et al. 2008). Expression of TWIST1 correlates with poor survival in various cancer types (Riaz et al. 2012; Wushou et al. 2014). Inhibition of TWIST1 has led to decreased tumor growth and formation of metastases in preclinical models (Finlay et al. 2015; Khan et al. 2015). TWIST1 is a major component of the Adnatest® EMT kit, which has been one of the first commercially available platforms for detection of cells with an EMT like phenotype. After enrichment of EPCAM, EGFR or HER2 positive cells by immunomagnetic nanobeads, mRNA is isolated and a reverse transcription PCR is performed for TWIST1, Akt2 and PI3Kalpha. Using this technology in patients with breast cancer, it could be demonstrated that especially in advanced breast cancer, a significant proportion of patients have CTC with mesenchymal characteristics (indicated by expression of TWIST1, Akt1 or PI3Kalpha) and that neoadjuvant chemotherapy might be ineffective in eliminating these CTC (Aktas et al. 2009; Mego et al. 2012). In patients with bladder cancer, we could show that 12.5% of patients with metastatic bladder cancer have CTC with expression of TWIST1 whereas no patient with non-metastatic bladder cancer (Todenhofer et al. 2016b). Papadaki et al. analyzed TWIST1 expression in CTC of patients with early and metastatic breast cancer by immunocytochemistry and observed, that not only the expression of TWIST1 but also the subcellular localization have important clinical implications. A nuclear localization was observed with higher frequency in the metastatic setting whereas cytoplasmatic TWIST1 expression was more typical for early breast cancer. Similar to Vimentin, TWIST1 has been also described to be expressed by white blood cells. Therefore, assessment of TWIST1 should be performed in combination with other markers (such as negative selection of CD45) to exclude false-positive test results (Li et al. 2010; Merindol et al. 2014).

11.2.3 PI3K/Akt

The PI3K/Akt/mTOR pathway is an attractive therapeutic target in a variety of malignancies including renal cell carcinoma. Being activated by PI3K, Akt has a broad variety of downstream effects leading to tumor cell growth, invasion and metastases (Fresno Vara et al. 2004). One of the main effects of Akt in the process of EMT is the suppression of E-cadherin (Barber et al. 2015; Larue and Bellacosa 2005). PI3Kalpha and Akt2 are major components of the above-mentioned Adnatest® assay for detection of CTCs (Todenhofer et al. 2016b). Expression of phospho-Akt and phospho-PI3K was detected in CTC of >80% of patients in a cohort of breast cancer patients with early and late stage breast cancer using immunocytochemistry. Schneck et al. assessed the mutational status of PIK3CA in CTC from breast cancer patients with 7 out of 44 patients showing a SNP within PIK3CA. In patients with metastatic colorectal cancer, Ning et al. observed a significantly inferior survival of patients with expression of PI3Kalpha or Akt2.

11.2.4 N-cadherin

N-cadherin is an adherens junction that is mainly expressed in mesenchymal cells. It is a broadly accepted marker of EMT. Similar to other EMT markers, its overexpression is associated with increased metastatic potential and poor prognosis (Hui et al. 2013; Nieman et al. 1999; Yi et al. 2014). There is only limited data on the role of N-cadherin in circulating tumor cells. Armstrong et al. could show in a small cohort of 10 patients with breast cancer and 10 patients with metastatic CRPC, that after enrichment for EpCAM positive cells, 84% (CRPC) and 82% of CTC express N-cadherin (Armstrong et al. 2011). However, in the majority of patient cells positive for N-cadherin showed also a significant level of E-cadherin expression indicating that these cells have features of an intermediate state EMT CTC. In a study assessing the expression of N-cadherin and the stem-cell marker CD133 in CTCs of 26 patients with metastatic breast cancer, N-cadherin expression assessed by immunocytochemistry was present in less than a third of CTC emphasizing the dependence of the expression of these markers not only on the patient cohorts but also the technique used for expression analysis and CTC enrichment (Bock et al. 2014).

11.2.5 Zeb1

Zeb 1 is a zinc finger and homeodomain transcription factor with high significance for processes related to tumor cell dissemination and EMT (Bourcy et al. 2016). Recent preclinical evidence suggests that the inhibition of Zeb1 significantly reduces the metastatic potential of tumor cells (Bourcy et al. 2016; Zhang et al. 2015). Recently, ZEB1 expression has been used to identify a subgroup of CTC with an EMT phenotype and overexpression of other EMT related genes (Gorges et al. 2016). In a study evaluating KRASmutations in pancreatic circulating tumor cells, Zeb1 expressing non-WBC were defined as CTC (after depletion of CD45 positive WBC) (Kulemann et al. 2016). Interestingly, the majority of these Zeb1 expressing CTC also expressed CK19 as an epithelial marker and only a low proportion of patients showed Zeb1 expression only. Although limited by a low number of patients, Zeb1 expression was associated with worse overall survival. CK-negative Zeb1-positive cells had a worse outcome than CK-positive Zeb1-positive cells. Using qPCR for RNA analysis of CD45 depleted PBMC, no CTC with Zeb1 expression were identified in a cohort of 102 patients with early breast cancer whereas other EMT-associated transcripts (such as SLUG) were present. Using qPCR of CD45 depleted PBMC from healthy donors, the authors could show that a background expression of Zeb1 is also present in benign cells. In accordance with this, another study in breast cancer showed that Zeb1 expression levels in EPCAM/CD326 positive CTC do not have higher levels of Zeb1 than CD45 positive WBC (Giordano et al. 2012). This has to be taken into consideration when interpreting the presence of Zeb1 expression in PBMC.

11.3 Stem Cells in Solid Cancers and CTCs

In normal tissue stem cells represent a rare, slow-cycling cell type that owns unique biological properties. Of particular importance are their abilities to self-renew and to differentiate into diverse tissue-specific cell types. In general, these processes enable stem cells maintaining the ability to undergo extensive proliferation, if required, while preserving the undifferentiated state (Clevers 2011). The well-established multistep model of tumor formation and progression also postulates a single long-lived cell as source of cancer formation in which accumulation of genetic alterations occurs (Fearon and Vogelstein 1990). From there, the cancer stem cell (CSC) hypothesis proposes that cancer might be driven by tumor cells with stem cell-like properties. In other words solid tumors might be comprised of cells that are functionally heterogeneous, with only a subset of cells being liable for maintenance and progression of the tumor (Clevers 2011). Because tumor cells that are classified as CSCs often express mesenchymal markers, it has furthermore been postulated that during tumorigenesis the multipotent stem cell-like phenotype could be acquired through EMT. Particularly metastasis-associated traits, like heightened motility and invasiveness, are also characteristics of CSCs (Singh and Settleman 2010). Thus, metastatic cancer cells, which have presumably gained epithelial to mesenchymal plasticity, may exhibit a CSC phenotype. The CSC concept raises important implications concerning the identification and characterization of CSCs as the biological and therapeutic relevant subpopulation of CTC.

11.3.1 Therapeutic Resistance

First of all the CSC concept provides major consequences on appraisal of therapeutic resistance and tumor recurrence, which both represent severe clinical problems. Chemo- and radiotherapy are widely used standard methods of treatment in many cancer entities. These therapeutic approaches predominantly aim to eliminate highly proliferating and replicating cells. One of the proposed key characteristics of the CSC population is in contrast a low proliferative activity. Accordingly, CSCs may largely be able to survive these therapeutic regimens and proliferate after chemotherapy withdrawal to allow for tumor recurrence in a clinical setting (Mitra et al. 2015a). Here the CSC concept explains convincingly that rare quiescent tumor cells might cause tumor recurrence, which is the almost-inevitable outcome of effective treatment of solid tumors. Therefore, identification and characterization of potential CSC subsets in the whole CTC population may yield valuable information about treatment efficacy and presence or development of therapy resistance. This could allow for better-informed approaches to treat cancer patient efficiently.

11.3.2 Metastasis

In general, metastatic outgrowth in secondary organs is the main cause of cancer related death of solid tumors and CTC that have dislodged from the primary tumor are the potential new seeds of a secondary tumor at the distant site (Braun et al. 2005). On the other hand, metastasis is a highly inefficient process, and the presence of CTC does not inevitably imply that metastases already exist. Even though mere CTC count is a reliable predictor of relapse in solid tumors like breast cancer (Rack et al. 2014), which suggest that presence of CTC is in fact associated with clinical manifestation of micro-metastases or at least the presence of disseminated tumor cell in secondary organs. The ability to initiate metastatic outgrowth is nevertheless a major bottleneck in cancer progression. Thus, only a very small number of cells present in the entire CTC population, are even capable of successfully forming overt metastasis in a secondary organ (Coumans et al. 2013). For that reason it has been postulated that metastases arise from a rare subset of CTC with stem cell-like traits. These metastasis initiating cells (MIC) are potentially the most dangerous cells in the whole CTC population, with self-renewal, multipotency and tumor initiating capabilities. From there identification and characterization of potential MICs in the whole CTC subpopulation from patient derived blood samples might help to predict in which patient metastasis formation is most likely to occur and also enable further investigation of metastasis relevant pathways.

11.3.3 Dormancy

Another unwieldy clinical phenomenon is cancer dormancy, which is defined as an unusually long time between removal of the primary tumor and subsequent distant relapse in a patient who has been clinically disease-free (Uhr and Pantel 2011). For instance, in breast cancer clinical data suggest that a majority of cancer survivors have residual cancer cells for decades but can remain clinically cancer-free for their lifetime (Karrison et al. 1999). It has been proposed that also here slow-cycling or even quiescent CSCs are the source of latent metastatic growth (Uhr and Pantel 2011). Hence, CTC that are shed into the circulation might contain a small proportion of stem-like cells which can lodge in secondary tissue and remain in a quiescent state for decades. Later, depending on external influences these initial cells or a differentiated subset of them might start to proliferate again and establish micro- and macro-metastases in the secondary tissue (Uhr and Pantel 2011). Interestingly, during the progression of cancer and formation of metastasis, CTC that have lodged in secondary organs can occupy stem cell niches, a specialized microenvironment that normally regulate stem cell behavior, like cell differentiation and cell-cycle entry, of local stem cells. In these niches the disseminated tumor cells have to resist and overcome a non-permissive environment to survive. Increasing evidence suggests that, these disseminated cells have to adopt stem-like properties in order to colonize the stem cell niches (Lander et al. 2012). Once settled in the niches they do not depend solely on cell-intrinsic events but instead rely heavily on the right microenvironment to control the dormant state as well as maintain proliferative activity and fitness. It has been proposed that signaling pathways that maintain CSCs represent attractive targets for novel therapeutic approaches. For instance substances that suspend interaction of quiescent cells with the stem cell niches could render these cells vulnerable for chemotherapy (Lander et al. 2012).

Taken together the CSC model has important implications for cancer therapy and tumor stratification and for the major clinical problems involving therapy resistance and distant metastasis formation. Thus, great attention has been paid on comprehensive analyses of CTC heterogeneity and identification of stem-like CTC sub-populations in blood samples taken from cancer patients.

11.4 Markers and Functional Analysis of Stem-Cell Like CTC

Driven by the apparent benefits to directly target CSC populations in cancer patients, different studies aimed to further prove the CSC hypothesis and also to functionally characterize CSCs. Studies of hematopoietic malignancies identified populations of CSC that could be serially transplanted into NOD-SCID mice and resulted in leukemia, whereas injection of more differentiated leukemic cells did not. These CSC populations can be prospectively identified and enriched by characteristic cell surface expression profiles. The general approach for the isolation of CSC is fractionation of tumor cells using cell-surface markers characteristic of stem cells, followed by their implantation into NOD-SCID mice to assess xenograft growth and cellular composition (Shipitsin and Polyak 2008). Based on this methodology researchers have succeeded in enriching subpopulations of tumor cells with stem cell-like features and with tumorigenic capabilities also from various solid tumor entities. Nevertheless, the differentiation hierarchy and expression pattern of putative stem cell populations from solid organs are to a lesser extend characterized than in the hematopoietic system (Shipitsin and Polyak 2008). Despite this fragmentary knowledge, the most commonly used surface markers to identify CSCs from solid tumors are CD24, CD44, CD133, and ALDH1. Initially in 2003, Al-Hajj and colleagues could show in a xenograft transplantation model that only a minority of breast cancer cells had the ability to form new tumors in immune-deficient mice. In their study they prospectively identified and isolated potential CSCs by flow-cytometric enrichment of CD44high/CD24low tumor cells. Based on cell surface marker expression they were able to distinguish the tumor initiating from the non-tumorigenic cancer cells. These findings are consistent with the proposed CSC phenotype and the CD44high/CD24low expression pattern of mammary stem cells with multipotent differentiation ability (Al-Hajj et al. 2003). Similar results were published by Patrawala and colleagues for a xenograft transplantation model of prostate cancer cells. Although these authors enriched cells solely based on CD44 expression, they could show that CD44high prostate cancer cells are more proliferative, clonogenic, tumorigenic, and metastatic than the CD44low cell population. Subsequent molecular studies demonstrated that the CD44high prostate cancer cells possess certain intrinsic properties of metastatic progenitor cells (Patrawala et al. 2006). While not completely appropriate for breast and prostate derived CSC enrichment, expression of CD133 can be used for isolation of stem-like cells from a variety of cancerous tissues including glioblastoma and colorectal tumors (Galli et al. 2004; O'Brien et al. 2007). Initially demonstrated by Ginestier and colleagues, also expression and activity of ALDH1 facilitates the identification and isolation of normal and malignant human mammary stem cells *in vitro*, *in vivo*, and *in situ* in fixed tissues (Ginestier et al. 2007).

Yet, all these studies enriched potential CSCs from primary tumor material or pleura effusions and not from blood samples as subpopulation of CTC. A pioneering study by Baccelli et al. aimed in contrast to specifically isolate MICs from blood samples of breast cancer patients to support the hypothesis that CTC contain subpopulation of highly aggressive CSCs that are capable to colonize secondary organs. In this study blood samples from luminal breast cancer patients with known CTC count were depleted for hematopoietic cells and potential CSCs were further enriched for cell surface marker expression of EPCAM, CD44, CD47 and MET. Subsequently a xenograft assay using the isolated CTC for implanting into the bone marrow cavity of sub-lethally irradiated mice showed that primary human luminal breast cancer CTC contain MICs that give rise to bone, lung and liver metastases in mice. Also in a small cohort of patients with metastases, the number of CTC, with positive EPCAM, CD44, CD47 and MET but not with merely EPCAM expression correlated with lower overall survival and increased number of metastatic sites. Thus, these results define functional circulating MICs among total CTC in patient derived blood samples (Baccelli et al. 2013). Another study published by Lu et al. aimed however to directly identify and enrich invasive CTC from blood samples of breast cancer patients. The authors applied a functional cell separation method based on collagen adhesion to isolate CTC with an invasive phenotype from patient-derived blood samples. Using this technique they were able to isolate viable CTC from blood of stage one to stage three breast cancer patients. Gene expression and multiplex flow cytometric analyses on functionally captured and invasive CTC demonstrated the existence of distinct populations including these of epithelial lineage and stem or progenitor cells (Lu et al. 2010). Recently, also a permanent cell line designated CTC-MCC-41 has been successfully established from CTCs out of the blood of a colorectal cancer patient. Thorough analysis showed that CTC-MCC-41 cells resemble characteristics of the original tumor cells in the patient with colon cancer and display a stable phenotype characterized by an intermediate epithelial/mesenchymal phenotype and stem cell-like properties. Functional studies showed that CTC-MCC-41 cells induced rapidly in vitro endothelial cell tube formation and in vivo tumors after xenografting in immune-deficient mice. Thus, the establishment of this first colon cancer CTC line allows now a wealth of functional studies on the biology of CTC as well as in vitro and in vivo drug testing (Cayrefourcq et al. 2015). Nevertheless, there is also evidence that the CSC concept does not universally account for all tumors. For instance, a proof-of-concept study for ex vivo culture and characterization of patient derived CTC, which aimed to noninvasively monitor the changing patterns of drug susceptibility in breast cancer patients, did not observe increased expression of defined stem cell related signatures in CTC cultures, although the majority of the established CTC cell lines were tumorigenic in xenograft assays and derived from metastatic patients (Yu et al. 2014).

11.5 Prognostic and Clinical Relevance of Stem-Cell Like CTCs

The CSC hypothesis raises several important implications for the prognostic and clinical relevance of stem-cell like cells CTC. Foremost, if a population of biologically unique CSCs really exists, then tumor cells lacking stem cell properties will not be able to initiate self-propagating tumors, regardless of their differentiation status or proliferative capacity. Also curative therapy will require complete elimination of the CSC population. Patients who show an initial response to treatment may ultimately relapse if even a small number of CSCs survive (Marsden et al. 2009). Thus, the detection of CTC expressing markers of stemness in peripheral blood samples may represent a useful, conservative, diagnostic tool to guide treatment decisions. Additionally also functional analysis of stem-like CTC could improve understanding the mechanisms of tumorigenesis, dormancy, and metastasis. From there signaling pathways that maintain CSCs represent attractive targets for the establishment of new therapeutic strategies (Lander et al. 2012). Several studies aimed to identify and further characterize a stem-like subfraction of CTC. These studies are summarized in Table 11.2. Following some of these studies from particular tumor entities are briefly delineated.

11.5.1 Breast Cancer

The first study that analyzed stem cell characteristics of CTC from breast cancer patients was published in 2009 by Aktas and colleagues. They evaluated 226 blood samples from 39 metastatic breast cancer patients during a follow-up of therapy for

Table 11.2 Markers for detection of stem-cell like circulating tumor cells (CTC) in patients with different tumor types

Tumor entity	Determined stem cell marker	Patients included	Enrichment of CTCs	Applied analysis	References
Breast	ALDH1	130	Density gradient centrifugation	IF staining	Papadaki et al. (2014)
Breast	ALDH1	39	Adna Kit	qRT-PCR	Aktas et al. (2009)
Breast	CD44	45	Density gradient centrifugation	Flow cytometry	Wang et al. (2012)
Breast	CD44	38	Multi-parametric FACS	Multiplexed qRT-PCR and IF staining	Vishnoi et al. (2015)
Breast	ALDH1	28	Density gradient centrifugation	ALDEFLUOR assay and flow cytometry	Giordano et al. (2012)
	CD44		CD326- and CD45-based depletion		
	CD133				
Breast	CD133	16	EpCAM-based enrichment	IF staining in Cellsearch	Armstrong et al. (2011)
Colon	AGR2	73	No enrichment, blood-based analysis	qRT-PCR	Valladares-Ayerbes et al. (2012)
	LGR5				
Colon	CD133	50	Density gradient centrifugation	qRT-PCR	Pilati et al. (2012)
Colon	CD133	7	Density gradient centrifugation	Flow cytometry	Malara et al. (2016)
Colon	CD133	197	No enrichment, blood-based analysis	qRT-PCR	Shimada et al. (2012)
Endometrium	ALDH1	34	EpCAM-based enrichment	qRT-PCR	Alonso-Alconada et al. (2014)
	CD44				
Stomach	CD44	45	Density gradient centrifugation	IF staining	Li et al. (2014)
Liver	ABCG2	123	CD45-based depletion	IF staining in Cellsearch qRT-PCR	Sun et al. (2013)
	CD133				
Lung	ALDH1	48	Adna Kit	qRT-PCR	Hanssen et al. (2016)
Ovary	ALDH1	3	Adna Kit	qRT-PCR	Blassl et al. (2016)
	CD44				

(continued)

Table 11.2 (continued)

Tumor entity	Determined stem cell marker	Patients included	Enrichment of CTCs	Applied analysis	References
Prostate	ABCG2	70	EpCAM-based enrichment	qRT-PCR	Chang et al. (2015)
	CD133				
	PSCA				
Prostate	CD133	35	EpCAM-based enrichment	IF staining in Cellsearch	Pal et al. (2015)
Prostate	CD133	41	EpCAM-based enrichment	IF staining in Cellsearch	Armstrong et al. (2011)
Kidney	CD44	25	EpCAM-based enrichment	RT-PCR	Gradilone et al. (2011)

the expression of the stem cell marker ALDH1 along with EMT markers and correlated results with the presence of CTC and response to therapy. In this study ALDH1 transcripts were detected in 14% of tested blood samples from CTC negative patients, whereas in the CTC positive group ALDH1 transcripts were detected in 69% of blood samples. In non-responders, ALDH1 expression was found in 44% of patients, in responders the rate was 5%, respectively. This data indicates that a major proportion of CTC of metastatic breast cancer patients indeed shows tumor stem cell characteristics (Aktas et al. 2009). Subsequently, further studies were published that evaluated expression and activity of ALDH1 in CTC from breast cancer patients. By using triple immunofluorescence staining of individual CTC with anti-cytokeratin, anti-ALDH1 and anti-TWIST antibodies, Papadaki et al. found that CTC from patients with metastatic breast cancer, frequently express high amounts of ALDH1 protein and show in parallel nuclear localization of the EMT-related TWIST protein. This suggests that these CTC own stem-like characteristics and may prevail during disease progression (Papadaki et al. 2014). Besides, in a prospective study published by Giordano et al. a comprehensive approach was utilized to assess CSC features of CTC in 28 patients with HER2 positive metastatic breast cancer. Here, CTCs were enriched from peripheral blood using CD326- and CD45-depletion. In addition to transcript analysis of EMT marker expression in purified cells, these cells were analyzed using multiparameter flow cytometry for ALDH activity and for CD24, CD44, and CD133 stem cell marker expression. It was found that the CD326- and CD45-depletion cell fraction of patients with elevated expression of EMT-related transcripts also had significantly higher percentage of ALDH and CD133 positive cells in their blood than did patients with normal EMT expression marker. This indicates that patients with HER2 positive metastatic breast cancer bear CTCs with EMT and CSC characteristics (Giordano et al. 2012). Also expression of CD44 and CD24 has been successfully utilized to enrich CTC subsets related to the CSC phenotype from blood samples of breast cancer patients. To particularly isolate CTC subsets related to tumor dormancy Vishnoi and colleagues enriched for EpCAM and CD24 negativity but positivity for CD44 expression from peripheral blood of patients diagnosed with or without breast cancer brain metastasis. They combined their analysis with assessment of uPAR and Integrin-β1 expression, two markers directly implicated in breast cancer dormancy mechanisms. CTCs that were isolated by this method were successfully cultured in vitro in three-dimensional tumorspheres. Interestingly, proliferative and invasive properties of these CTC cultures were distinctive upon combinatorial expression of uPAR and Integrin-β1. Thus, this approach may enhance abilities to prospectively identify patients who may be at high risk of developing breast cancer brain metastasis (Vishnoi et al. 2015).

11.5.2 Colorectal Cancer

Studies on colonic crypt stem cells have contributed substantially to the understanding of stem cell biology of epithelial tissues and LGR5 expression is as a well-established marker for stem cells in the small intestine and colon (Barker et al. 2007). The prognostic significance of LGR5 transcript expression as biomarker in peripheral blood of colorectal cancer patients was evaluated by Valladares-Ayerbes and colleagues in 54 patients and 19 controls. It was found that LGR5 mRNA were significantly increased in blood samples from colorectal cancer patients compared to healthy controls. Moreover, heightened LGR5 expression in these blood samples correlated with metastasis, high-grade and poor overall. These findings indicate that the assessment of LGR5 in peripheral blood might reflect the presence of stem cell like CTCs in blood samples taken from colorectal cancer patients (Valladares-Ayerbes et al. 2012). Also expression of CD133 is a well-established stem cell marker for colorectal CSCs and has successfully been used to enrich and characterize potential CSC subsets in CTCs from colorectal cancer patients. Malara and colleagues separated heterogeneous CTC populations, which derived from whole blood samples of seven colorectal cancer patients. It was possible to distinguish two distinct subgroups of CTCs which were also associated with different clinical outcome. Thus, patients with prevalence of putative circulating cancer stem cells showing CD133 expression have a lower overall survival (Malara et al. 2016). Besides, Pierluigi et al. retrospectively evaluated prospectively collected preoperative blood samples to identify applicable circulating biomarkers in patients undergoing complete resection of metastatic colorectal cancer to the liver. Among seven analyzed genes the expression of CD133 was determined to be the only independent predictor of patient survival. The authors concluded that CD133-positive CTCs may represent a suitable prognostic marker to stratify the risk of patients who undergo liver resection for CRC metastasis, which opens the avenue to identifying and potentially monitoring the patients who are most likely to benefit from adjuvant treatments (Pilati et al. 2012).

11.5.3 Prostate Cancer

Similar results were obtained from studies analyzing blood samples of prostate cancer patients. In such a study published by Armstrong et al. expression of the stem-cell marker CD133 was assessed together with expression of EMT markers by immunocytochemistry in CTCs from 41 patients with castration-resistant prostate cancer. It was shown that the majority of these CTCs co-express the stem cell marker CD133 together with epithelial proteins such as EpCAM, cytokeratins, and E-cadherin and with mesenchymal proteins including vimentin, N-cadherin and O-cadherin. Based on these results it was suggested that stem-like CTCs may be highly prevalent among patients with metastatic epithelial tumors which might account for therapy resistance (Armstrong et al. 2011). Also Chang and colleagues set up a quantitative PCR method to detect EMT and stem cell gene expression status in peripheral blood derived from metastatic prostate cancer patients to validate whether this method could complement plain CTC enumeration. They collected and analyzed peripheral blood from 70 patients and enumerated CTC in these blood samples using CellSearch system. In parallel mRNA expression of prostate stem cell-related genes ABCG2, CD133 and PSCA and EMT-related genes TWIST1 and vimentin was assessed. In this setting positive stem cell gene expression indicated poor prognosis, whereas EMT related expression did not. Also for 40 patients categorized into the favorable CTC enumeration group, positive stem cell gene expression suggested poor prognosis. As a result, detection of peripheral blood stem cell gene expression could complement CTC enumeration in predicting overall survival and treatment effects in metastatic prostate cancer patients (Chang et al. 2015).

11.5.4 Other Cancer Entities

Also in blood samples taken from patients with endometrial cancer putative CSC subpopulations coexpressing EMT and stem cell markers have been identified. EpCAM-based isolation detected CTC in high-risk endometrial cancer patients and CTC characterization indicated a remarkable plasticity phenotype defined by the expression of the EMT markers and expression of stem cell markers ALDH and CD44 (Alonso-Alconada et al. 2014). Likewise in blood samples taken from hepatocellular carcinoma patients, EpCAM positive CTCs with stem cell-like phenotypes were identified. CTCs displayed expression of cancer stem cell markers CD133 and ABCG2 as well as expression of EMT markers. Additionally this phenotype was also associated with Wnt pathway activation, high tumorigenic potential and low apoptotic propensity. Hence, these EpCAM positive CTCs may constitute the tumor-initiating subpopulation in hepatocellular carcinoma specimens which may serve as a real-time parameter for monitoring treatment response (Sun et al. 2013). EpCAM based enrichment of stem cell-like CTC from hepatocellular carcinoma patients has also been utilized by Schulze et al. Their study demonstrates frequent presence of EpCAM-positive, stem-like CTCs in patients with intermediate or advanced hepatocellular carcinoma. Here, detection of these cells had prognostic value for overall survival with possible implications for future treatment stratification (Schulze et al. 2013). Recently, also in 86% of blood samples taken from non-small cell lung cancer patients ALDH1 expression was detected, indicating that in NSCLC a large fraction of CTCs are of stemness character (Hanssen et al. 2016).

In summary, several studies covering different entities of solid tumors have analyzed expression of stem cell associated genes in CTCs and in peripheral blood samples, respectively. Generally, the detection of increased expression of CSC markers like CD133, CD44 and ALDH1 was associated with poor patient outcome. This indicated that a rare CSC subpopulation among total CTCs really exists. Nevertheless, there is also evidence that CSC concept does apply to progression of all tumors. For instance, in one study analyzing whether melanoma is hierarchically organized into phenotypically distinct subpopulations of tumorigenic and nontumorigenic cells, the authors were unable to find any large subpopulation of melanoma cells that lacked tumorigenic potential. None of 22 heterogeneously expressed markers enriched tumorigenic cells and many markers appeared to be reversibly expressed by tumorigenic melanoma cells (Quintana et al. 2010). Moreover, the precise contribution of tumor initiating cells that express the defined stem cell marker is ill defined. As such, it was shown that CD133 expression does not identify the entire population of epithelial and tumor-initiating cells in human metastatic colon cancer. Both CD133+ and CD133- metastatic tumor subpopulations formed colonospheres in in vitro cultures and were capable of long-term tumorigenesis in a serial xenotransplantation model, suggesting that CD133 expression is not restricted to intestinal stem or cancer-initiating cells (Shmelkov et al. 2008). Furthermore, recent studies that were all based on genetic lineage tracing, describe various strategies employed by normal epithelial stem cell hierarchies to replace damaged or lost stem cells (Greulich and Simons 2016). As the CSC model of tumor cell hierarchies propose that commitment and differentiation occur unidirectional, these findings challenge the classification of a CSC and highlight that plasticity within a tumor cell population might be more common than appreciated in the classical CSC concept. The identification of rare but highly aggressive CTC subsets in peripheral blood is nevertheless of high clinical interest. Monitoring the outcome of systemic cancer therapies by sequential assessment of potential CSC or MIC subpopulation is feasible, but an appropriate methodology faces even more challenges regarding specificity and sensitivity than mere CTC enumeration. The recently launched and EU-funded CANCER-ID innovative medicine initiative aims to develop new, less invasive ways of capturing cancer cells and genetic material from tumors from blood samples and analyzing them for clues to what treatment is needed and how well drugs are working. Accurate CSC identification are in any case needed to implement the CSC concept into clinical practice and validated protocols for liquid biopsies could pave the way for interventional clinical studies on treatment stratification.

References

Aktas B, Tewes M, Fehm T et al (2009) Stem cell and epithelial-mesenchymal transition markers are frequently overexpressed in circulating tumor cells of metastatic breast cancer patients. Breast Cancer Res 11(4):R46

Al-Hajj M, Wicha MS, Benito-Hernandez A et al (2003) Prospective identification of tumorigenic breast cancer cells. Proc Natl Acad Sci U S A 100(7):3983–3988

Alix-Panabieres C, Bartkowiak K, Pantel K (2016) Functional studies on circulating and disseminated tumor cells in carcinoma patients. Mol Oncol 10(3):443–449

Alix-Panabieres C, Pantel K (2014a) The circulating tumor cells: liquid biopsy of cancer. Klinicheskaia laboratornaia diagnostika 4:60–64

Alix-Panabieres C, Pantel K (2014b) Technologies for detection of circulating tumor cells: facts and vision. Lab Chip 14(1):57–62

Alonso-Alconada L, Muinelo-Romay L, Madissoo K et al (2014) Molecular profiling of circulating tumor cells links plasticity to the metastatic process in endometrial cancer. Mol Cancer 13:223

Andreopoulou E, Yang LY, Rangel KM et al (2012) Comparison of assay methods for detection of circulating tumor cells in metastatic breast cancer: AdnaGen AdnaTest BreastCancer Select/Detect versus Veridex CellSearch system. Int J Cancer 130(7):1590–1597

Armstrong AJ, Marengo MS, Oltean S et al (2011) Circulating tumor cells from patients with advanced prostate and breast cancer display both epithelial and mesenchymal markers. Mol Cancer Res MCR 9(8):997–1007

Baccelli I, Schneeweiss A, Riethdorf S et al (2013) Identification of a population of blood circulating tumor cells from breast cancer patients that initiates metastasis in a xenograft assay. Nat Biotechnol 31(6):539–544

Barber AG, Castillo-Martin M, Bonal DM et al (2015) PI3K/AKT pathway regulates E-cadherin and Desmoglein 2 in aggressive prostate cancer. Cancer Med 4(8):1258–1271

Barker N, van Es JH, Kuipers J et al (2007) Identification of stem cells in small intestine and colon by marker gene Lgr5. Nature 449(7165):1003–1007

Barriere G, Fici P, Gallerani G et al (2014) Circulating tumor cells and epithelial, mesenchymal and stemness markers: characterization of cell subpopulations. Annal Transl Med 2(11):109

Blassl C, Kuhlmann JD, Webers A et al (2016) Gene expression profiling of single circulating tumor cells in ovarian cancer – establishment of a multi-marker gene panel. Mol Oncol 10 (7):1030–1042

Bock C, Rack B, Huober J et al (2014) Distinct expression of cytokeratin, N-cadherin and CD133 in circulating tumor cells of metastatic breast cancer patients. Future Oncol 10(10):1751–1765

Bourcy M, Suarez-Carmona M, Lambert J et al (2016) Tissue factor induced by epithelial-mesenchymal transition triggers a procoagulant state that drives metastasis of circulating tumor cells. Cancer Res 76(14):4270–4282

Braun S, Vogl FD, Naume B et al (2005) A pooled analysis of bone marrow micrometastasis in breast cancer. N Engl J Med 353(8):793–802

Cayrefourcq L, Mazard T, Joosse S et al (2015) Establishment and characterization of a cell line from human circulating colon cancer cells. Cancer Res 75(5):892–901

Chang K, Kong YY, Dai B et al (2015) Combination of circulating tumor cell enumeration and tumor marker detection in predicting prognosis and treatment effect in metastatic castration-resistant prostate cancer. Oncotarget 6(39):41825–41836

Clevers H (2011) The cancer stem cell: premises, promises and challenges. Nat Med 17 (3):313–319

Coumans FA, Siesling S, Terstappen LW (2013) Detection of cancer before distant metastasis. BMC Cancer 13:283

De Craene B, Berx G (2013) Regulatory networks defining EMT during cancer initiation and progression. Nat Rev Cancer 13(2):97–110

Dinney CPNM, Melnikova VO, Pretzsch SM, Garza M, Wu W, Davis DW, Anderes KL (2014) Heterogeneity of circulating tumor cells isolated from bladder cancer patients using ApoStream and biomarkers of epithelial-mesenchymal transition. ASCO Meet Abstr 32:349

Fearon ER, Vogelstein B (1990) A genetic model for colorectal tumorigenesis. Cell 61 (5):759–767

Finlay J, Roberts CM, Lowe G et al (2015) RNA-based TWIST1 inhibition via dendrimer complex to reduce breast cancer cell metastasis. Biomed Res Int 2015:382745

Freidin MB, Tay A, Freydina DV et al (2014) An assessment of diagnostic performance of a filter-based antibody-independent peripheral blood circulating tumour cell capture paired with cytomorphologic criteria for the diagnosis of cancer. Lung Cancer 85(2):182–185

Fresno Vara JA, Casado E, de Castro J et al (2004) PI3K/Akt signalling pathway and cancer. Cancer Treat Rev 30(2):193–204

Galli R, Binda E, Orfanelli U et al (2004) Isolation and characterization of tumorigenic, stem-like neural precursors from human glioblastoma. Cancer Res 64(19):7011–7021

Ginestier C, Hur MH, Charafe-Jauffret E et al (2007) ALDH1 is a marker of normal and malignant human mammary stem cells and a predictor of poor clinical outcome. Cell Stem Cell 1 (5):555–567

Giordano A, Gao H, Anfossi S et al (2012) Epithelial-mesenchymal transition and stem cell markers in patients with HER2-positive metastatic breast cancer. Mol Cancer Ther 11 (11):2526–2534

Gorges TM, Kuske A, Rock K, Mauermann O, Müller V, Peine S, Verpoort K, Novosadova V, Kubista M, Riethdorf S, Pantel K (2016) Accession of tumor heterogeneity by multiplex transcriptome profiling of single circulating tumor cells. Clin Chem 62(11):1504–1515

Gradilone A, Iacovelli R, Cortesi E et al (2011) Circulating tumor cells and "suspicious objects" evaluated through CellSearch(R) in metastatic renal cell carcinoma. Anticancer Res 31 (12):4219–4221

Greulich P, Simons BD (2016) Dynamic heterogeneity as a strategy of stem cell self-renewal. Proc Natl Acad Sci U S A 113(27):7509–7514

Gupta V, Jafferji I, Garza M et al (2012) ApoStream(), a new dielectrophoretic device for antibody independent isolation and recovery of viable cancer cells from blood. Biomicrofluidics 6 (2):24133

Hanssen A, Wagner J, Gorges TM et al (2016) Characterization of different CTC subpopulations in non-small cell lung cancer. Sci Rep 6:28010

Hegemann M, Stenzl A, Bedke J et al (2016) Liquid biopsy: ready to guide therapy in advanced prostate cancer? BJU Int 118(6):855–863

Howard TD, Paznekas WA, Green ED et al (1997) Mutations in TWIST, a basic helix-loop-helix transcription factor, in Saethre-Chotzen syndrome. Nat Genet 15(1):36–41

Hu L, Lau SH, Tzang CH et al (2004) Association of Vimentin overexpression and hepatocellular carcinoma metastasis. Oncogene 23(1):298–302

Hui L, Zhang S, Dong X et al (2013) Prognostic significance of twist and N-cadherin expression in NSCLC. PLoS One 8(4):e62171

Hvichia GE, Parveen Z, Wagner C et al (2016) A novel microfluidic platform for size and deformability based separation and the subsequent molecular characterization of viable circulating tumor cells. Int J Cancer 138(12):2894–2904

Hyun KA, Koo GB, Han H et al (2016) Epithelial-to-mesenchymal transition leads to loss of EpCAM and different physical properties in circulating tumor cells from metastatic breast cancer. Oncotarget 7(17):24677–24687

Kallergi G, Papadaki MA, Politaki E et al (2011) Epithelial to mesenchymal transition markers expressed in circulating tumour cells of early and metastatic breast cancer patients. Breast Cancer Res 13(3):R59

Karrison TG, Ferguson DJ, Meier P (1999) Dormancy of mammary carcinoma after mastectomy. J Natl Cancer Inst 91(1):80–85

Khan MA, Tania M, Wei C et al (2015) Thymoquinone inhibits cancer metastasis by downregulating TWIST1 expression to reduce epithelial to mesenchymal transition. Oncotarget 6(23):19580–19591

Konigsberg R, Obermayr E, Bises G et al (2011) Detection of EpCAM positive and negative circulating tumor cells in metastatic breast cancer patients. Acta Oncol 50(5):700–710

Krawczyk N, Meier-Stiegen F, Banys M et al (2014) Expression of stem cell and epithelial-mesenchymal transition markers in circulating tumor cells of breast cancer patients. Biomed Res Int 2014:415721

Kreso A, Dick JE (2014) Evolution of the cancer stem cell model. Cell Stem Cell 14(3):275–291

Kulemann B, Liss AS, Warshaw AL et al (2016) KRAS mutations in pancreatic circulating tumor cells: a pilot study. Tumour Biol J Int Soc Oncodevelop Biol Med 37(6):7547–7554

Lamouille S, Xu J, Derynck R (2014) Molecular mechanisms of epithelial-mesenchymal transition. Nat Rev Mol Cell Biol 15(3):178–196

Lander AD, Kimble J, Clevers H et al (2012) What does the concept of the stem cell niche really mean today? BMC Biol 10:19

Larue L, Bellacosa A (2005) Epithelial-mesenchymal transition in development and cancer: role of phosphatidylinositol 3' kinase/AKT pathways. Oncogene 24(50):7443–7454

Li M, Zhang B, Zhang Z et al (2014) Stem cell-like circulating tumor cells indicate poor prognosis in gastric cancer. Biomed Res Int 2014:981261

Li X, Marcondes AM, Gooley TA et al (2010) The helix-loop-helix transcription factor TWIST is dysregulated in myelodysplastic syndromes. Blood 116(13):2304–2314

Lindsay CR, Le Moulec S, Billiot F et al (2016) Vimentin and Ki67 expression in circulating tumour cells derived from castrate-resistant prostate cancer. BMC Cancer 16:168

Lu J, Fan T, Zhao Q et al (2010) Isolation of circulating epithelial and tumor progenitor cells with an invasive phenotype from breast cancer patients. Int J Cancer 126(3):669–683

Malara N, Trunzo V, Foresta U et al (2016) Ex-vivo characterization of circulating colon cancer cells distinguished in stem and differentiated subset provides useful biomarker for personalized metastatic risk assessment. J Transl Med 14(1):133

Marie-Egyptienne DT, Lohse I, Hill RP (2013) Cancer stem cells, the epithelial to mesenchymal transition (EMT) and radioresistance: potential role of hypoxia. Cancer Lett 341(1):63–72

Marsden CG, Wright MJ, Pochampally R et al (2009) Breast tumor-initiating cells isolated from patient core biopsies for study of hormone action. Methods Mol Biol 590:363–375

Mascalchi M, Falchini M, Maddau C et al (2016) Prevalence and number of circulating tumour cells and microemboli at diagnosis of advanced NSCLC. J Cancer Res Clin Oncol 142 (1):195–200

Mathenge EG, Dean CA, Clements D et al (2014) Core needle biopsy of breast cancer tumors increases distant metastases in a mouse model. Neoplasia 16(11):950–960

Mego M, Mani SA, Lee BN et al (2012) Expression of epithelial-mesenchymal transition-inducing transcription factors in primary breast cancer: the effect of neoadjuvant therapy. Int J Cancer 130(4):808–816

Merindol N, Riquet A, Szablewski V et al (2014) The emerging role of Twist proteins in hematopoietic cells and hematological malignancies. Blood Cancer J 4:e206

Mitra A, Mishra L, Li S (2015a) EMT, CTCs and CSCs in tumor relapse and drug-resistance. Oncotarget 6(13):10697–10711

Mitra A, Satelli A, Xia X et al (2015b) Cell-surface Vimentin: a mislocalized protein for isolating csVimentin(+) CD133(−) novel stem-like hepatocellular carcinoma cells expressing EMT markers. Int J Cancer 137(2):491–496

Mohme M, Riethdorf S, Pantel K (2016) Circulating and disseminated tumour cells – mechanisms of immune surveillance and escape. Nat Rev Clin Oncol

Nastaly P, Ruf C, Becker P et al (2014) Circulating tumor cells in patients with testicular germ cell tumors. Clin Cancer Res 20(14):3830–3841

Nieman MT, Prudoff RS, Johnson KR et al (1999) N-cadherin promotes motility in human breast cancer cells regardless of their E-cadherin expression. J Cell Biol 147(3):631–644

O'Brien CA, Pollett A, Gallinger S et al (2007) A human colon cancer cell capable of initiating tumour growth in immunodeficient mice. Nature 445(7123):106–110

Pal SK, He M, Wilson T et al (2015) Detection and phenotyping of circulating tumor cells in high-risk localized prostate cancer. Clin Genitourin Cancer 13(2):130–136

Pantel K, Alix-Panabieres C (2016) Functional Studies on Viable Circulating Tumor Cells. Clin Chem 62(2):328–334

Pantel K, Deneve E, Nocca D et al (2012) Circulating epithelial cells in patients with benign colon diseases. Clin Chem 58(5):936–940

Papadaki MA, Kallergi G, Zafeiriou Z et al (2014) Co-expression of putative stemness and epithelial-to-mesenchymal transition markers on single circulating tumour cells from patients with early and metastatic breast cancer. BMC Cancer 14:651

Pardal R, Clarke MF, Morrison SJ (2003) Applying the principles of stem-cell biology to cancer. Nat Rev Cancer 3(12):895–902

Park S, Ang RR, Duffy SP et al (2014) Morphological differences between circulating tumor cells from prostate cancer patients and cultured prostate cancer cells. PLoS One 9(1):e85264

Patrawala L, Calhoun T, Schneider-Broussard R et al (2006) Highly purified CD44+ prostate cancer cells from xenograft human tumors are enriched in tumorigenic and metastatic progenitor cells. Oncogene 25(12):1696–1708

Pilati P, Mocellin S, Bertazza L et al (2012) Prognostic value of putative circulating cancer stem cells in patients undergoing hepatic resection for colorectal liver metastasis. Ann Surg Oncol 19(2):402–408

Poruk KE, Valero V 3rd, Saunders T et al (2016) Circulating tumor cell phenotype predicts recurrence and survival in pancreatic adenocarcinoma. Annal Surg 264(6):1073–1081

Powell AA, Talasaz AH, Zhang H et al (2012) Single cell profiling of circulating tumor cells: transcriptional heterogeneity and diversity from breast cancer cell lines. PLoS One 7(5): e33788

Quintana E, Shackleton M, Foster HR et al (2010) Phenotypic heterogeneity among tumorigenic melanoma cells from patients that is reversible and not hierarchically organized. Cancer Cell 18(5):510–523

Rack B, Schindlbeck C, Juckstock J et al (2014) Circulating tumor cells predict survival in early average-to-high risk breast cancer patients. J Natl Cancer Inst 106(5)

Riaz M, Sieuwerts AM, Look MP et al (2012) High TWIST1 mRNA expression is associated with poor prognosis in lymph node-negative and estrogen receptor-positive human breast cancer and is co-expressed with stromal as well as ECM related genes. Breast Cancer Res BCR 14(5): R123

Satelli A, Brownlee Z, Mitra A et al (2015a) Circulating tumor cell enumeration with a combination of epithelial cell adhesion molecule- and cell-surface vimentin-based methods for monitoring breast cancer therapeutic response. Clin Chem 61(1):259–266

Satelli A, Mitra A, Brownlee Z et al (2015b) Epithelial-mesenchymal transitioned circulating tumor cells capture for detecting tumor progression. Clin Cancer Res Offic J Am Assoc Cancer Res 21(4):899–906

Satelli A, Mitra A, Cutrera JJ et al (2014) Universal marker and detection tool for human sarcoma circulating tumor cells. Cancer Res 74(6):1645–1650

Schilling D, Todenhofer T, Hennenlotter J et al (2012) Isolated, disseminated and circulating tumour cells in prostate cancer. Nat Rev Urol 9(8):448–463

Schulze K, Gasch C, Staufer K et al (2013) Presence of EpCAM-positive circulating tumor cells as biomarker for systemic disease strongly correlates to survival in patients with hepatocellular carcinoma. Int J Cancer 133(9):2165–2171

Shimada R, Iinuma H, Akahane T et al (2012) Prognostic significance of CTCs and CSCs of tumor drainage vein blood in Dukes' stage B and C colorectal cancer patients. Oncol Rep 27 (4):947–953

Shipitsin M, Polyak K (2008) The cancer stem cell hypothesis: in search of definitions, markers, and relevance. Lab Investig 88(5):459–463

Shmelkov SV, Butler JM, Hooper AT et al (2008) CD133 expression is not restricted to stem cells, and both CD133+ and CD133- metastatic colon cancer cells initiate tumors. J Clin Invest 118 (6):2111–2120
Singh A, Settleman J (2010) EMT, cancer stem cells and drug resistance: an emerging axis of evil in the war on cancer. Oncogene 29(34):4741–4751
Sun YF, Xu Y, Yang XR et al (2013) Circulating stem cell-like epithelial cell adhesion molecule-positive tumor cells indicate poor prognosis of hepatocellular carcinoma after curative resection. Hepatology 57(4):1458–1468
Thiery JP (2002) Epithelial-mesenchymal transitions in tumour progression. Nat Rev Cancer 2 (6):442–454
Todenhofer T, Hennenlotter J, Faber F et al (2015) Significance of apoptotic and non-apoptotic disseminated tumor cells in the bone marrow of patients with clinically localized prostate cancer. Prostate 75(6):637–645
Todenhofer T, Azad A, Stewart C et al (2016a) AR-V7 transcripts in whole blood RNA of patients with metastatic castration resistant prostate cancer correlate with response to Abiraterone acetate. J Urol
Todenhofer T, Hennenlotter J, Dorner N et al (2016b) Transcripts of circulating tumor cells detected by a breast cancer-specific platform correlate with clinical stage in bladder cancer patients. J Cancer Res Clin Oncol 142(5):1013–1020
Todenhofer T, Park ES, Duffy S et al (2016c) Microfluidic enrichment of circulating tumor cells in patients with clinically localized prostate cancer. Urol Oncol 34(11):483.e9–483.e16
Uhr JW, Pantel K (2011) Controversies in clinical cancer dormancy. Proc Natl Acad Sci U S A 108 (30):12396–12400
Valladares-Ayerbes M, Blanco-Calvo M, Reboredo M et al (2012) Evaluation of the adenocarcinoma-associated gene AGR2 and the intestinal stem cell marker LGR5 as biomarkers in colorectal cancer. Int J Mol Sci 13(4):4367–4387
Van der Auwera I, Peeters D, Benoy IH et al (2010) Circulating tumour cell detection: a direct comparison between the CellSearch System, the AdnaTest and CK-19/mammaglobin RT-PCR in patients with metastatic breast cancer. Br J Cancer 102(2):276–284
Vesuna F, van Diest P, Chen JH et al (2008) Twist is a transcriptional repressor of E-cadherin gene expression in breast cancer. Biochem Biophys Res Commun 367(2):235–241
Vishnoi M, Peddibhotla S, Yin W et al (2015) The isolation and characterization of CTC subsets related to breast cancer dormancy. Sci Rep 5:17533
Wang N, Shi L, Li H et al (2012) Detection of circulating tumor cells and tumor stem cells in patients with breast cancer by using flow cytometry: a valuable tool for diagnosis and prognosis evaluation. Tumour Biol 33(2):561–569
Weissenstein U, Schumann A, Reif M et al (2012) Detection of circulating tumor cells in blood of metastatic breast cancer patients using a combination of cytokeratin and EpCAM antibodies. BMC Cancer 12:206
Wu S, Liu S, Liu Z et al (2015) Classification of circulating tumor cells by epithelial-mesenchymal transition markers. PLoS One 10(4):e0123976
Wushou A, Hou J, Zhao YJ et al (2014) Twist-1 up-regulation in carcinoma correlates to poor survival. Int J Mol Sci 15(12):21621–21630
Yang MH, Imrali A, Heeschen C (2015) Circulating cancer stem cells: the importance to select. Chinese J Cancer Res = Chung-kuo yen cheng yen chiu 27(5):437–449
Ye LY, Chen W, Bai XL et al (2016) Hypoxia-induced epithelial-to-mesenchymal transition in hepatocellular carcinoma induces an immunosuppressive tumor microenvironment to promote metastasis. Cancer Res 76(4):818–830
Yi S, Yang ZL, Miao X et al (2014) N-cadherin and P-cadherin are biomarkers for invasion, metastasis, and poor prognosis of gallbladder carcinomas. Pathol Res Pract 210(6):363–368
Yoshida GJ, Saya H (2016) Therapeutic strategies targeting cancer stem cells. Cancer Sci 107 (1):5–11

Yu M, Bardia A, Aceto N et al (2014) Cancer therapy. Ex vivo culture of circulating breast tumor cells for individualized testing of drug susceptibility. Science 345(6193):216–220

Zelenko Z, Gallagher EJ, Tobin-Hess A et al (2016) Silencing vimentin expression decreases pulmonary metastases in a pre-diabetic mouse model of mammary tumor progression. Oncogene

Zhang L, Huang G, Li X et al (2013) Hypoxia induces epithelial-mesenchymal transition via activation of SNAI1 by hypoxia-inducible factor -1alpha in hepatocellular carcinoma. BMC Cancer 13:108

Zhang P, Sun Y, Ma L (2015) ZEB1: at the crossroads of epithelial-mesenchymal transition, metastasis and therapy resistance. Cell Cycle 14(4):481–487

Zhu P, Stanton ML, Castle EP et al (2016a) Detection of tumor-associated cells in cryopreserved peripheral blood mononuclear cell samples for retrospective analysis. J Transl Med 14(1):198

Zhu QQ, Ma C, Wang Q et al (2016b) The role of TWIST1 in epithelial-mesenchymal transition and cancers. Tumour Biol J Int Soc Oncodev Biol Med 37(1):185–197

Chapter 12
Mesenchymal-Epithelial Transition and Circulating Tumor Cells in Small Cell Lung Cancer

Gerhard Hamilton and Barbara Rath

Abstract Cancer patients die of metastatic disease but knowledge regarding individual steps of this complex process of intravasation, spread and extravasation leading to secondary lesions is incomplete. Subpopulations of tumor cells are supposed to undergo an epithelial-mesenchymal transition (EMT), to enter the bloodstream and eventually establish metastases in a reverse process termed mesenchymal-epithelial transition (MET). Small cell lung cancer (SCLC) represents a unique model to study metastatic spread due to early dissemination and relapse, as well as availability of a panel of circulating cancer cell (CTC) lines recently. Additionally, chemosensitive SCLC tumor cells switch to a completely resistant phenotype during cancer recurrence. In advanced disease, SCLC patients display extremely high blood counts of CTCs in contrast to other tumors, like breast, prostate and colon cancer. Local inflammatory conditions at the primary tumor site and recruitment of macrophages seem to increase the shedding of tumor cells into the circulation in processes which may proceed independently of EMT. Since millions of cells are released by tumors into the circulation per day, analysis of a limited number of CTCs at specific time points are difficult to be related to the development of metastatic lesions which may occur approximately one year later. We have obtained a panel of SCLC CTC cell line from patients with relapsing disease, which share characteristic markers of this malignancy and a primarily epithelial phenotype with unique formation of large tumorospheres, containing quiescent and hypoxic cells. Although smoking and inflammation promote EMT, partial expression of vimentin indicates a transitional state with partial EMT in these cell lines at most. The CTC lines exhibit high expression of EpCAM, absent phosphorylation of β-catenin and background levels of Snail. Provided that these tumor cells had ever undergone EMT, here in advanced disease MET seem to have occurred already in the peripheral circulation. Alternative explanations for the expression of mesenchymal markers of the CTC lines are the heterogeneity of SCLC cells, cooperative migration or altered gene expression in response to the

G. Hamilton (✉) • B. Rath
Society for Research on Biology and Treatment of Cancer (SRBTC), A-1160 Vienna, Austria
e-mail: Hamilton.SRBTC@gmx.org; gerhard.hamilton@meduniwien.ac.at

M.J.M. Magbanua, J.W. Park (eds.), *Isolation and Molecular Characterization of Circulating Tumor Cells*, Advances in Experimental Medicine and Biology 994,
DOI 10.1007/978-3-319-55947-6_12

inflammatory tumor microenvironment allowing for tumor spread without EMT/MET.

Keywords Small cell lung cancer • Circulating tumor cells • Metastasis • Mesenchymal-epithelial transition • Tumorosphere

12.1 Classical Model of Tumor Dissemination

Mortality of cancer patients is in most cases caused by metastatic disease and many steps of this complex process are characterized insufficiently (Wan et al. 2013). Tumor cells of the primary lesion increase their mobility by switching to cellular programs that allow several modes of invasion. For carcinomas, a standard model of the metastatic progression has been proposed (Fig. 12.1; Steeg 2016). These tumors derive from epithelia which form polarized layers of cells that are connected laterally via several types of cellular junctions. Additionally, epithelial cells are bound to the underlying basement membranes via hemidesmosomes which further connect with the epithelial-specific cytokeratin intermediate filaments. For metastatic spread, cancer cells must leave these cellular structures and gain mobility. Primary tumors are known to constantly shed a large number of cancer cells into the circulation, after cell subpopulations have presumably undergone an epithelial-mesenchymal transition (EMT) (Nieto et al. 2016). The precise mechanism of how tumor cells cross the endothelial barrier is largely unknown. E-cadherin is regarded as a gatekeeper of the epithelial state and, therefore, during EMT E-cadherin expression is downregulated through gene repression, promoter methylation and protein degradation in response to various signals (Tsai and Yang 2013). A partial loss of E-cadherin is associated with carcinoma progression and poor prognosis in various human tumor types (Thiery and Lim 2013).

Intermediate filaments switch from cytokeratins to vimentin during EMT and nonepithelial cadherins, such as N-cadherin, are induced (Nieto et al. 2016). In contrast to epithelial cells, mesenchymal cells embed themselves inside the extracellular matrix (ECM) and rarely establish tight contact with neighboring cells. EMT-promoting factors comprise growth factors, inflammatory cytokines and acidic/hypoxic conditions in the tumor microenvironment. In particular, the EMT is executed in response to pleiotropic signaling factors that induce specific transcription factors (TFs) called EMT-TFs (e.g., Snail, ZEB, Twist, and others) and miRNAs together with epigenetic and post-translational regulators, many of which are involved in embryonic development, wound healing, fibrosis and cancer metastasis (Cano et al. 2000; Thiery 2002). Cells could linger in intermediary stages and may frequently undergo a partial EMT program.

Eventually, some of the surviving cells may arrest in the vascular lumen and extravasate through the capillary endothelium into the parenchyma of distant organs. In the new stromal environment, an even smaller subset of tumor cells establish micrometastases with the potential to develop into fully malignant,

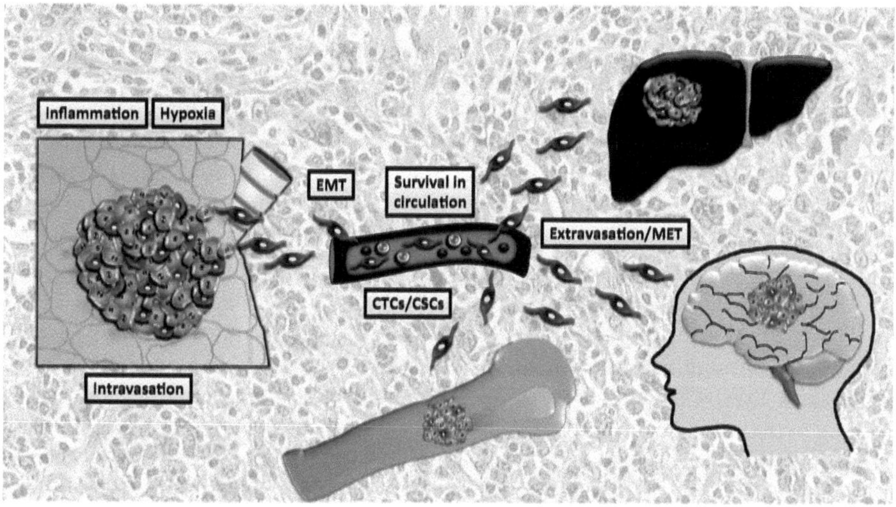

Fig. 12.1 Classical model of tumor dissemination. Scheme of primary tumor formation in the lung is shown at the *left side* of the figure. The tumor consists of a heterogeneous mixture of cells including a subpopulation of cells with higher motility (*dark colour*) and protease expression which are able to intravasate into the bloodstream. Inflammatory conditions in the tumor micro-environment together with an acidic and hypoxic milieu seem to enhance aggressiveness of the cancer cells and provide immune protection. Migration of the tumor cells and their intravasation is supposed to be related to an epithelial-mesenchymal transition (EMT) program. In the blood-stream a small fraction of these circulating tumor cells (CTCs) which may exhibit cancer stem cell characteristics, survive and spread to generate secondary lesions, in the case of SCLC preferentially in liver, brain and bone. Since metastases recapitulate the epithelial phenotype of the primary tumor, the EMT trait must be reversed in a process termed mesenchymal-epithelial transition (MET) for colonization of affected distal organs. Whether MET takes place already in the circulation or after extravasation is not known. This proposed model may vary for different tumors and conditions

secondary tumors that are clinically detectable and eventually fatal (Thiery 2002; Kalluri and Weinberg 2009). Since metastases exhibit an epithelial phenotype again, the migratory and invasive EMT cells need to reverse this process with a loss of this motile properties, adoption of an apico-basal polarization and reexpression of junctional complexes in a so-called mesenchymal-epithelial transition (MET) (Thiery et al. 2009).

12.2 Significance of Epithelial-Mesenchymal Transition (EMT) in Dissemination

Cancer-associated EMT was predominatly studied using cell lines or experimental animal models (Nieto et al. 2016). Most commonly markers for the epithelial phenoptype are E-cadherin, EpCAM, occludins, and cytokeratins, and for the mesenchymal cell type N-cadherin and vimentin, respectively (Thiery and Sleeman 2006; Thiery et al. 2009). Originally, a complete switch from epithelial to mesenchymal markers was regarded as a confirmation of EMT but such a total change was not detectable in patients (Huang et al. 2013; Yu et al. 2013). This failure to prove a full EMT made the whole concept and the significance of this transition in tumor spread questionable (Tarin et al. 2005). However, intermediate hybrid epithelial and mesenchymal phenotypes were observed in association with fibrosis and cancer processes (Grande et al. 2015; Lovisa et al. 2015; Grigore et al. 2016; Huang et al. 2013; Jordan et al. 2011). Tumor cells which exhibit such a hybrid phenotype have been referred to as "metastable" (Lee et al. 2006; Tam and Weinberg 2013; Nieto et al. 2016).

The regulation of classical EMT centers on the transcriptional suppression of E-cadherin through activities of major EMT-TFs, such as SNAI1, SNAI2, ZEB1, ZEB1, and TWIST1 (Peinado et al. 2007; Thiery et al. 2009; Lamouille et al. 2014). Mesenchymal traits in a hybrid state in a partial EMT may be limited to a decrease of epithelial properties like apico-basal polarity and a remodeling of junctional complexes (Nieto et al. 2016; Huang et al. 2012). Acquisition of true mesenchymal traits may comprise a wide range of different characteristics characteristic and markers. Functional programs associated with EMT, such as invasion, increased survival or decreased proliferation have to be taken into account. Whether EMT plays a crucial role in cancer metastasis in human patients and in some animal model systems is still under debate (Zheng et al. 2015), largely due to the lack of the ability to track the occurrence of EMT and to follow the fate of cells undergoing EMT in clinical settings. Especially, the diversity of the EMT program that can elude detection using a single EMT marker or reporter in animal models.

12.3 Circulating Tumor Cells

Tumors that are disseminated as CTCs may settle to selected protected niches [e.g., as disseminated tumor cells (DTCs) in the bone marrow] and can persist in a dormant state for extended time periods (Alix-Panabières and Pantel 2016). While CTCs can potentially be detected in essentially all human cancers, the CellSearch system (Veridex, Raritan, NJ) has only been approved for enumeration of these cells in metastatic breast, colon and colon cancer. CTCs serve as an independent predictor of progression free survival and overall survival (Cohen et al. 2008; Alix-Panabières and Pantel 2016). Such CTCs are defined as nucleated EpCAM- and cytokeratin-positive cells lacking a leukocyte marker, and a cutoff of 5 CTCs/7.5 ml blood separates patient populations with high and low risk of progression. Results showed that, with an increasing number of CTCs, the risks of cancer progression (hazard ratio of progression-free survival) and death (hazard ratio of overall survival) increases continuously. A linear relationship was demonstrated with a small number of CTCs (<5), however, both risks tapered beyond 5 CTCs/7.5 ml blood (Hong and Zu 2013). CTCs having undergone EMT would not be detected using methods which depend on epithelial markers, and such techniques may miss the most important tumor cells responsible for metastasis

(Gorges et al. 2012). Indeed, by using more sensitive detection approaches than the Cell Search system, the presence of at least a 30–100-fold higher number of CTCs was found in a variety of cancer patients (Flores et al. 2010).

There are a number of questions remaining for the detection of CTCs and their relationship to their parent bulk tumors. The frequency of the CTC population measured in an aliquot may not be a statistical representative of the entire sample. Based on the Poisson distribution, the probability of collecting ≥ 1 CTCs in one aliquot of 7.5 mL blood from a patient with 500 CTCs is 50% (Tibbe et al. 2007; Allan and Keeney 2010; Hong and Zu 2013). Twenty mL of whole blood would have to be assessed if the cell event was elevated for lower frequency at 1 CTC in 10^7 leukocytes (Rosenblatt et al. 1997). CTCs are shed from solid tumors at a daily rate of 3.2 to 4.1×10^6 per gram of tissue, based on a rat model (Butler and Gullino 1975). Half of these CTCs perish within 2.4 h, although longer half-lives were reported for a clinical setting (Meng et al. 2004). It is estimated that only <0.02% of disseminated tumor cells (DTCs) are able to successfully seed metastases (Chambers et al. 2002). An extended gap time often exists between the formation of the primary tumor and clinical manifestations of metastasis (Vanharanta and Massague 2013).The high attrition rate of CTCs during metastasis points to the existence of a rare and unique population of metastasis-initiating cells (MICs). Therefore, MICs are defined as cancer cells capable of seeding clinically significant metastatic colonies in secondary organs. MICs might exist at the primary tumors or emerge during the metastatic cascade. MICs seem to be distinguished by favorable traits, conferring cellular plasticity, metabolic reprogramming, ability to hide in dormancy, resistance to apoptosis, immune evasion, and cooperation with stromal cells (Celià-Terrassa and Kang 2016). These cells form the link between the primary tumor and subsequent metastasis but are exceedingly difficult to identify, track, and characterize. CTCs in short term culture are used to test chemoresistance and their enumeration in patients is discussed as surrogate marker for response to therapeutic agents. However, CTCs are specialized tumor cells and their chemosensitivity is not expected to be representative for the whole tumor and, in particular, they may be chemosensitive in the circulation and resistant due to protection in an inflammatory environment or as member of large tumorospheres (Hamilton et al. 2016a, b, c, d).

12.4 EMT in Circulating Tumor Cells

So far, only a limited number of studies using mouse tumor models examined the relationship of EMT to CTCs directly. For the capturing of CTCs that have fully undergone EMT, the current isolation methods which rely on using epithelial markers, such as EpCAM, are not suitable and newly developed methods for enrichment based on size, rigidity or surface charge need to be employed (Hong and Zu 2013; Alix-Panabières and Pantel 2016). Clinically, the CTCs in breast cancers with a triple-negative molecular subtype (ER–/PR–/HER2–) tend to have a more mesenchymal phenotype (Yu et al. 2013). The proportion of carcinoma cells with EMT features in primary breast tumors does not exceed 3% in estrogen receptor (ER)-positive tumors and 10–15% in ER-negative tumors. These mesenchymal CTCs isolated from breast cancer patients were found clustered with platelet cells, which produce TGFβ that in turn induces EMT (Yu et al. 2013). Furthermore, the EMT status consistently predicts overall survival (OS) and disease-free survival (DFS) (Tan et al. 2014). Importantly, cancer therapy affects CTC number and phenotype, with refractory patients having more mesenchymal-like CTCs and patients who are responding to treatment demonstrating significantly fewer CTCs and a more epithelial-like phenotype (Bonnomet et al. 2012; Yu et al. 2013).

EMT may be a focal event at the tumor margin, which occurs in response of cancer cells to their local microenvironment. Macrophages participate in EMT induction within primary tumors in transgenic mouse models, orthotopic xenografts, and primary human breast carcinomas (Wyckoff et al. 2004; Robinson et al. 2009). Therefore, macrophages may be also critical for local intravasation and, actually, we observed recruitment of macrophages by SCLC CTCs lines *in vitro* (Hamilton et al. 2015a). However, most CTCs are heterogenous and express both epithelial and mesenchymal markers leading to the interpretation of an ongoing EMT process during dissemination of carcinoma cells (Thiery and Lim 2013; Yu et al. 2013; Khoo et al. 2015). In support of this finding, after transient amplification of breast cancer CTCs the cells exhibit a full range of EMT phenotypes (Khoo et al. 2015). However, the majority of CTCs in breast cancer exhibit an intermediate EMT phenotype.

For lung cancer, there is some indirect evidence for the induction of an EMT phenotype in normal lung and transformed cells (Galván et al. 2014) Various groups of active compounds found in cigarette smoke, such as polycyclic aromatic hydrocarbons (PAH), nicotine-derived nitrosamine ketone (NNK), and reactive oxygen species (ROS) can induce EMT through different signaling pathways linked to biological responses to cigarette smoke, such as hypoxia, inflammation, and oxidative damage (Vu et al. 2016). EMT has been also found to be increased human bronchial epithelial cells of patients with chronic obstructive pulmonary disease (COPD) (Milara et al. 2013). The coexistence of lung cancer and COPD is commonly detected in smokers, and the risk of developing lung cancer in smoking patients is significantly increased in the presence of COPD (Sohal and Walters 2013). In general, the tumor microenvironment induces EMT and contributes to immune suppression and drug resistance (Mittal 2016). STAT3 is also reported to be elevated in lung biopsies from patients with idiopathic pulmonary fibrosis and may be a key molecule in inflammation associated with SCLC (Hamilton et al. 2015b). STAT3 is a downstream mediator of TGFβ signaling and induces EMT by increasing Snail expression in cancer cells (Saitoh et al. 2016). Furthermore, the inflammatory cytokine TNFα can stabilize Snail1 via NF-kB activation and induce Twist1 expression via IKK-b and NF-kB p65 activation. Inflammation seems to increase the EMT-rate in pancreatic cancer (Jolly et al. 2015; Rhim et al. 2012). Cytokines in the tumor microenvironment can also activate Stat3 via JAK kinases to induce Twist1 expression (Lo et al. 2007). Essential, all SCLC cells exhibit mutations of p53 and the loss of p53 causes a decrease in miR-200c, thereby increasing EMT, with a concomitant increase in the stem cell population (Chang et al. 2011).

12.5 Significance of MET in Dissemination

Cancer cells in metastatic outgrowths are clearly epithelial-like, and they can be identified morphologically and molecularly as having been derived from the primary tumor (Nieto et al. 2016). Thus, mesenchymal cells must revert to the epithelial phenotype to invade secondary organs in a reversal of EMT, called mesenchymal-epithelial transition (MET) or reverse EMT (rEMT). Several investigations have suggested that MET may be important for metastatic colonization by reactivating cell signaling pathways and/or facilitating attachment to heterologous cells within the healthy tissue (Gunasinghe et al. 2012). Whether CTCs only undergo transitions after reaching the metastatic site or if MET can also occur in the bloodstream is not clear at present. Vimentin-positive CTCs might have undergone MET to form vimentin-negative macrometastasis by loss of an EMT-inducing signal at the distant site (Tsuji et al. 2008; Tsai and Yang 2013). E-cadherin re-expression imparted by a partial MET at the secondary site increases survival of the metastatic cancer cell and increase chemoresistance as tumor spheroids (Chao et al. 2012). Studies in cell culture showed that induction of EMT by Snail1 and ZEB2 directly represses cell division and activation of Twist1 was found to be associated with reduced tumor cell proliferation (Tsai and Yang 2013; Yu et al. 2013). Since colonization demands tumor cells to restart proliferation upon extravasation into a foreign microenvironment, reversion of EMT may be required to provide such growth advantage. Interestingly, circulating tumor clusters are more effective in colonizing secondary sites than single mesenchymal CTCs (Aceto et al. 2014). Again, this highlights the requirement for mesenchymal cancer cells to at least partially reverse to the epithelial state for metastatic growth (Nieto 2013). However, both MET-dependent and MET–independent metastatic cascades were found in models involving carcinosarcoma and prostate carcinoma metastasis (Somarelli et al. 2016). In good agreement, MET-independent metastasis was reported from analysis of bone metastases from patients with castration-resistant prostate cancer. In conclusion, the processes leading to the formation of epithelial-type metastases during tumor spread from EMT cancer cells are poorly characterized so far.

12.6 Small Cell Lung Cancer (SCLC) as Tumor Dissemination Model

Despite numerous experimental studies using tissue cultures and animal models, many steps of tumor spread in patients are not fully characterized so far (Wan et al. 2013). An ideal malignancy to study tumor dissemination would comprise early metastasis in the majority of cases, rapid disease progression and access to tumor cells responsible for the establishment of secondary lesions. Clearly, this is not feasible in most tumor types exhibiting unpredictable progression after extended time periods of dormancy and low levels of circulating or disseminated tumor cells

(CTCs/DTCs). In contrast, SCLC may be suitable as metastatic tumor model due to high dissemination, predictable relapses within approximately one year and, recently, access to a panel of CTCs in unlimited amounts in tissue culture (Hamilton et al. 2015c).

SCLC is an aggressive neuroendocrine cancer characterized by rapid growth and early development of widespread metastases accompanied by drug resistance (Kalemkerian 2014; Byers and Rudin 2015; Pietanza et al. 2015). This tumor type accounts for approximately 15% of all lung cancers and represents a major cause of cancer mortality, with little progress in therapy for the last decades (Koinis et al. 2016). SCLC is associated with heavy tobacco exposure and the percentage of SCLC cases in women is arising due to the differences in smoking patterns in contrast to declining incidence and mortality in men (Jiménez et al. 2012). In the majority of cases SCLC is found disseminated at first presentation and surgery is limited to a small subgroup of patients with confined diseases (Hamilton et al. (2016b). Although a mostly chemotherapy- and radiation-sensitive disease initially, SCLC typically recurs rapidly after primary treatment with cisplatin (carboplatin)/etoposide combination chemotherapy, with poor further survival (Pillai and Owonikoko 2014; Byers and Rudin 2015). The single drug approved for second-line treatment of SCLC, namely topotecan, yields response of short duration in a small fraction of patients (Asai et al. 2014). For patients with extended stage disease (ED-SCLC), the median survival is around 10 months. In contrast to continuously increased 5-year survival rates from colon, rectal, and breast cancers, therapeutic options for SCLC have remained unchanged for the last decades, with stagnant clinical success (Coleman and Allemani 2015). Thus, almost invariably, patients exhibit therapeutic failure and tumor progression. In almost all cases of SCLC, p53 and RB1 are mutated thus inactivating two tumor suppressors (Rudin et al. 2012). SCLC shares mutations of p53, CDKN2A PIK3CA, PTEN with squamous and adenocarcinoma as well as of FGFR1 and SOX2 with squamous cell carcinoma (Rudin et al. 2012; Peifer et al. 2012). However, SCLC is not broadly characterized by targetable driver oncogenes, rather transcriptional deregulation may have a more important role. Although half of the SCLC cases may harbor at least one actionable alteration to personalize the therapy, so far each of the clinical trials has yielded negative results (Pietanza and Ladanyi 2012; Semenova et al. 2015; Koinis et al. 2016).

Thus, investigations of the underlying mechanisms responsible for the rapid tumor dissemination and development of chemoresistance of SCLC are urgently needed to develop new modes of treatment. Since the majority of patients present with advanced disease, diagnosis is confirmed by small biopsies leaving insufficient material for research. So-called liquid biopsies in form of CTCs or free tumor-derived DNA have proven to substitute for a limited range of studies (Rolfo et al. 2014). Furthermore, SCLC is distinguished by extremely high numbers of circulating tumor cells (CTCs), exceeding blood counts of other tumor entities up to several hundredfold (Yu et al. 2015). Actually, enriched CTCs have been used to generate xenografts in immunocompromised mice which mirror the drug sensitivity of the original tumors. However, *ex vivo* expansion of CTCs at our institution allows for a detailed cell biological characterization of these cells for the first time (Hamilton et al. 2015c). In fact, we were able to establish seven permanent SCLC CTC cell lines from blood samples of patients with extended disease and use expanded in vitro cultures for characterization of markers, receptor kinases, proteases and interactions with cells of the immune system (Hamilton et al. 2015a). Therefore, SCLC represents an excellent model to study tumor dissemination and the role and phenotype of the CTCs involved.

Acquisition of the invasive phenotype is thought to involve EMT to gain migratory potential and capability to survive in the circulation (Tsai and Yang 2013, Mitra et al. 2015). Thus, CTCs in initial stages are assumed to express an EMT phenotype and show a corresponding reduction in cell proliferation which may eventually result in a dormant state for extended periods of time. In mouse models for SCLC, the tumors were often composed of phenotypically different cells with either a neuroendocrine or a mesenchymal marker profile (Calbo et al. 2011). When engrafted as a mixed population, the mesenchymal cells endowed the neuroendocrine cells with metastatic capacity. The large non-neuroendocrine cells expressed a range of mesenchymal markers including nestin, vimentin, Sca1, Bmp4 and CD44. When morphologically different subpopulations of SCLC cell lines were analyzed for EMT and epigenetic features in another study, adherent subpopulations were found to express high levels of mesenchymal markers such as vimentin and fibronectin and very low levels of epithelial markers like E-cadherin and Zona Occludens 1 (ZO-1) (Krohn et al. 2014). Furthermore, expression of EMT-related transcription factors and cellular functions like migration, invasion, matrix metalloproteases secretion, and resistance to chemotherapeutic drugs all differed between these sublines. Correspondingly, nuclear snail expression among lung cancers was seen in 20% of cases, this being strongest in SCLC, and positive snail expression was associated with poor survival (Merikallio et al. 2012). In contrast, among clinical specimens of SCLC ($n = 38$) investigated for EMT markers E-cadherin, cytokeratins 8, 18, and 19, vimentin, and c-MET, patients bearing SCLC with a mesenchymal-like phenotype (c-MET^{High} E-cadherin^{Low}) had longer survival and a trend toward lower CTCs (Pore et al. 2016). Therefore, cells composing an SCLC primary may themselves exhibit a range of epithelial and mesenchymal traits. Tumor cells involved in extravasation and formation of metastases are characterized by expression of epithelial markers, most easily explained by MET (Nieto et al. 2016). In SCLC, most patients have one metastatic site, but multiple lesions affecting up to five sites are observed (Nakazawa et al. 2012). Sole liver metastasis is common and other sites comprise bone, brain, lung and adrenal glands. The majority of metastatic lesions in SCLC patients proved to be EpCam-positive (Spizzo et al. 2011). MET has not been possible to study in SCLC due to the fact that the large number of CTCs is heterogeneous with unknown functional significance and patients with extended disease are usually not subject to invasive procedures as surgery and biopsies.

12.7 Insights from SCLC CTC Cell Lines

SCLC patients featuring high CTC counts (> several hundred CTCs/7.5 ml blood) were suitable as source of circulating cells to induced xenotransplants (CDX) in immunocompromised mice (Hodgkinson et al. 2014). Expansion of CTCs in vitro has been demonstrated in a few instances in breast and one colon cancer (Hamilton et al. 2015c). Within the last years we have obtained seven permanent CTC cell lines from advanced and relapsed SCLC and initiated a full cell biologic characterization. All cell lines have unique p53 mutations and express typical markers of SCLCs, such as CD56, chromogranin and synaptophysin and the first two lines were found to induce tumors with SCLC markers in immunocompromised mice. They are distinguished from permanent SCLC tumor cell lines by spontaneous formation of large tumorospheres reaching diameters of 1–2 mm with necrotic cores in regular tissue culture (Hamilton et al. 2016c). Pluripotent stem cell markers were tested using Human Profiler Arrays (R&D systems, Minneapolis, MN, USA) and the cell lines found highly positive for EpCam and E-cadherin, negative for OCT-3/4 and Nanog with background levels of Snail1 (Hamilton et al. 2016c). Vimentin was highly expressed in the BHGc7 CTC line, with other lines showing significant but low expression. All four cell lines display a high EpCAM/vimentin protein expression ratio. The role of EpCAM in breast cancer strongly depends on the epithelial or mesenchymal phenotype of the tumor cells. Cancer cells with epithelial phenotype need EpCAM as a growth- and invasion-promoting mediator, whereas tumor cells with a mesenchymal phenotype are independent of EpCAM (Martowicz et al. 2012). In summary, four SCLC CTCs established from patients with advanced disease display mixed mesenchymal and epithelial markers. CTCs commonly display significant heterogeneity in terms of the degree of EMT/MET phenotype that probably reflects differential invasive potential (Polioudaki et al. 2015). Our results indicate, that the CTC SCLC cell lines have undergone almost complete or partial MET, provided that there was an EMT in the first place. Although the lines seem to express a typical partial EMT/MET they form large, organized tumorospheres with tight cell-cell contacts, typical for epithelial tissues (Hamilton et al. 2016b and c). Single cells of these SCLC CTC cell lines attach to the tissue culture plates and grow connected to the other cells but not usually in an elongated mesenchymal-like shape. Furthermore, CTCs may include a subpopulation of cells with self-renewal, multipotency and tumor initiating capabilities designated circulating cancer stem cells (CSCs) which may hold the highest malignant potential (Barriere et al. 2014). In good correspondence, the SCLC CTC overexpress mediators of the noncanonical WNT pathway (Hamilton et al. 2015d).

The goal in characterization of CTCs is to differentiate specific subgroups of that are truly responsible for metastasis, e.g. MICs (Hong and Zu 2013; Cellà-Terrassa and Kang 2016). Of all the CTCs initially shed by the primary tumor, the SCLC CTC lines seem to represent the MICs which have survived in the circulation and lead to the demise of the advanced and refractory SCLC patients. The quiescent and hypoxic cells of the tumorospheres seem to be responsible for the chemoradioresistant phenotype of the cancer cells of the relapsing patients (Weiswald et al. 2015). Furthermore, the tumorospheres exclude chemotherapeutics, such leaving the extended spectrum of drugs tried in SCLC ineffective.

12.8 Conclusion

The role of EMT in metastasis remains controversial although this transition has been postulated as a requirement for tumor invasion (Tarin et al. 2005; Chui 2013). Many cell culture and mouse tumor model studies have corroborated the significance of EMT in tumor progression but EMT, if present, remains difficult to prove in patients. Of course, in absence of EMT, MET is not necessary and absent during tumor spread. As a consequence, it was suggested that malignant cells can metastasize without radical changes in their cellular phenotype (Tarin et al. 2005). Markers used in EMT studies were suspected to become expressed due to inherent genetic instability of tumors. In carcinomas which derive from epithelial tissues, epithelial morphology and gene expression are always retained to some degree (Chui 2013). Most cancers seem to invade and travel through lymphatic and blood vessels via cohesive epithelial migration, rather than going through the EMT-MET sequence. Snail, Slug and Twist have traditionally been thought of as inducers of EMT but they also mediate dedifferentiation and maintenance of the stem cell state. Despite fundamental support for the EMT-MET concept (Thiery et al. 2009; Lamouille et al. 2014; Ye and Weinberg 2015), more recent data suggest notes of caution on the true role of EMT in cancer progression (Fischer et al. 2015; Zheng et al. 2015). The description of the tumor invasive front as being functionally distinct from the main tumor bulk (Brabletz et al. 2001, 2005) points to the heterogeneous nature of the EMT program executed within the tumor mass. Thus, there is probably an EMT gradient from focal full expression, to partial expression during intravasation, to absence in the main tumor bulk (Huang et al. 2013). Although important for invasion and the formation of CTCs, EMT is reported to be not required for metastatic colonization (Ocana et al. 2012; Tsai and Yang 2013). The induction of both EMT and stemness at the invasive fronts of tumors was first suggested to explain how cancer stem cells (CSCs) disseminate and seed fully heterogeneous tumors at secondary sites (Brabletz et al. 2005). Induction of pluripotency is also relevant to the persistence of CSCs and enhanced features of EMT (Kong et al. 2010). As an alternative model to intravasation of cells with EMT traits, EMT cells may be responsible for degrading the tumor stroma to enable intravasation of both EMT and non-EMT cells. Only non-EMT cells that have entered the blood stream are able to re-establish colonies in the secondary sites (Tsuji et al. 2008). This proposed mechanismus has been termed collective migration and, thereby, EMT may facilitate the invasion and intravasation of other cells that retain their epithelial character. As such, even if EMT were more limited than anticipated, it would still be required for tumor progression to the metastatic state (Li and Kang 2016).

Intravasation has been the least studied process in the metastatic cascade and the possibility of cancer epithelial cells being able themselves to efficiently intravasate cannot be excluded (Fischer et al. 2015; Zheng et al. 2015). Simply leakiness of the tumor vessels may be sufficient to allow intravasation of epithelial cell clusters observable in the circulation (Aceto et al. 2014). Additionally, the recent proposal that tumor-associated macrophages and vascular mimicry acquired by carcinoma cells may be involved in intravasation (Harney et al. 2015; Wagenblast et al. 2015; Benes et al. 2006). In the absence of a reliable proof for EMT for specific tumors and conditions, the claim to have cancer cells with a MET phenotype is difficult to substantiate. Thus, data regarding the point in the lifespan of a CTC at which the cell undergoes a MET-like process either already in the bloodstream or after extravasation presumes occurrence of MET at first.

The first report on EMT markers in CTCs was published by Kallergi et al. (2011; Hensler et al. 2015) in 2011. Two EMT markers, Twist and vimentin, in CTCs of breast cancer patients were found with higher frequency in metastatic breast cancer patients than in patients with early stages (Kallergi et al. 2011; Kölbl et al. 2016). Furthermore, CTCs coexpressing variable proportions of epithelial, EMT and cancer stem cell (CSC) markers were found in patients with metastatic diseases (Armstrong et al. 2011; Blassl et al. 2016). In almost 90% of the CTCs at least one EMT-associated transcription factor was upregulated, pointing towards the presence of a high number of EMT-CTCs (Giordano et al. 2012). In SCLC, mechanisms of tumor spread may be different from the best-characterized clinical model, namely breast cancer. Although the SCLC CTC lines express variable amounts of vimentin, the formation of organized tumorospheres with close cell-cell contacts represent a typical epithelial feature. Whether the expression of mesenchymal markers by the CTC cell lines indicate a previous EMT is not clear; vimentin may stem from the heterogeneous expression by SCLC tumor cells, or be acquired in inflammatory processes involving tumor-associated macrophages in the tumor microenvironment, or the consequence of deregulated gene expression in SCLC cells exhibiting a host of mutations. EMT confers resistance to cell death induced through various means in cancer cells (Vega et al. 2004; Thiery et al. 2009), including chemotherapy (Singh and Settleman 2010). Even in studies that find a limited contribution of cells that have undergone EMT to established metastases, the role of EMT in conferring chemoresistance is clear (Fischer et al. 2015; Zheng et al. 2015). EGFR-mutated NSCLC switches EGFR to Axl receptor tyrosine kinase in association with a mesenchymal phenotype (Gjerdrum et al. 2010; Byers et al. 2013; Schmalhofer et al. 2009). A similar overexpression of Axl and the noncanonical WNT pathway was found in the CTC cell lines (Hamilton et al. 2015d). However, our SCLC CTC lines are highly chemosensitive to topotecan and epirubicin in form of single cell suspensions obviously lacking a chemoresistant phenotype supposed to be conferred by a possible EMT (Hamilton et al. 2015d). In conclusion, marker expression of the SCLC CTC cell lines may be interpreted as a hybrid EMT phenotype; however, formation of tumorospheres, chemosensitivity and relative high expression of EpCAM and E-cadherin are compatible with direct shedding of epithelial-type cancer cells by primary or metastatic lesions capable of induction of metastases without requirement of an EMT-MET cycle.

References

Aceto N, Bardia A, Miyamoto DT et al (2014) Circulating tumor cell clusters are oligoclonal precursors of breast cancer metastasis. Cell 158(5):1110–1122

Alix-Panabières C, Pantel K (2016) Clinical applications of circulating tumor cells and circulating tumor DNA as liquid biopsy. Cancer Discov 6(5):479–491

Allan AL, Keeney M (2010) Circulating tumor cell analysis: technical and statistical considerations for application to the clinic. J Oncol 2010:426218

Armstrong AJ, Marengo MS, Oltean S et al (2011) Circulating tumor cells from patients with advanced prostate and breast cancer display both epithelial and mesenchymal markers. Mol Cancer Res 9(8):997–1007

Asai N, Ohkuni Y, Kaneko N et al (2014) Relapsed small cell lung cancer: treatment options and latest developments. Ther Adv Med Oncol 6(2):69–82

Barriere G, Fici P, Gallerani G et al (2014) Circulating tumor cells and epithelial, mesenchymal and stemness markers: characterization of cell subpopulations. Ann Transl Med 2(11):109

Benes P, Macecková V, Zdráhal Z et al (2006) Role of vimentin in regulation of monocyte/macrophage differentiation. Differentiation 74(6):265–276

Blassl C, Kuhlmann JD, Webers A et al (2016) Gene expression profiling of single circulating tumor cells in ovarian cancer—establishment of a multi-marker gene panel. Mol Oncol 10 (7):1030–1042

Bonnomet A, Syne L, Brysse A et al (2012) A dynamic in vivo model of epithelial-to-mesenchymal transitions in circulating tumor cells and metastases of breast cancer. Oncogene 31 (33):3741–3753

Brabletz T, Jung A, Reu S et al (2001) Variable beta-catenin expression in in colorectal cancers indicates tumor progression driven by the tumor environment. Proc Natl Acad Sci U S A 98 (18):10356–10361

Brabletz T, Jung A, Spaderna S et al (2005) Opinion: migrating cancer stem cells – an integrated concept of malignant tumour progression. Nat Rev Cancer 5(9):744–749

Butler TP, Gullino PM (1975) Quantitation of cell shedding into efferent blood of mammary adenocarcinoma. Cancer Res 35(3):512–516

Byers LA, Rudin CM (2015) Small cell lung cancer: where do we go from here? Cancer 121 (5):664–672

Byers LA, Diao L, Wang J et al (2013) An epithelial-mesenchymal transition gene signature predicts resistance to EGFR and PI3K inhibitors and identifies Axl as a therapeutic target for overcoming EGFR inhibitor resistance. Clin Cancer Res 19(1):279–290

Calbo J, van Montfort E, Proost N et al (2011) A functional role for tumor cell heterogeneity in a mouse model of small cell lung cancer. Cancer Cell 19(2):244–256

Cano A, Perez-Moreno MA, Rodrigo I et al (2000) The transcription factor snail controls epithelial-mesenchymal transitions by repressing E-cadherin expression. Nat Cell Biol 2 (2):76–83

Celià-Terrassa T, Kang Y (2016) Distinctive properties of metastasis-initiating cells. Genes Dev 30(8):892–908

Chambers AF, Groom AC, MacDonald IC (2002) Dissemination and growth of cancer cells in metastatic sites. Nat Rev Cancer 2:563–572

Chang CJ, Chao CH, Xia W et al (2011) p53 regulates epithelial-mesenchymal and stem cell properties through modulating miRNAs. Nat Cell Biol 13(3):317–323

Chao Y, Wu Q, Shepard C, Wells A (2012) Hepatocyte induced re-expression of E-cadherin in breast and prostate cancer cells increases chemoresistance. Clin Exp Metastasis 29(1):39–50
Chui MH (2013) Insights into cancer metastasis from a clinicopathologic perspective: epithelial–mesenchymal transition is not a necessary step. Int J Cancer 132(7):1487–1495
Cohen SJ, Punt CJ, Iannotti N et al (2008) Relationship of circulating tumor cells to tumor response, progression-free survival, and overall survival in patients with metastatic colorectal cancer. J Clin Oncol 26(19):3213–3221
Coleman MP, Allemani C (2015) Cancer: the elephant in the room. Lancet 385(9973):1047–1048
Fischer KR, Durrans A, Lee S et al (2015) Epithelial-to-mesenchymal transition is not required for lung metastasis but contributes to chemoresistance. Nature 527(7579):472–476
Flores LM, Kindelberger DW, Ligon AH et al (2010) Improving the yield of circulating tumour cells facilitates molecular characterisation and recognition of discordant HER2 amplification in breast cancer. Br J Cancer 102(10):1495–1502
Galván JA, Astudillo A, Vallina A et al (2014) Prognostic and diagnostic value of epithelial to mesenchymal transition markers in pulmonary neuroendocrine tumors. BMC Cancer 14:855
Giordano A, Gao H, Anfossi S et al (2012) Epithelial-mesenchymal transition and stem cell markers in patients with HER2-positive metastatic breast cancer. Mol Cancer Ther 11 (11):2526–2534
Gjerdrum C, Tiron C, Høiby T et al (2010) Axl is an essential epithelial-to-mesenchymal transition-induced regulator of breast cancer metastasis and patient survival. Proc Natl Acad Sci USA 107(3):1124–1129
Gorges TM, Tinhofer I, Drosch M et al (2012) Circulating tumour cells escape from EpCAM-based detection due to epithelial-to-mesenchymal transition. BMC Cancer 12:178
Grande MT, Sanchez-Laorden B, Lopez-Blau C et al (2015) Snail1-induced partial epithelial-to-mesenchymal transition drives renal fibrosis in mice and can be targeted to reverse established disease. Nat Med 21(9):989–097
Grigore AD, Jolly MK, Jia D, Farach-Carson MC, Levine H (2016) Tumor budding: the name is EMT. Partial EMT. J Clin Med 5(5). pii: E51
Gunasinghe NP, Wells A, Thompson EW et al (2012) Mesenchymal-epithelial transition (MET) as a mechanism for metastatic colonisation in breast cancer. Cancer Metastasis Rev 31 (3–4):469–478
Hamilton G, Rath B, Klameth L et al (2015a) Small cell lung cancer: recruitment of macrophages by circulating tumor cells. Oncoimmunology 5(3):e1093277
Hamilton G, Rath B, Klameth L et al (2015b) Receptor tyrosine kinase expression of circulating tumor cells in small cell lung cancer. Oncoscience 2(7):629–634
Hamilton G, Burghuber O, Zeillinger R (2015c) Circulating tumor cells in small cell lung cancer: ex vivo expansion. Lung 193(3):451–452
Hamilton G, Rath B, Ulsperger E (2015d) How to target small cell lung cancer. Oncoscience 2 (8):684–692
Hamilton G, Moser D, Hochmeier M (2016a) Metastasis: circulating tumor cells in small cell lung cancer. Trend Cancer 2:159–160
Hamilton G, Rath B, Ulsperger E (2016b) A review of the role of surgery for small cell lung cancer and the potential prognostic value of enumeration of circulating tumor cells. Eur J Surg Oncol 42(9):1296–1302
Hamilton G, Hochmair M, Rath B et al (2016c) Small cell lung cancer: circulating tumor cells of extended stage patients express a mesenchymal-epithelial transition phenotype. Cell Adhes Migr 26:1–8
Hamilton G, Rath B, Holzer S et al (2016d) Second-line therapy for small cell lung cancer: exploring the potential role of circulating tumor cell. Transl Lung Cancer Res 5(1):71–77
Harney AS, Arwert EN, Entenberg D et al (2015) Real-time imaging reveals local, transient vascular permeability, and tumor cell intravasation stimulated by TIE2hi macrophage-derived VEGFA. Cancer Discov 5(9):932–943

Hensler M, Vancurova I, Becht E et al (2015) Gene expression profiling of circulating tumor cells and peripheral blood mononuclear cells from breast cancer patients. Oncoimmunology 5(4): e1102827
Hodgkinson CL, Morrow CJ, Li Y et al (2014) Tumorigenicity and genetic profiling of circulating tumor cells in small-cell lung cancer. Nat Med 20(8):897–903
Hong B, Zu Y (2013) Detecting circulating tumor cells: current challenges and new trends. Theranostics 3(6):377–394
Huang RY, Guilford P, Thiery JP (2012) Early events in cell adhesion and polarity during epithelial-mesenchymal transition. J Cell Sci 125(Pt 19):4417–4422
Huang RY, Wong MK, Tan TZ et al (2013) An EMT spectrum defines an anoikis-resistant and spheroidogenic intermediate mesenchymal state that is sensitive to e-cadherin restoration by a src-kinase inhibitor, saracatinib (AZD0530). Cell Death Dis 4:e915
Jiménez Ruiz CA, Ramos Pinedo A, Cicero Guerrero A et al (2012) Characteristics of COPD smokers and effectiveness and safety of smoking cessation medications. Nicotine Tob Res 14 (9):1035103–1035109
Jolly MK, Boareto M, Huang B et al (2015) Implications of the hybrid epithelial/mesenchymal phenotype in metastasis Front. Oncologia 5:155
Jordan NV, Johnson GL, Abell AN (2011) Tracking the intermediate stages of epithelial-mesenchymal transition in epithelial stem cells and cancer. Cell Cycle 10(17):2865–2873
Kalemkerian GP (2014) Advances in pharmacotherapy of small cell lung cancer. Expert Opin Pharmacother 15(16):2385–2396
Kallergi G, Papadaki MA, Politaki E et al (2011) Epithelial to mesenchymal transition markers expressed in circulating tumour cells of early and metastatic breast cancer patients. Breast Cancer Res 13(3):R59
Kalluri R, Weinberg RA (2009) The basics of epithelial–mesenchymal transition. J Clin Invest 119 (6):1420–1428
Khoo BL, Lee SC, Kumar P et al (2015) Short-term expansion of breast circulating cancer cells predicts response to anti-cancer therapy. Oncotarget 6(17):15578–15593
Koinis F, Kotsakis A, Georgoulias V (2016) Small cell lung cancer (SCLC): no treatment advances in recent years. Transl Lung Cancer Res 5(1):39–50
Kölbl AC, Jeschke U, Andergassen U (2016) The significance of epithelial-to-mesenchymal transition for circulating tumor cells. Int J Mol Sci 17(8)
Kong D, Banerjee S, Ahmad A et al (2010) Epithelial to mesenchymal transition is mechanistically linked with stem cell signatures in prostate cancer cells. PLoS One 5(8):e12445
Krohn A, Ahrens T, Yalcin A et al (2014) Tumor cell heterogeneity in Small Cell Lung Cancer (SCLC): phenotypical and functional differences associated with Epithelial-Mesenchymal Transition (EMT) and DNA methylation changes. PLoS One 9(6):e100249
Lamouille S, Xu J, Derynck R (2014) Molecular mechanisms of epithelial- mesenchymal transition. Nat Rev Mol Cell Biol 15(3):178–196
Lee JM, Dedhar S, Kalluri R et al (2006) The epithelialmesenchymal transition: new insights in signaling, development, and disease. J Cell Biol 172(7):973–981
Li W, Kang Y (2016) Probing the fifty shades of EMT in metastasis. Trend Cancer 2(2):65–67
Lo HW, Hsu SC, Xia W, Cao X, Shih JY, Wei Y et al (2007) Epidermal growth factor receptor cooperates with signal transducer and activator of transcription 3 to induce epithelial-mesenchymal transition in cancer cells via up-regulation of TWIST gene expression. Cancer Res 67(19):9066–9076
Lovisa S, LeBleu VS, Tampe B, Sugimoto H, Vadnagara K, Carstens JL et al (2015) Epithelial-to-mesenchymal transition induces cell cycle arrest and parenchymal damage in renal fibrosis. Nat Med 21(9):998–1009
Martowicz A, Spizzo G, Gastl G et al (2012) Phenotype-dependent effects of EpCAM expression on growth and invasion of human breast cancer cell lines. BMC Cancer 12:501
Meng S, Tripathy D, Frenkel EP et al (2004) Circulating tumor cells in patients with breast cancer dormancy. Clin Cancer Res 10(24):8152–8162

Merikallio H, Turpeenniemi-Hujanen T, Pääkkö P et al (2012) Snail promotes an invasive phenotype in lung carcinoma. Respir Res 13:104

Milara J, Peiró T, Serrano A, Cortijo J (2013) Epithelial to mesenchymal transition is increased in patients with COPD and induced by cigarette smoke. Thorax 68(5):410–420

Mitra A, Mishra L, Li S (2015) EMT, CTCs and CSCs in tumor relapse and drug-resistance. Oncotarget 26(13):10697–10711

Mittal V (2016) Epithelial mesenchymal transition in aggressive lung cancers. Adv Exp Med Biol 890:37–56

Nakazawa K, Kurishima K, Tamura T et al (2012) Specific organ metastases and survival in small cell lung cancer. Oncol Lett 4(4):617–620

Nieto MA (2013) Epithelial plasticity: a common theme in embryonic and cancer cells. Science 342(6159):1234850

Nieto MA, Huang RY, Jackson RA et al (2016) EMT: 2016. Cell 166(1):21–45

Ocana OH, Corcoles R, Fabra A et al (2012) Metastatic colonization requires the repression of the epithelial-mesenchymal transition inducer Prrx1. Cancer Cell 22(6):709–724

Peifer M, Fernández-Cuesta L, Sos ML et al (2012) Integrative genome analyses identify key somatic driver mutations of small-cell lung cancer. Nat Genet 44(10):1104–1110

Peinado H, Olmeda D, Cano A (2007) Snail, Zeb and bHLH factors in tumour progression: an alliance against the epithelial phenotype? Nat Rev Cancer 7(6):415–428

Pietanza MC, Byers LA, Minna JD et al (2015) Small cell lung cancer: will recent progress lead to improved outcomes? Clin Cancer Res 21(10):2244–2255

Pietanza MC, Ladanyi M (2012) Bringing the genomic landscape of small-cell lung cancer into focus. Nat Genet 44(10):1074–1075

Pillai RN, Owonikoko TK (2014) Small cell lung cancer: therapies and targets. Semin Oncol 41 (1):133–142

Polioudaki H, Agelaki S, Chiotaki R et al (2015) Variable expression levels of keratin and vimentin reveal differential EMT status of circulating tumor cells and correlation with clinical characteristics and outcome of patients with metastatic breast cancer. BMC Cancer 15:399

Pore M, Meijer C, de Bock GH et al (2016) Cancer stem cells, epithelial to mesenchymal markers, and circulating tumor cells in small cell lung cancer. Clin Lung Cancer S1525-7304(16):30131

Rhim AD, Mirek ET, Aiello NM et al (2012) EMT and dissemination precede pancreatic tumor formation. Cell 148(1–2):349–361

Robinson BD, Sica GL, Liu YF et al (2009) Tumor microenvironment of metastasis in human breast carcinoma: a potential prognostic marker linked to hematogenous dissemination. Clin Cancer Res 15(7):2433–2441

Rolfo C, Castiglia M, Hong D et al (2014) Liquid biopsies in lung cancer: the new ambrosia of researchers. Biochim Biophys Acta 1846(2):539–546

Rosenblatt JI, Hokanson JA, McLaughlin SR et al (1997) Theoretical basis for sampling statistics useful for detecting and isolating rare cells using flow cytometry and cell sorting. Cytometry 27 (3):233–238

Rudin CM, Durinck S, Stawiski EW et al (2012) Comprehensive genomic analysis identifies SOX2 as a frequently amplified gene in small-cell lung cancer. Nat Genet 44(10):1111–1116

Saitoh M, Endo K, Furuya S et al (2016) STAT3 integrates cooperative Ras and TGF-beta signals that induce Snail expression. Oncogene 35(8):1049–1057

Schmalhofer O, Brabletz S, Brabletz T (2009) E-cadherin, beta-catenin, and ZEB1 in malignant progression of cancer Cancer. Metastasis Rev 28(1–2):151–166

Semenova EA, Nagel R, Berns A (2015) Origins, genetic landscape, and emerging therapies of small cell lung cancer. Genes Dev 29(14):1447–1462

Singh A, Settleman J (2010) EMT, cancer stem cells and drug resistance: an emerging axis of evil in the war on cancer. Oncogene 29(34):4741–4751

Sohal SS, Walters EH (2013) Role of epithelial mesenchymal transition (EMT) in chronic obstructive pulmonary disease (COPD). Respir Res 14:120

Somarelli JA, Schaeffer D, Marengo MS et al (2016) Distinct routes to metastasis: plasticity-dependent and plasticity-independent pathways. Oncogene 35(33):4302–4311
Spizzo G, Fong D, Wurm M et al (2011) EpCAM expression in primary tumour tissues and metastases: an immunohistochemical analysis. J Clin Pathol 64(5):415–420
Steeg PS (2016) Targeting metastasis. Nat Rev Cancer 16(4):201–218
Tam WL, Weinberg RA (2013) The epigenetics of epithelial-mesenchymal plasticity in cancer. Nat Med 19(11):1438–1449
Tan TZ, Miow QH, Miki Y et al (2014) Epithelial-mesenchymal transition spectrum quantification and its efficacy in deciphering survival and drug responses of cancer patients. EMBO Mol Med 6(10):1279–1293
Tarin D, Thompson EW, Newgreen DF (2005) The fallacy of epithelial mesenchymal transition in neoplasia. Cancer Res 65(14):5996–6000
Thiery JP (2002) Epithelial-mesenchymal transitions in tumour progression. Nat Rev Cancer 2 (6):442–454
Thiery JP, Sleeman JP (2006) Complex networks orchestrate epithelial-mesenchymal transitions. Nat Rev Mol Cell Biol 7(2):131–142
Thiery JP, Acloque H, Huang RY et al (2009) Epithelial mesenchymal transitions in development and disease. Cell 139(5):871–890
Thiery JP, Lim CT (2013) Tumor dissemination: an EMT affair cancer. Cell 23(3):272–273
Tibbe AG, Miller MC, Terstappen LW (2007) Statistical considerations for enumeration of circulating tumor cells. Cytometry A 71(3):154–162
Tsai JH, Yang J (2013) Epithelial-mesenchymal plasticity in carcinoma metastasis. Genes Dev 27 (20):2192–2206
Tsuji T, Ibaragi S, Shima K et al (2008) Epithelial-mesenchymal transition induced by growth suppressor p12CDK2-AP1 promotes tumor cell local invasion but suppresses distant colony growth. Cancer Res 68(24):10377–10386
Vanharanta S, Massague J (2013) Origins of metastatic traits. Cancer Cell 24:410–421
Vega S, Morales AV, Ocana OH et al (2004) Snail blocks the cell cycle and confers resistance to cell death. Genes Dev 18(10):1131–1143
Vu T, Jin L, Datta PK (2016) Effect of cigarette smoking on Epithelial to Mesenchymal Transition (EMT) in lung cancer. J Clin Med 5(4):E44
Wagenblast E, Soto M, Gutierrez-Angel S et al (2015) A model of breast cancer heterogeneity reveals vascular mimicry as a driver of metastasis. Nature 520(7547):358–362
Wan L, Pantel K, Kang Y (2013) Tumor metastasis: moving new biological insights into the clinic. Nat Med 19:1450–1464
Weiswald LB, Bellet D, Dangles-Marie V (2015) Spherical cancer models in tumor biology. Neoplasia 17(1):1–15
Wyckoff J, Wang W, Lin EY et al (2004) A paracrine loop between tumor cells and macrophages is required for tumor cell migration in mammary tumors. Cancer Res 64(19):7022–7029
Ye X, Weinberg RA (2015) Epithelial-mesenchymal plasticity: a central regulator of cancer progression trends. Cell Biol 25(11):675–686
Yu M, Bardia A, Wittner BS et al (2013) Circulating breast tumor cells exhibit dynamic changes in epithelial and mesenchymal composition. Science 339(6119):580–584
Yu N, Zhou J, Cui F, Tang X (2015) Circulating tumor cells in lung cancer: detection methods and clinical applications. Lung 193(2):157–171
Zheng X, Carstens JL, Kim J et al (2015) Epithelial-to-mesenchymal transition is dispensable for metastasis but induces chemoresistance in pancreatic cancer. Nature 527(7579):525–530

Chapter 13
Clinical Relevance of a Candidate Stem Cell Marker, p75 Neurotrophin Receptor (p75NTR) Expression in Circulating Tumor Cells

Tomoyuki Okumura, Tetsuji Yamaguchi, Toru Watanabe, Takuya Nagata, and Yutaka Shimada

Abstract Despite advances in its diagnosis and multimodal therapies, the prognosis of esophageal squamous cell carcinoma (ESCC) patients remains poor, because of high incidences of metastasis. Recent reports suggested that circulating tumor stem cells (CTSCs), rather than circulating tumor cells (CTCs), were more accurate diagnostic marker for metastasis, because tumor stem cells or cancer stem cells (CSCs) are more responsible for metastasis through processes such as epithelial mesenchymal transition (EMT) and tumor initiation. A neurotrophin receptor p75 (p75NTR) is expressed in a candidate CSCs in ESCC, which possess enhanced tumorigenicity along with strong expression of EMT-related genes. Our recent report using two-color flow cytometry demonstrated that CTC counts based on a combined expression of epithelial cell adhesion molecule (EpCAM) and p75NTR was significantly higher in peripheral blood samples of ESCC patients than healthy controls. In addition, EpCAM + p75NTR+, but not EpCAM + p75NTR- CTC counts, correlated with clinically diagnosed distant metastasis and pathological venous invasion in surgically resected primary ESCC tumors. Malignant cytology of the isolated EpCAM + p75NTR+ cells was microscopically confirmed as well. These results demonstrated that EpCAM + p75NTR+ CTC count was a more accurate diagnostic marker than EpCAM+ CTC count, suggesting the highly metastatic potential of CTCs with p75NTR expression.

T. Okumura (✉) • T. Yamaguchi • T. Watanabe • T. Nagata
Department of Surgery and Science, Graduate School of Medicine and Pharmaceutical Sciences, University of Toyama, 2630 Sugitani, Toyama City, Toyama 930-0194, Japan
e-mail: okumura@med.u-toyama.ac.jp; tetsuji-yama@blue.ocn.ne.jp; toruwatanabetoru@yahoo.co.jp; naga0103@med.u-toyama.ac.jp

Y. Shimada
Department of Nanobio Drug Discovery, Graduate School of Pharmaceutical Sciences, Kyoto University, 46-29 Yoshida-Shimo-Adachi-cho, Sakyo-ku, Kyoto 606-8501, Japan
e-mail: yshimada@pharm.kyoto-u.ac.jp

M.J.M. Magbanua, J.W. Park (eds.), *Isolation and Molecular Characterization of Circulating Tumor Cells*, Advances in Experimental Medicine and Biology 994,
DOI 10.1007/978-3-319-55947-6_13

Investigation using the isolated EpCAM + p75NTR+ CTCs to assess their stem cell properties may shed light on their roles in tumor metastasis in ESCC.

Further investigations based on large-scale prospective studies with long term follow up may provide us with evidences for its clinical use.

Keywords Esophageal cancer • Circulating tumor cells • Cancer stem cells • Flow cytometry • p75NTR

13.1 Esophageal Squamous Carcinoma (ESCC)

Recent progress in multimodal therapies, such as preoperative chemo- or chemoradiotherapy followed by radical surgery, has facilitated an improved postoperative prognosis in patients with locally advanced esophageal squamous cell carcinoma (ESCC) (Thallinger et al. 2011; van Hagen et al. 2012). However, many of the patients still exhibit postoperative tumor recurrence with a 5-year progression free survival rate of about 40% (Ando et al. 2012; Hara et al. 2013), indicating the presence of chemo-resistant micrometastasis, which were undetectable at the time of surgery (Kell et al. 2000). Therefore, innovative strategies to detect micrometastasis may provide us with a more accurate diagnosis to determine indications for therapies.

13.2 Detection of CTCs

In recent years, reports have demonstrated circulating tumor cells (CTCs) as an early detection marker for cancer metastasis (Hughes and King 2012). Quantification of CTCs revealed that CTCs were an independent prognostic factor in patients with various types of tumors, such as colorectal (Cohen et al. 2008), breast (Cristofanilli et al. 2004), and prostate cancer (de Bono et al. 2008).

The most widely reported CTC detection has been based on immunomagnetic enrichment with epithelial cell adhesion molecule (EpCAM) antibodies and subsequent immunological identification using cytokeratin (CK) antibodies (Ross et al. 1986; Mostert et al. 2009). EpCAM is broadly expressed in most of the epithelial cells and carcinomas (Ross et al. 1986; Mostert et al. 2009). CKs are also used as markers for tumor cells of epithelial origin (Moll et al. 1982; Osborn et al. 1986).

On the other hand, recent studies suggested a clinical significance of a subpopulation of CTCs with cancer stem cell (CSC) properties, such as self-renew, tumorigenicity, drug resistance and metastasis (Clarke et al. 2006; Reya et al. 2001), which were named circulating tumor stem cells (CTSCs) (Grover et al. 2014). Compared with CTCs, CTSCs are considered to be a more accurate prognostic factor because CSCs are responsible for metastasis through processes such as epithelial mesenchymal transition (EMT), invasion into vessels, circulation, and tumor initiation in the metastatic sites (Dean et al. 2005; Schatton and Frank 2008; Wicha and Hayes 2011). In reports, CSC markers of the primary tumor, such as CD44 or CD133, have been used to detect CTSCs in breast (Baccelli et al. 2013), colon (Pilati et al. 2012) and hepatocellular carcinoma (Sun et al. 2013).

13.3 p75 Neurotrophin Receptor (p75NTR) Is a Candidate Stem Cell Marker in ESCC

In ESCC, p75 neurotrophin receptor (p75NTR or CD271) has been reported to be a candidate CSC marker (Okumura et al. 2006; Huang et al. 2009). p75NTR is expressed in mitotically quiescent basal cells in normal esophageal epithelium and infiltrative margin of the tumor in ESCC (Okumura et al. 2015; Yamaguchi et al. 2016a) (Fig. 13.1). A recent report from our laboratory further demonstrated that p75NTR positive cells isolated by flow cytometry from ESCC cell lines showed significantly higher colony formation, enhanced tumor formation in mice, and greater chemo resistance, along with stronger expression of EMT-related genes (Yamaguchi et al. 2016a). Molecularly, p75NTR is a 75-kDa cell-surface receptor glycoprotein, which is a member of the tumor necrosis factor receptor superfamily (Rodriguez-Tebar et al. 1992) and involved in regulation of malignant phenotypes in various types of cancer. For example, the NGF/proNGF/p75NTR axis was demonstrated to play a critical role in regulating the self-renewal of quiescent CSC, as well as promoting EMT, in breast cancer (Tomellini et al. 2015). Overexpression of NGF and its autocrine loop was also shown to enhance cell proliferation and migration in ESCC cell lines (Tsunoda et al. 2006), suggesting that p75NTR is critically involved in metastasis in ESCC.

13.4 Flow Cytometric Detection of CTCs Based on the Expression of p75NTR and Its Clinical Relevance in ESCC

In a recent report from our laboratory, we used flow cytometry to detect CTCs, which enabled us to analyze the expression of multiple cell surface markers in viable cells (Yamaguchi et al. 2016b). Investigation using peripheral blood samples of ESCC patients revealed that the EpCAM+ cell count was significantly higher than that of healthy controls, with cell counts (average $\pm$ SD) of 2.3 ± 2.5 and 34.0 ± 35.8, respectively ($p = 0.011$), indicating successful detection of CTCs using flow cytometry. Then our two-color flow cytometric detection demonstrated that EpCAM+ p75NTR+ cell count was significantly higher in ESCC patients than healthy controls, with cell counts (average $\pm$ SD) of 0.4 ± 0.9 and 16.0 ± 18.3,

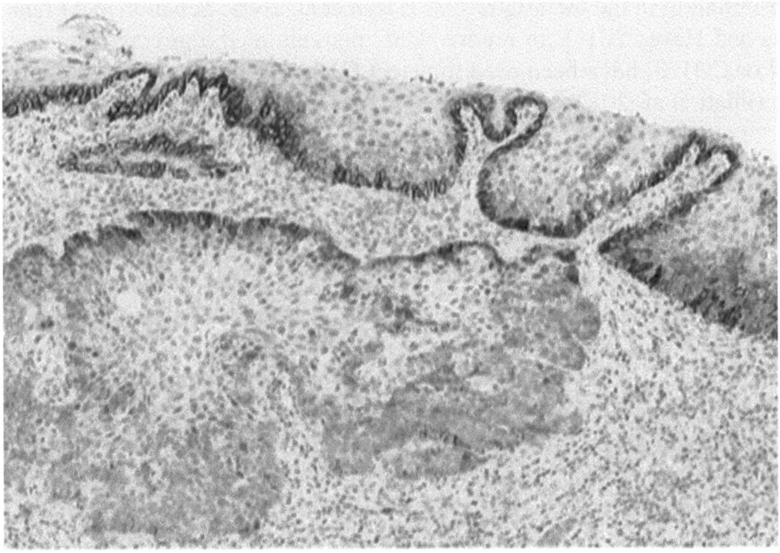

Fig. 13.1 A representative photograph of immunohistochemical staining for p75NTR in ESCC specimens (Reproduced from Yamaguchi et al. (2016b) with permission from BioMed Central)

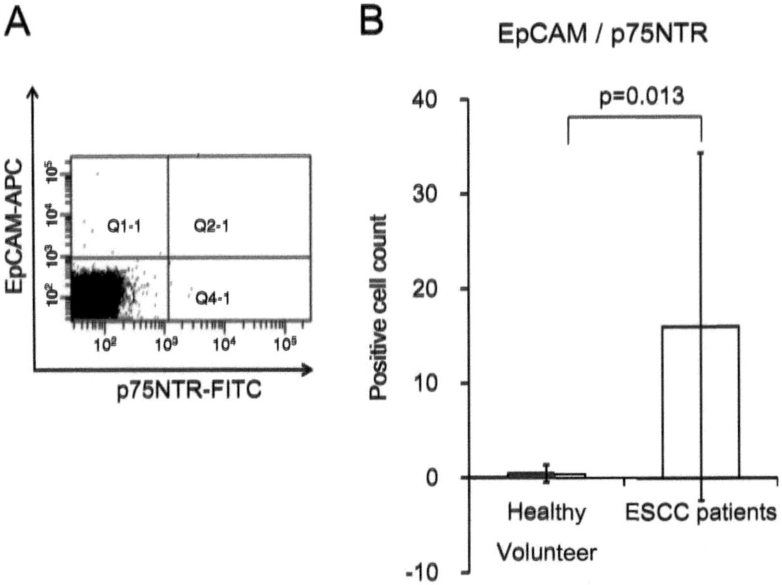

Fig. 13.2 Detection of CTCs in ESCC patients based on p75NTR expression A: Mononuclear cells from 3 mL peripheral blood of an ESCC patient were co-stained with anti-EpCAM-APC and anti-p75NTR-FITC, and analyzed by two-color flow cytometry. Quadrant markers were set according to isotype-matched controls. B: Mean numbers of p75NTR+ CTCs from 3 mL peripheral blood of ESCC patients and controls. Error bars represent the standard error of the mean. (Reproduced from Yamaguchi et al. (2016b) with permission from BioMed Central)

Table 13.1 Relationship between the clinicopathological features and mean EpCAM + p75NTR+ or EpCAM + p75NTR- CTC counts in patients who underwent surgery

Characteristics	n	EpCAM + p75NTR+ (Average ± SD)	p-value	EpCAM + p75NTR- (Average ± SD)	p-value
pT 0–2/3–4	4/6	2.0 ± 2.8/26.2 ± 29.3	0.146	27.0 ± 50.1/2.0 ± 4.9	0.246
pN 0/1–3	7/3	14.9 ± 27.7/20.3 ± 23.1	0.773	0.8 ± 2.3/38.0 ± 55.7	0.090
ly 0/1–2	7/3	14.9 ± 27.7/20.3 ± 23.1	0.773	0.8 ± 2.3/38.0 ± 55.7	0.090
v 0/1–2	7/3	5.0 ± 4.2/43.3 ± 35.6	*0.016	0.8 ± 2.3/38.0 ± 55.7	0.090
pStage 1–2/3–4	7/3	15.7 ± 27.2/18.3 ± 25.1	0.891	15.4 ± 38.2/4.0 ± 6.9	0.632

Reproduced from Yamaguchi et al. (2016b) with permission from BioMed Central
CTC circulating tumor cell, *ly* lymphatic invasion, *v* venous invasion, *SD* standard deviation. *p < 0.05

respectively (p = 0.013, Fig. 13.2a, b). The proportion of EpCAM+ p75NTR+ cells in EpCAM+ cells (average ± SD) was 56.7 ± 39.6% (range 5.6–100.0%).

More importantly, EpCAM + p75NTR+, but not EpCAM + p75NTR- CTC counts, correlated with clinically diagnosed distant metastasis (p = 0.003, Table 13.1) and pathological venous invasion in surgically resected primary ESCC tumors (p = 0.016, Table 13.2).

These results demonstrated that CTC detection with a combination of EpCAM and p75NTR was more accurate diagnostic marker than EpCAM alone, suggesting the highly metastatic potential of CTCs with p75NTR expression.

Investigations based on large-scale prospective studies with long term follow up may provide us with evidences for its clinical use.

13.5 Isolation and Molecular Characterization of p75NTR-Positive CTCs

Due to technical limitations in their sensitively, specifically and viability, it has been challenging to characterize CTCs in most of the reported CTC detection strategies (van der Toom EE et al. 2016).

In our previous report (Yamaguchi et al. 2016b), immunocytochemical double staining using EpCAM-APC and p75NTR-FITC confirmed the expression of EpCAM and p75NTR in viable cells isolated from the peripheral blood of ESCC patients (Fig. 13.3). The cell was a mononuclear cell, 35 μm in diameter with a high nucleocytoplasmic ratio, with a diagnosis of malignant cytology.

To assess the biological properties of the cells, we seeded EpCAM+ p75NTR+ cells sorted from 23 of advanced ESCC patients with cell number (average ± SD)

Table 13.2 Relationship between the clinical features and mean EpCAM + p75NTR+ or EpCAM + p75NTR- CTC counts in patients who received chemotherapy or chemoradio therapy

Characteristics	n	EpCAM + p75NTR+ (Average ± SD)	p-value	EpCAM + p75NTR- (Average ± SD)	p-value
T 0–2/3–4	1/12	7.0/16.4 ± 13.0	0.501	0/23.9 ± 30.6	0.468
N 0/1–3	1/12	7.0/16.4 ± 13.0	0.501	0/23.9 ± 30.6	0.468
M 0/1	8/5	7.1 ± 5.9/29.4 ± 6.4	*0.003	19.5 ± 20.8/26.2 ± 43.7	0.713
Stage1–2/3–4	1/12	7.0/16.4 ± 13.0	0.501	0/23.9 ± 30.6	0.468

Reproduced from Yamaguchi et al. (2016b) with permission from BioMed Central
CTC circulating tumor cell, *SD* standard deviation *$p < 0.05$

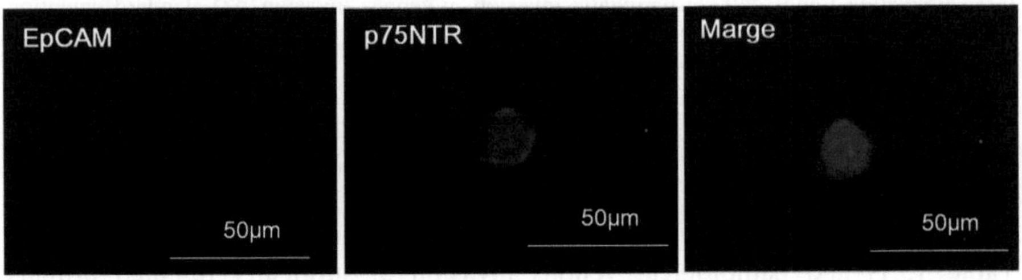

Fig. 13.3 Image of a representative EpCAM+ and p75NTR+ cell sorted from 3 mL peripheral blood in a patient with ESCC using flow cytometer. The images show an overlay of DAPI (*Blue*), p75NTR (*Green*), and EpCAM (*Red*) (Reproduced from Yamaguchi et al. (2016b) with permission from BioMed Central)

of 16.0 ± 18.3, onto cell culture condition, however, we could not obtain primary culture of the cells.

A possible reason of the failure was that the numbers of the isolated cells were too small. A recent report from our laboratory demonstrated that minimally 100 cells were required to establish colonies in vitro, using p75NTR+ cells isolated from cultured ESCC cell lines (Yamaguchi et al. 2016a). In addition, a previous report demonstrated that even using resected primary tumor, esophageal cancer cell lines were established only 21 of 50 (42.0%) ESCC patients under the same culture condition which we used in this study (Shimada et al. 1992).

Improvement of CTC isolation procedure with higher yield and higher viability may enable us biological characterization of the EpCAM+ p75NTR+ CTCs in ESCC.

13.6 Conclusion

Flow cytometric detection of CTCs based on combined expression of EpCAM and p75NTR was demonstrated to be a more accurate diagnostic marker than EpCAM alone in patients with ESCC. Large-scale prospective studies with long term follow up may provide us with evidences for its clinical use. Investigation using the isolated EpCAM+ and p75NTR+ CTCs to assess their stem cell properties may shed light on their roles in tumor metastasis in ESCC as well.

Conflicts of Interest Disclosure None of the authors has any financial relationships to disclose.

References

Ando N, Kato H, Igaki H et al (2012) A randomized trial comparing postoperative adjuvant chemotherapy with cisplatin and 5-fluorouracil versus preoperative chemotherapy for localized advanced squamous cell carcinoma of the thoracic esophagus (JCOG9907). Ann Surg Oncol 19(1):68–74

Baccelli I, Schneeweiss A, Riethdorf S et al (2013) Identification of a population of blood circulating tumor cells from breast cancer patients that initiates metastasis in a xenograft assay. Nat Biotechnol 31(6):539–544

Clarke MF, Dick JE, Dirks PB et al (2006) Cancer stem cells-perspectives on current status and future directions: AACR workshop on cancer stem cells. Cancer Res 66(19):9339–9344

Cohen SJ, Punt CJ, Iannotti N et al (2008) Relationship of circulating tumor cells to tumor response, progression-free survival, and overall survival in patients with metastatic colorectal cancer. J Clin Oncol 26(19):3213–3221

Cristofanilli M, Budd GT, Ellis MJ et al (2004) Circulating tumor cells, disease progression, and survival in metastatic breast cancer. N Engl J Med 351(8):781–791

de Bono JS, Scher HI, Montgomery RB et al (2008) Circulating tumor cells predict survival benefit from treatment in metastatic castration-resistant prostate cancer. Clin Cancer Res 14 (19):6302–6309

Dean M, Fojo T, Bates S (2005) Tumour stem cells and drug resistance. Nat Rev Cancer 5 (4):275–284

Grover PK, Cummins AG, Price TJ et al (2014) Circulating tumour cells: the evolving concept and the inadequacy of their enrichment by EpCAM-based methodology for basic and clinical cancer research. Ann Oncol 25(8):1506–1516

Hara H, Tahara M, Daiko H et al (2013) Phase II feasibility study of preoperative chemotherapy with docetaxel, cisplatin, and fluorouracil for esophageal squamous cell carcinoma. Cancer Sci 104(11):1455–1460

Huang SD, Yuan Y, Liu X-H et al (2009) Self-renewal and chemotherapy resistance of p75NTR positive cells in esophageal squamous cell carcinomas. BMC Cancer 9:9

Hughes AD, King MR (2012) Nanobiotechnology for the capture and manipulation of circulating tumor cells. Wiley Interdiscip Rev Nanomed Nanobiotechnol 4(3):291–309

Kell MR, Winter DC, O'Sullivan GC et al (2000) Biological behaviour and clinical implications of micrometastases. Br J Surg 87(12):1629–1639

Moll R, Franke WW, Schiller DL et al (1982) The catalog of human cytokeratins: patterns of expression in normal epithelia, tumors and cultured cells. Cell 31(1):11–24

Mostert B, Sleijfer S, Foekens JA et al (2009) Circulating tumor cells (CTCs): detection methods and their clinical relevance in breast cancer. Cancer Treat Rev 35(5):463–474

Okumura T, Tsunoda S, Mori Y et al (2006) The biological role of the low-affinity p75 neurotrophin receptor in esophageal squamous cell carcinoma. Clin Cancer Res 12 (17):5096–5103

Okumura T, Shimada Y, Sakurai T et al (2015) Abnormal cell proliferation in the p75NTR-positive basal cell compartment of the esophageal epithelium during squamous carcinogenesis. Dis Esophagus 28(7):634–643

Osborn M, van Lessen G, Weber K et al (1986) Differential diagnosis of gastrointestinal carcinomas by using monoclonal antibodies specific for individual keratin polypeptides. Lab Investig 55(4):497–504

Pilati P, Mocellin S, Bertazza L et al (2012) Prognostic value of putative circulating cancer stem cells in patients undergoing hepatic resection for colorectal liver metastasis. Ann Surg Oncol 19(2):402–408

Reya T, Morrison SJ, Clarke MF et al (2001) Stem cells, cancer, and cancer stem cells. Nature 414 (6859):105–111

Rodriguez-Tebar A, Dechant G, Gotz R et al (1992) Binding of neurotrophin-3 to its neuronal receptors and interactions with nerve growth factor and brainderived neurotrophic factor. EMBOJ 11(3):917–922

Ross AH, Herlyn D, Iliopoulos D et al (1986) Isolation and characterization of a carcinoma-associated antigen. Biochem Biophys Res Commun 135(1):297–303

Schatton T, Frank MH (2008) Cancer stem cells and human malignant melanoma. Pigment Cell Melanoma Res 21(1):39–55

Shimada Y, Imamura M, Wagata T et al (1992) Characterization of 21 newly established esophageal cancer cell lines. Cancer 69(2):277–284

Sun YF, Xu Y, Yang XR et al (2013) Circulating stem cell-like epithelial cell adhesion molecule-positive tumor cells indicate poor prognosis of hepatocellular carcinoma after curative resection. Hepatology 57(4):1458–1468

Thallinger CM, Raderer M, Hejna M (2011) Esophageal cancer: a critical evaluation of systemic second-line therapy. J Clin Oncol 29(35):4709–4714

Tomellini E, Touil Y, Lagadec C et al (2015) Nerve growth factor and proNGF simultaneously promote symmetric self-renewal, quiescence, and epithelial to mesenchymal transition to enlarge the breast cancer stem cell compartment. Stem Cells 33(2):342–353

van der Toom EE, Verdone JE, Gorin MA et al (2016) Technical challenges in the isolation and analysis of circulating tumor cells. Oncotarget Aug 10. [Epub ahead of print]

van Hagen P, Hulshof MC, van Lanschot JJ et al (2012) Preoperative chemoradiotherapy for esophageal or junctional cancer. N Engl J Med 366(22):2074–2084

Tsunoda S, Okumura T, Ito T et al (2006) Significance of nerve growth factor overexpression and its autocrine loop in esophageal squamous cell carcinoma. Br J Cancer 95(3):322–330

Wicha MS, Hayes DF (2011) Circulating tumor cells: not all detected cells are bad and not all bad cells are detected. J Clin Oncol 29(15):1508–1511

Yamaguchi T, Okumura T, Hirano K et al (2016a) p75 neurotrophin receptor expression is a characteristic of the mitotically quiescent cancer stem cell population present in esophageal squamous cell carcinoma. Int J Oncol 48(5):1943–1954

Yamaguchi T, Okumura T, Hirano K et al (2016b) Detection of circulating tumor cells by p75NTR expression in patients with esophageal cancer. World J Surg Oncol 14(1):40

Chapter 14
Personalized Treatment Through Detection and Monitoring of Genetic Aberrations in Single Circulating Tumor Cells

Swee Jin Tan, Trifanny Yeo, Sarvesh Abhay Sukhatme, Say Li Kong, Wan-Teck Lim, and Chwee Teck Lim

Abstract Circulating tumor cells (CTCs) present a viable alternative to access tumor materials other than primary biopsies in cancer. This disease is among the most widespread in the world and is difficult to target because of its complex nature, challenges in getting quality samples and dynamic temporal changes in response to treatment. Conventional methods of detection and monitoring the disease profile do not suffice to be able to target the heterogeneity that exists at the cellular level. CTCs have been identified as a possible substitute for tumor tissue samples, and can be

---

S.J. Tan • T. Yeo
Clearbridge Accelerator Pte Ltd, 81 Science Park Drive, The Chadwick, #02-03, Singapore Science Park 1, Singapore 118257, Singapore
e-mail: tansweejin@gmail.com; trifanny@clearbridgeaccelerator.com

S.A. Sukhatme
Mechanobiology Institute of Singapore, 5A Engineering Drive 1, Singapore 117411, Singapore
e-mail: mbisas@nus.edu.sg

S.L. Kong
Genome Institute of Singapore, 60, Biopolis Street, #02-01, Genome, Singapore 138672, Singapore
e-mail: kongsl@gis.a-star.edu.sg

W.-T. Lim
Division of Medical Oncology, National Cancer Centre Singapore, 11 Hospital Drive, Singapore 169610, Singapore

Institute of Molecular and Cell Biology, 61 Biopolis Drive, Proteos, Singapore 138673, Singapore
e-mail: dmolwt@nccs.com.sg

C.T. Lim (✉)
Mechanobiology Institute of Singapore, 5A Engineering Drive 1, Singapore 117411, Singapore

Department of Biomedical Engineering, National University of Singapore, 9 Engineering Drive 1, Block EA, #03-12, Singapore 117575, Singapore
e-mail: ctlim@nus.edu.sg

M.J.M. Magbanua, J.W. Park (eds.), *Isolation and Molecular Characterization of Circulating Tumor Cells*, Advances in Experimental Medicine and Biology 994,
DOI 10.1007/978-3-319-55947-6_14

used to complement current disease management. Challenges in CTCs molecular analysis lie in the purity of the sample, which is masked by the presence of large quantities of white blood cells (WBCs). In this chapter, we present a microfluidic biochip platform that performs secondary purification to isolate single CTCs efficiently. Studying single CTCs will allow for sensitive detection of critical mutations and addressing intercellular variances that will be otherwise missed easily due to low mutation frequencies when evaluating bulk cell retrieval. Using the biochip, we isolated single CTCs, and conducted personalized integrated *EGFR* mutational analysis using conventional polymerase chain reaction (PCR) and Sanger sequencing. We also demonstrated that high quality next generation sequencing (NGS) libraries can be readily generated from these samples. In our initial study, we revealed that the dominant *EGFR* mutations such as L858R and T790M could be detected in Non Small Cell Lung Cancer (NSCLC) patients with low CTC counts. We envision the biochip will enable efficient isolation of rare single cells from samples. This technology coupled with downstream molecular characterization of CTCs will aid in realizing the personalized medicine for cancer patients.

Keywords Cancer • Liquid biopsy • Drug resistance • Clonal heterogeneity • Single cell analysis

14.1 Introduction

Cancer is a global healthcare burden and drug resistance by the cancer cells is a major obstacle in eradicating the disease (Saunders et al. 2012). The disease is complex and differs from patient to patient even though these patients may be diagnosed with the same type of cancer. Several key genes have been discovered to play key roles in cancer progression. Over or under expression of these genes have been found to drive tumor growth. Inter-individual variation in the genetic composition of the disease may also influence the response to treatment (Kessler et al. 2014). Some individuals are also at a greater predisposition to cancer because of hereditary factors such as *BRCA1* for breast cancer, which results in a higher risk of developing the disease (Andrykowski et al. 1996). Hence, the genetic composition plays a significant role in the diagnosis and prognosis of cancer.

The diagnosis of cancer is frequently an amalgamation of different tests. Central to this problem is how to obtain ample tumor tissue for definitive pathological diagnosis. Additional molecular tests are carried out on the gross sample where indicated (e.g. *EGFR* mutation testing in lung cancer). These conventional methods of molecular analysis use average cell population data collected from tissues, however these methods lack the information regarding genetic variations present at the cellular level. This can lead to false negative calls for key genetic mutations if they exist at low frequencies. This problem can be overcome by increasing the purity and representation of tumor tissue (e.g. using laser capture microdissection) or increasing the sensitivity of the tests to pick up the rare variants (e.g. targeted resequencing). The need for a test with high sensitivity emphasizes the rare nature of these tumor cells in the background matrix of normal or stromal cells. These challenges are amplified when we utilize blood-based biopsy for enumeration of rare circulating tumor cells (CTCs).

Since their discovery (Ashworth 1869), CTCs are being extensively studied for detection and monitoring cancer progression (Maheswaran and Haber 2010; Kling 2012; Alix-Panabières and Pantel 2013). Particularly, due to their significant role in metastasis, great progress has been made to effectively isolate and study CTCs from various different cancer types in patient's blood (Aceto et al. 2014; Pierga et al. 2008). Further molecular analysis of CTCs provides rich information about the omics of the disease, which can be translated into a better prognosis (Cristofanilli et al. 2004a). The number of CTCs in blood is rare (Williams 2013) and highly dependent on the type of cancer, treatment given and stage of the disease (Allard et al. 2004). Typically, patients in the advanced disease stages have greater CTC counts (Fan et al. 2009). Enumeration of CTCs itself can provide prognostic value for identifying patients with better overall survival outcome (Cohen et al. 2008; Cristofanilli et al. 2005). Because CTCs are obtained from blood, this method is less invasive and simply requires a routine draw of blood specimens and hence termed "liquid biopsy".

CTCs present a viable substitute for conventional tissue biopsy but purity within blood samples is a limiting factor. Traditional molecular profiling essentially produces a mean response and does not suffice in such rare cell events. Furthermore, studying population averages are insufficient to address intercellular variances that can be critical to disease profiling (Schubert 2011). Single cell analysis allow probing of the real cellular variance and provides more accurate representation of the disease complexity (Wang and Bodovitz 2010). In this chapter, we describe a microfluidic biochip that enables the selective recovery of single cells with minimal losses coupled with morphology and immuno-cytochemistry. It fulfills for single cell analysis the critical need in the sample preparation of mix cells populations for various downstream assays as depicted in Fig. 14.1. We describe the sample output integration process with conventional polymerase chain reaction (PCR) and next-generation sequencing (NGS) library preparation. Here, we demonstrate the essential need of single cell analysis in the detection of *EGFR* mutations within late stage non-small cell lung cancer (NSCLC) samples.

14.2 Microfluidics and the Need for Isolating Single Cells

Micro and nano-devices offer great potential for sample and fluid manipulation at a small scale. One great example is microfluidics technology (Autebert et al. 2012; Whitesides 2006) which harnesses the laminar characteristics of fluid flow in the microdevices. Microfluidics can lead to improved sensitivity (Chin et al. 2007), provides integration of biological assays (Paguirigan and Beebe 2008) and cater for multiplex capabilities (Thorsen et al. 2002). A variety of functionalities such as

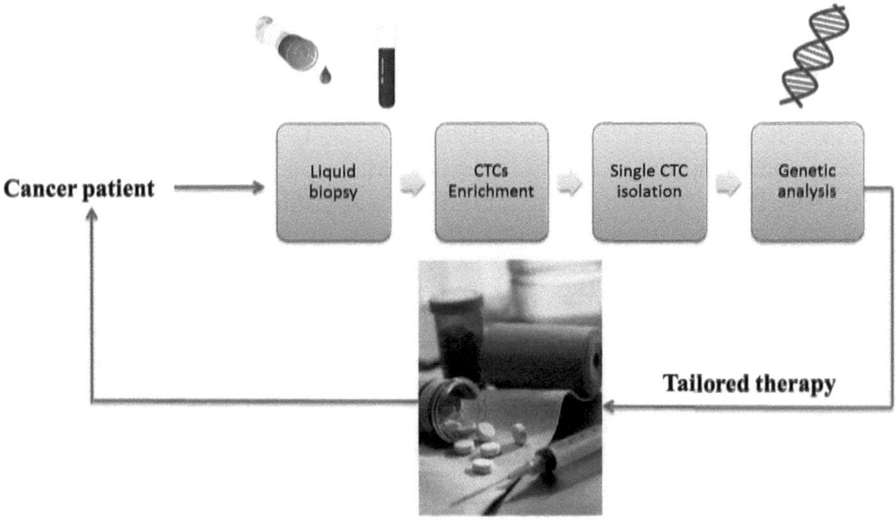

Fig. 14.1 Personalized approach to the treatment of cancer

DNA sequencing (Kartalov and Quake 2004), enzyme-linked immunosorbent assay (ELISA) (Eteshola and Balberg 2004) and blood analysis (VanDelinder and Groisman 2006) have been implemented on microfluidic platforms with efficiencies greater than that of conventional available systems, higher throughput and more cost-effective as it only requires nano-scale liter of less of reagents volume (Mark et al. 2010).

14.2.1 Microfluidics and CTCs Enrichment

Microfluidics plays an important role in the advancement of CTC detection and analysis (Dong et al. 2013). The main technical challenge has been the excessive amounts of accompanying white blood cells (WBCs) in each specimen (Budd 2009; Powell et al. 2012). In a healthy adult, 1 ml of blood contains approximately in the order of 10^6 leukocytes and 10^9 erythrocytes. Therefore sensitive methods are required for obtaining CTCs directly from blood. Numerous platforms have been developed to enrich for rare CTCs from the blood of mixed cells populations based on antibody affinity (Nagrath et al. 2007; Ozkumur et al. 2013; Reategui et al. 2015), size based separation (Hou et al. 2013; Tan et al. 2009) and flow based assays (Karabacak et al. 2014; Mach et al. 2011). These technologies have achieved relatively good results in CTCs detection and analysis (Fig. 14.2). Cancer cell recovery rates from spiked cell experiments were as high as 95% and enumeration data from clinical specimens were correlated to treatment and disease outcome (Cristofanilli et al. 2004b). However, the contaminating WBCs still pose a major technical challenge for molecular analysis. Abundant copies of wild type DNA

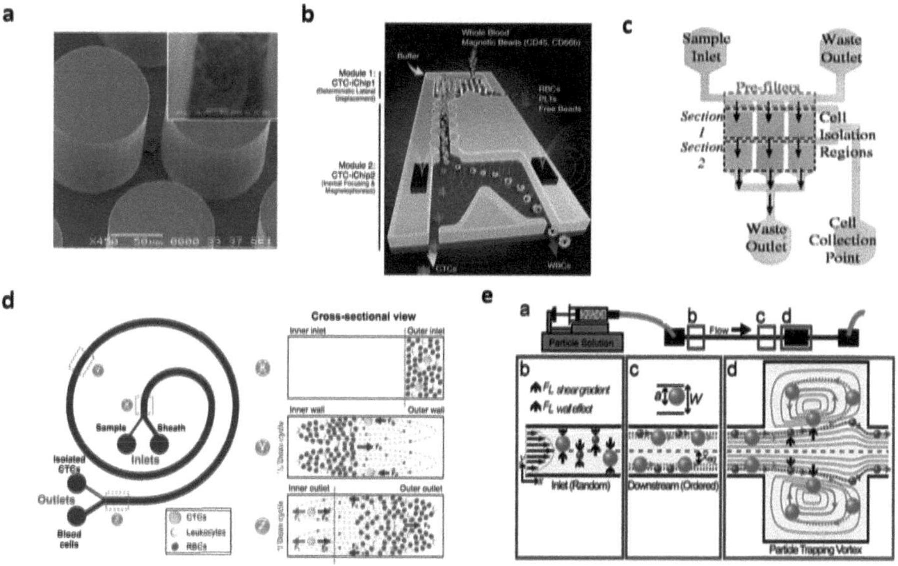

Fig. 14.2 CTC enrichment using microfluidic technologies based on different cellular properties. (**a**) Antibody based CTC selection (Nagrath et al. 2007). (**b**) Combinatory flow based and antibody affinity separation (Karabacak et al. 2014). (**c**) Size and cellular deformability based separation (Tan et al. 2009). (**d**) Label free inertial flow separation (Hou et al. 2013). (**e**) Cell separation via laminar microvortices (Mach et al. 2011)

hinder the accurate detection of low frequency mutations (Punnoose et al. 2010) even after primary enrichment using these CTC platforms. This can result in mutant signatures being marginalized in pooled CTC sample studies. For example, in a clinical trial to detect *EGFR* mutations in NSCLC patients by Punnoose et al. (2012), it reported low concordance rates of 12.5% between CTCs and the matching corresponding primary tumor. Hence, the need to remove background signals is paramount for the successful analysis of these rare cells.

Single cell analysis offers great promise to enhance the sensitivity of mutation detection assays by pre-filtering of unwanted background cells. As such, only tumor cells are selected for examination of disease related analysis. Cell to cell variability can also be better addressed, which is important to capture critical driver mutations and avoid false negative results. In order to retrieve these rare single CTCs, it is necessary to remove the contaminating WBCs from the enriched blood specimens obtained from cell enrichment devices. As the absolute CTC number is considered small, conventional methods using fluorescence activated cell sorters (FACS) (Swennenhuis et al. 2013; Neves et al. 2014) or micropipette aspiration (Dey et al. 2015; Stoecklein et al. 2008) are inadequate or tedious. In a study done using FACS to capture single CTCs, it was determined that losses could exceed more than 50% (Swennenhuis et al. 2013). The process of micropipette aspiration is tedious as it involves massive number of cells that need to be surveyed in a CTC specimen and hence increases the risk of human errors. The cell losses and laborious procedures make these methods less desirable and difficult to be implemented in a clinical setting. Microfluidics has had some successes in single cell preparation and analysis. Various such systems have shown to have different capabilities in integrating NGS analysis in its workflow (White et al. 2011; Yang et al. 2015; Swennenhuis et al. 2015). These include massive large scale sorting by magnetic separation (Robert et al. 2011) and dielectrophoretic (DEP) separation (Stoecklein et al. 2008) for the precise selection of single cells. However, cell losses and limited capacity remained the major obstacles associated with these integrated technologies (Peeters et al. 2013; Hyun and Jung 2014). Nonetheless, the need for single cell preparation of rare cell samples is escalating for numerous applications such as CTCs detection and molecular analysis. Our proposed device fills the gap and prepares single CTC samples with high fidelity and minimal losses for downstream single cell analysis.

14.2.2 Development of a Single Cell Isolation Microfluidic Biochip

The biochip (Yeo et al. 2016) that was developed to address single cell sorting and recovery works on the principle of hydrodynamic focusing for efficient cell isolation and interrogation, immuno-fluorescence detection for cell selection and active fluid control for selective cell recovery. The schematic layout of the biochip design is illustrated in Fig. 14.3, which demonstrates a high-speed capture of the precise cancer cell movement into the cell chamber. Briefly, the design of the biochip encompasses numerous temporary holding chambers for single cells that are positioned along a curved portion of the microfluidic channel. This allows for multiplexing in terms of retaining and viewing numerous cells at the same time. Further throughput enhancement can be achieved by increasing the number of cell chambers. We employ hydrodynamic focusing to ensure cells are flowing close to these chambers. The nett resultant force directed towards these chambers favored the entry of a single cell into an unoccupied chamber (Fig 14.3b). This ensured the efficiency in cell capture and minimal losses of target cells in the samples. Cells in the chambers will be pre-stained with an identifying marker for either positive selection or negative depletion. Desired single cells can then be recovered by activating a dedicated control line attached to the chamber to push out the cell. Such an active mechanism allows for separation of desired or selected cells. This biochip is flexible enough to pool all of the desired cells in the recovery channel or to extract them as single cells for downstream molecular profiling.

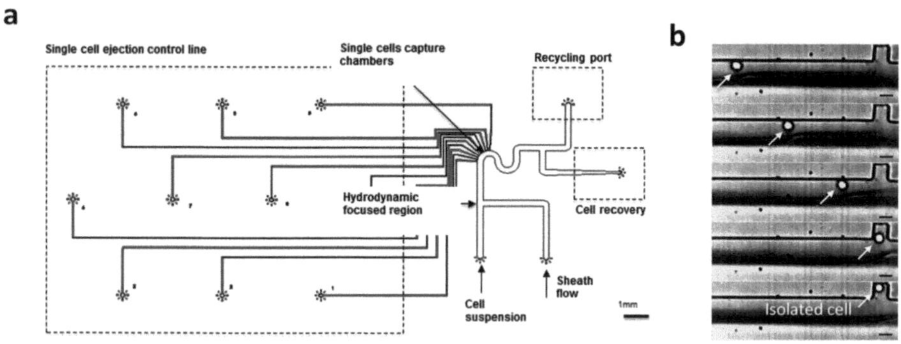

Fig. 14.3 (**a**) Device schematic showing cell and sheath flow entry, hydrodynamic focusing region and cell recovery. Scale bar represents 1 mm. (**b**) High speed imaging of single MCF-7 cell isolation captured at 27,000 fps. Scale bar represents 20 μm

14.2.2.1 Fast Processing Time

One of the key limitations of conventional single cell isolation methodologies such as micropipette aspiration is the tedious and time-consuming nature of the procedure. Using the biochip, we have designed the operations in such a way that cells can be easily trapped in these chambers. With polystyrene beads as a model sample, the device was shown to allow for rapid capture of single beads in the chambers as indicated in Fig 14.4a. It took a mere 2 s to fully load the biochip at a flow rate of 50 μl/min. Sample concentrations were tested in the range of 50,000 to 100,000 beads/ml that simulated a blood specimen. The fast processing time allows a rapid turnover of samples and the ability to address hundreds and thousands of cells at a relatively short amount of time. Using clinical CTC samples that involve 7.5–8 ml of whole blood, it takes approximately 3 h to complete the single cell recovery process.

14.2.2.2 Precise Cell Selection and Perfect Cell Separation

Cells are selected within the system based on antibody-antigen labeling or physical characteristics of the cell. As the biochip is integrated into an existing microscope, it provides the flexibility for image analysis as shown in Fig 14.4b. Cells can be selected in these cell chambers based on a positive or negative marker akin to flow cytometry or by physical characteristics such as size or nucleus to cytoplasmic ratio based on optical imaging. The flexibility is required for CTC samples, as that will maximize the yield of these circulating cells from each blood specimen. This also ensures that we capture the entire range of CTCs, which might be missed when only using a single positive biomarker. The precise cell selection within this biochip is achieved with the dedicated flow control lines attached to each chamber. Only cells that pass the selection criteria are routed to recovery. We have demonstrated using spiked controls with MCF-7, a breast adenocarcinoma cell line, in an abundance of

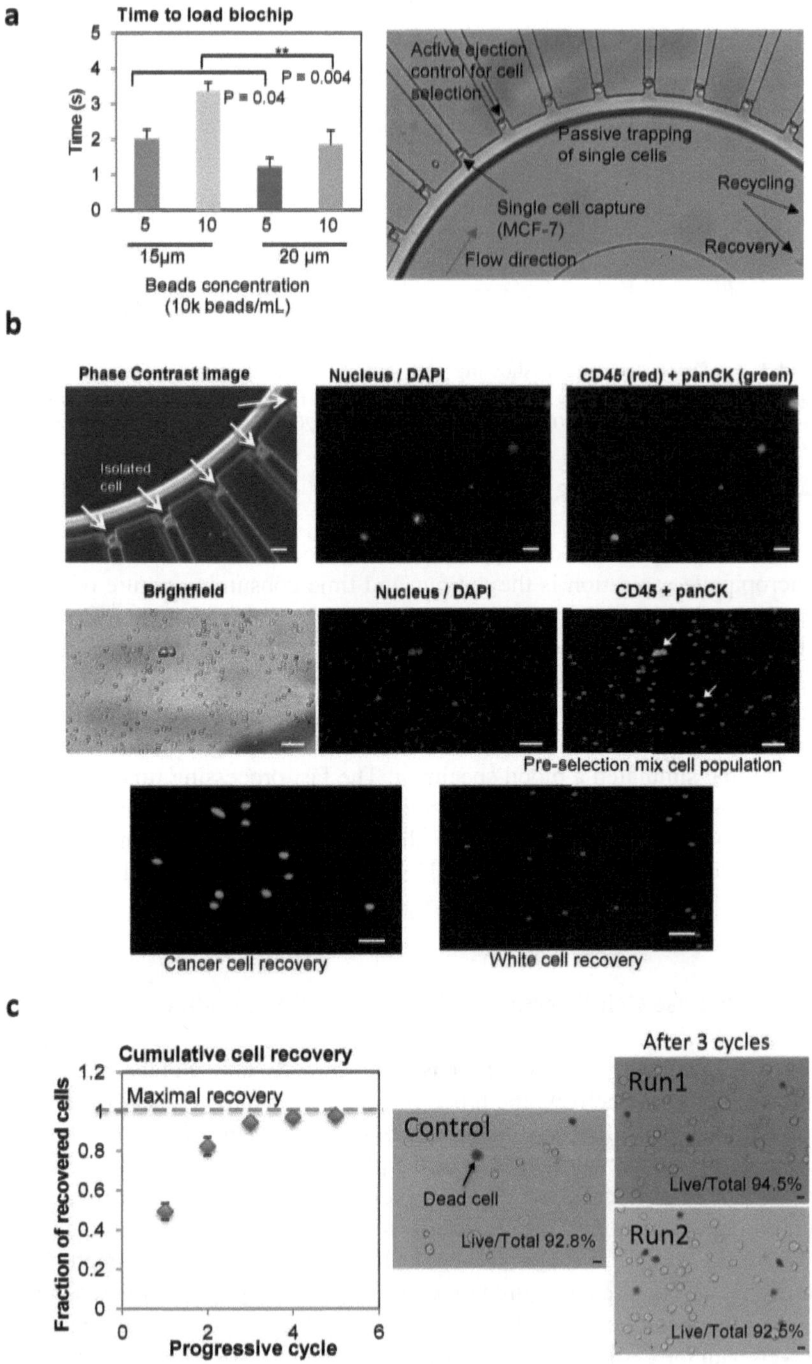

Fig. 14.4 Single cell biochip characterisitcs and efficiency. (**a**) Sample loading characterization showing rapid cell loading for selection. (**b**) Immuno-cytochemistry for cell selection to ensure perfect separation at the recovery. (**c**) Cell loss measurements indicating three cycles of processing are desired for each sample. Cell integrity after biochip processing shows that the cell viability remaining similar to input control

WBCs to achieve perfect cell separation using both positive (cytokeratin) and negative (CD45) selection. Cytokeratin are intermediate filaments found in the cytoplasmic region of epithelial cells. CTCs that are disseminated from tumor tissues may have this signature present, which can be utilized as a marker for positive selection. In our own trials, we also ensured cell integrity as a criterion for recovery, as our goal is to pipe these single cell samples for downstream molecular profiling assays. The intactness of the cells is important for the subsequent PCR step used to amplify the genetic locus of interest.

14.2.2.3 Minimal Losses and Viable Cellular Output

Optimal cell recovery is another important parameter that affects the sensitivity and specificity of using CTCs in disease profiling. Using this biochip, we ascertained that the cell losses could be reduced to a negligible amount by incorporating multiple processing cycles of every specimen. This operational procedure allowed the system to isolate any remaining CTCs and achieve higher capture efficiency. As shown in Fig 14.4c, the sample recovery was more than 99% after three cycles. The biochip characterization trials were performed five times independently. This feature is crucial for CTC applications, as CTCs exist in extremely low numbers in comparison to the accompanying blood cells. Extending further, we determined that the effects of flow and active selection did not compromise the viability of these cells. Using a Trypan blue test, we showed that there was no statistical significance in the total viable cells before and after sample processing. This affirms the gentleness of the cell sorting procedure.

14.2.3 Integration of Downstream Methods

The biochip allows for single cell preparation with high efficiency and minimal disturbances to the integrity of the sample. We further verified numerous downstream analysis methods as depicted in Fig 14.5a that draws the single cell samples from the biochip. Our verification experiments showed that integration with various molecular downstream assays is straightforward.

In our design specifications, we had integrated immuno-cytochemistry into the cell-sorting phase. Cells can be pre-stained with the desired antibodies prior to loading into the biochip and imaged under the microscope. An example is shown in Fig 14.5b where the cancer cell had been stained for cytokeratin and the hoechst nucleus stain. Concurrent antibodies staining can be performed to gauge the quantity of different cancer subpopulations within each sample. This can also be an effective way to study the expression levels of a particular protein within each single cell. In addition, the number of CTCs has been linked to disease outcome (Cristofanilli et al. 2004b) and this method provides a rapid means to enumerate each sample for CTCs.

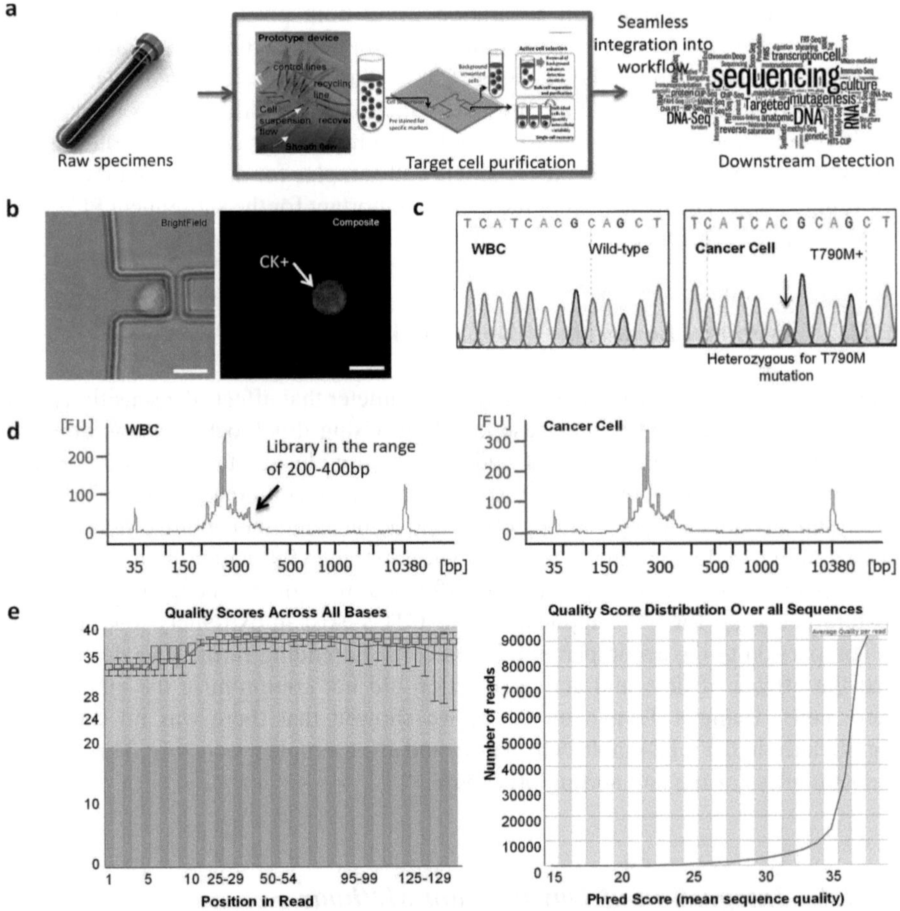

Fig. 14.5 Integrated downstream analysis for single cells capture on the biochip. (**a**) Sample processing workflow. (**b**) Immuno-cytochemistry performed on cell suspension prior to loading into the biochip. (**c**) Conventional genetic mutation detection using PCR and Sanger Sequencing. (**d**) Quality control on NGS library generated from single cells isolated from NSCLC patients. (**e**) Phred scores from an Illumina sequencing run demonstrating good quality reads

The gold standard for mutation analysis in current practice is verification using Sanger sequencing (Tsiatis et al. 2010). Single cells that are identified for recovery during sorting in the biochip can be retrieved into any compatible laboratory receptacles such as well plates and PCR tubes. In a proof of value trial, we negatively depleted WBCs from enriched CTC samples and placed each single cell into 0.2 ml PCR tubes containing lysis buffer to extract its genomic DNA. The lysis step used the Ambion Single Cell Lysis Kit (Thermo Fisher Scientific, USA) and followed procedures recommended by the manufacturer with slight modification for DNA extraction (Yeo et al. 2016). The PCR master mix containing both

EGFR L858R and T790M primer sets were then added. The primers designed for detection of *EGFR* L858R and T790M mutations are as follows:

L858R

Forward: 5′- CTAACGTTCGCCAGCCATAAGTCC-3′
Reverse: 5′- GCTGCGAGCTCACCCAGAATGTCTGG-3′

T790M

Forward: 5′-TGTAAAACGACGGCCAGTCCATGAGTACGTATTTTGAAAC TC-3′
Reverse: 5′-CAGGAAACAGCTATGACCCATATCCCCATGGCAAACTCTT GC-3′

Thermocycling conditions were as follows: 94 °C for 2 min, 40 cycles of 94 °C for 15 s, 56 °C for 30 s, 72 °C for 45 s, one cycle of 72 °C for 7 min and hold at 4 °C. The amplicons were purified and Sanger sequencing was performed. Figure 14.5c shows the electropherograms of a typical single cell that were positive for the mutations. In our validation experiments with 100 different single cells, we had shown that the loss of material was insignificant and the success rate of extracting information from the single cells that were obtained from our biochip was 98%. The high efficiency was attributed to the improved single lysis and PCR steps where the chances of cell losses were the highest.

The allure of NGS to examine massive number of genes in parallel has made it an important tool in clinical diagnosis. Its enhanced sensitivity in DNA mutation testing as compared to the conventional Sanger sequencing has demonstrated its potential for medical use. We had integrated the process to create quality NGS libraries from each of the single cells that were isolated from CTC samples. Briefly, whole genome amplification (WGA) was performed on the single cells using REPLI-g® Single Cell kit (Qiagen, USA) following the manufacturer's protocol. The denaturating buffer was added to the single cell followed by a 10min incubation at 65 °C. The denaturation was terminated by adding a neutralization buffer. The DNA amplification was carried out in a reaction mix consisting of reaction buffer and DNA polymerase for 8 h at 30 °C followed by DNA polymerase inactivation at 65 °C for 3 min. The amplified DNA was purified using AMPure XP beads (Beckman Coulter, USA) and DNA was quantified using Quant-iT™ PicoGreen® dsDNA reagent kit (Thermo Fisher Scientific, USA) on Infinite F200 PRO plate reader (Tecan, USA). We employed a targeted sequencing panel from the GeneRead™ DNAseq Targeted Panels (Qiagen, USA) to cover regions of interest. Input DNA templates taken from the amplified DNA of single cell were used to perform multiplex GeneRead™ Panel PCR and subjected to library construction using GeneRead™ DNA Library Core kit (Qiagen, USA). Each library was barcoded with an unique index and quantified using KAPA Library Quantification kit (Kapa Biosystems, USA). The library product was visualized on the Bioanalyzer (Agilent, USA) using a High Sensitivity DNA Chip (Fig 14.5d). The library with appropriate amplicon sizes indicated a successful NGS library construction. Multiple libraries were pooled together for a 150 bp paired-end sequencing run on NextSeq (Illumina, USA). Figure 14.5e shows the sequence quality from one of our clinical samples on breast cancer single cells. Average sequence quality per base were high and mean sequence quality showed consistently good quality reads. As inferred from the results, the accuracy of base calls were more than 99.9% that were indicative of a successful sequencing run.

14.3 Single Cell Analysis for Cancer Monitoring

The purpose of this chapter is to highlight the key advances in using a microfluidic biochip for single cell analysis. Liquid biopsy is potentially a valuable tool for screening as well as disease monitoring. The aims for single cell analysis using CTCs in cancer are to address the issues of the complexity of the disease and have a deeper understanding of the intra-tumor and inter-cellular heterogeneity. This can directly affect a patient's drug therapy and survival outcomes. It is clear that traditional biological assays that averages the contents of the entire sample population, under-represents the biological complexity (Blainey and Quake 2013; Wang et al. 2012; Bendall and Nolan 2012; Spencer and Sorger 2011). Single cell analysis can play an important role to probe the disease genetic heterogeneity and will provide a more accurate disease profile.

14.3.1 Single Cell Influence on Various Cancer Types

The significance of single cell analysis has been demonstrated in various cancer types. Detection and monitoring of genetic changes have been extensively investigated. In our own clinical validation, we have demonstrated that it is vital to separate out these single cells for an accurate profiling of the *EGFR* status of NSCLC patients. In other examples in cancer, single cell studies have been used to address cellular heterogeneity more effectively. For instance, Xu and colleagues performed exome sequencing of single clear cell renal cell carcinoma (ccRCC) and revealed that the same type of mutation may not be commonly shared among ccRCC patients (Xu et al. 2012). At the single cellular level, a patient presented intercellular variances with several other mutations discovered at different frequencies. Importantly, 70% of the mutations found in the analysis were unique and cell specific. All the cells commonly shared the remaining 30% of the detected mutations. These studies highlighted the extent of spatial heterogeneity in tumors and importance of single cell analysis in unraveling this complexity.

Besides RCC, breast cancer has also benefit greatly from the detailed molecular profiling at the single cell level. With the annual rate of breast cancer cases rising every year, it is a cause for concern (Hussain et al. 2005). Despite mortality in developed countries being lowered since the discovery of systemic adjuvant therapy, resistance to therapy still remains a challenge in advanced stages (Peto et al. 2000; Nahta et al. 2006). In a single cell study on breast cancer tumor heterogeneity, Powell et al. investigated the reliability of cell lines on drug development (Powell et al. 2012). Due to exposure of cells to long term culture states and not the tumor microenvironment, the genetic and epigenetic profiles of cancer cells may have been altered in response to environmental cues. The genetic profiles of breast cancer cell lines and CTCs from breast cancer patients were vastly different. A lack of growth factors at the transcriptional level was found in CTCs and not cell lines. In treatment targeted at proliferating cells, it may not be sufficient in eliminating metastatic disseminated CTCs (Powell et al. 2012). We now understand that drugs initially designed to target a subset of cancer may have lower significant response to patients due to a different cancer genotype (Garnett et al. 2012; Rask-Andersen et al. 2011). Thus, it is important that a complete molecular profile of the patient be available during systemic therapy, which could be tailored accordingly in the hope of reducing recurrences and prolonging survival.

In prostate cancer, the use of single CTCs presents an opportunity to provide a minimally invasive procedure to probe the mutational landscape. Lohr et al. for instance developed a systematic means to examine somatic single-nucleotide variants (SSNVs) of single prostate CTC using whole exome sequencing (Lohr et al. 2014). Applying their technique to various castration-resistant prostate cancer (CRPC) patients, it was determined that there was a strong correlation and concordance in the number of SSNVs found in CTCs and matched primary tumor or lymph node metastasis. More important, their study also uncovered that CTC sequencing can reveal early trunk mutations involved in tumor evolution that could be traced to the primary tumor and shared among metastatic sites. This confirms that CTCs are indeed genetically related to the primary and metastatic prostate cancer, hence the study of single CTCs provides a window into the metastatic process of these CRPC patients.

14.3.2 Clinical Validation Using the Single Cell Biochip in NSCLC Specimens

In lung cancer, detecting mutations that causes drug resistance in a promptly manner is crucial in selecting the appropriate treatment for the patients. In particular, lung cancer patients with sensitizing *EGFR* mutations in exon 19, 20 and 21 will demonstrate good initial response to tyrosine kinase inhibitor (TKI) therapy (Bell et al. 2005; Gazdar 2009). Indeed, TKIs are now the recommended 1st line treatment for patients diagnosed with *EGFR* mutations (Ettinger et al. 2015). Drugs such as Gefitinib and Erlotinib are promising at the start of therapy but ultimately, cancer cells acquires resistances through secondary *EGFR* mutations such as T790M. Third generation TKIs in combination with other therapy have demonstrated to be relatively effective to overcome resistance induced by *EGFR* T790M mutation. Hence targeting and monitoring *EGFR* profiles in NSCLC patients is important to capture the dynamic temporal changes of the disease in response to therapy.

Our clinical validation centers upon single CTCs in late stage NSCLC patients and comparing the *EGFR* mutation profiles with its matched tumor biopsy. CTCs are favored for being less invasive than tissue biopsy and hence open up possibilities for long term serial monitoring of the treatment efficacy. We sought to establish basic genetic relations of CTCs with late stage NSCLC patients and showed that single CTC analysis provided the sensitivity needed for detection. We randomly selected seven patients of varying *EGFR* mutation profiles (detected from primary tissue) and processed their blood specimens. All patients provided informed consent to participate in the trial and procedures for blood extraction and sample processing followed guidelines approved by the institutional review board (IRB). Briefly, 5.9–7.5 ml of blood specimens were drawn in either EDTA or Streck blood tubes. The samples were first enriched using ClearCell FX® enrichment platform (Clearbridge Biomedics, Singapore). Sample outputs contained approximately 20,000 WBCs together with CTCs. The output sample was stained with CD45 antibody that identified WBCs prior to single tumor cell isolation on the biochip. Selection was based on depleting WBCs from the bulk sample and recovering CD45 negative cells. Each sample was passed through the biochip three times to ensure most of the tumor cells were captured. Table 14.1 highlights the number of CTCs associated with each sample. Cumulatively, a total of 0–9 single CTCs were recovered, which is in good agreement to previous enumeration studies on NSCLC (Boshuizen et al. 2012; Muinelo-Romay et al. 2014). This strongly suggested the need for secondary purification step before any downstream molecular analysis, as sample purity can be as low as 0.005% (1 CTC in 20,000 WBCs) after the first enrichment process. In our model cell line experiments with PC9 lung cancer line cells, it was observed that the acquired *EGFR* T790M mutation were all heterozygous in nature. This adds further difficulties for detection as in a heterozygous cell, the mutant DNA content within these patients samples will be as low as 0.0025% without removing the background cells.

In the single CTC PCR and subsequent Sanger sequencing results for *EGFR* L858R and T790M mutations, we observed good concordance between CTCs and matched tumor biopsy for six of the patients (Table 14.1). Using the Cohen's Kappa Coefficient, κ was 0.70 for T790M and 0.59 for L858R. If the sample without CTCs was excluded from the calculations, the concordance rate was 100% matching with the primary tumor profile. All internal controls using single WBC extracted from the same patients' blood showed wildtype characteristics. This demonstrated the excellent specificity of the assay. An added benefit over classical pooled CTC analysis is that the single cell test provides quantification for the proportion of tumor cells harboring these critical mutations. This is clear evidence of the heterogeneity of tumor cells in circulation, which can have significant value in disease prognosis. The clinical validation work lays the foundation for larger scale clinical studies to use single cell assays for predictive and prognostic analysis. The close

Table 14.1 CTC analysis from a single time point of late stage NSCLC patients

Patient details				Primary mutational analyses		CTC single cell analyses				
	Tumor site	Stage	Gender	T790M	L858R	CTC enumeration	Blood volume tested	T790M[b]	L858R[b]	Concordant
1	NSCLC	IV	F	+	+	0	5.9	NA	NA	NA
2	NSCLC	IV	F	–	–	2	7.5	0 (–)	0 (–)	Yes
3	NSCLC	IV	F	+	–	4	7.5	2 (+)	0 (–)	Yes
4	NSCLC	IV	F	+	–	9	6	3 (+)	0 (–)	Yes
5	NSCLC	IV	M	+	–	2	7.5	2 (+)	0 (–)	Yes
6	NSCLC	IV	F	–	+	8	7.5	0 (–)	4 (+)	Yes
7	NSCLC	IV	F	+	–	1	7.5	1 (+)	0 (–)	Yes
	Healthy volunteer	NA	M	NA	NA	0	Nil	NA	NA	NA
							κ^a	0.70	0.59	

Yeo et al. (2016)

Primary mutational analyses derived from tumor re-biopsies at point of resistance; *CTC* circulating tumor cell; CTC enumeration is achieved by analyzing CD45- cells recovered from the system

[a]Cohen's kappa was calculated with patient1 being negative for both tested sites

[b]The number of positive cells are listed in this column

correlations to primary tumor suggested it could complement disease management regimes for monitoring changes to the genetic profiles. This will allow swift treatment changes needed for patients who display positive mutant signatures in the hope of better clinical outcome. Our proposed single cell assay can also aid clinicians in clinical decision-making where tumor samples are inadequate or unavailable without the need to perform further invasive surgical procedures.

14.4 Conclusions

The role of single cell detection and analysis in the next generation of personalized medicine cannot be overemphasized. The assay sensitivity and vast amount of genetics information that it provides will allow better understanding of the disease and tailored drug regimes. In CTC processing, the main technical challenge is the rarity of cells and current technologies are not adequate to extract single CTCs efficiently. We developed a microfluidic biochip to reliably recover these rare cells from blood specimens. In our clinical example, we integrated various molecular detection methods to address different aspects of measuring the disease profile. Results from an early clinical validation showed good sensitivity and specificity in detecting key *EGFR* mutations in late stage NSCLC patients, which lays the groundwork for treatment monitoring and prognostic applications. We foresee great value in using NGS to cover a larger gene panel for concurrent measurements that will bring much needed information to combat drug resistance and allow better personalized treatment for cancer patients. NGS will also open new possibilities to characterize the disease based on SSNVs, CNVs and gene expressions that will aid in drug design and predictive capabilities for better clinical outcome.

References

Aceto N, Bardia A, Miyamoto DT et al (2014) Circulating tumor cell clusters are oligoclonal precursors of breast cancer metastasis. Cell 158(5):1110–1122

Alix-Panabières C, Pantel K (2013) Circulating tumor cells: liquid biopsy of cancer. Clin Chem 59 (1):110–118

Allard WJ, Matera J, Miller MC et al (2004) Tumor cells circulate in the peripheral blood of all major carcinomas but not in healthy subjects or patients with nonmalignant diseases. Clin Cancer Res 10(20):6897–6904

Andrykowski MA, Munn RK, Studts JL (1996) Interest in learning of personal genetic risk for cancer: a general population survey. Prev Med 25(5):527–536

Ashworth TR (1869) A case of cancer in which cells similar to those in the tumours were seen in the blood after death. Aust Med J 14(3):146–149

Autebert J, Coudert B, Bidard FC et al (2012) Microfluidic: an innovative tool for efficient cell sorting. Methods 57(3):297–307

Bell DW, Gore I, Okimoto RA et al (2005) Inherited susceptibility to lung cancer may be associated with the T790M drug resistance mutation in EGFR. Nat Genet 37(12):1315–1316

Bendall SC, Nolan GP (2012) From single cells to deep phenotypes in cancer. Nat Biotechnol 30 (7):639–647
Blainey PC, Quake SR (2013) Dissecting genomic diversity, one cell at a time. Nat Methods 11 (1):19–21
Boshuizen R, Kuhn P, van den Heuvel M (2012) Circulating tumor cells in non-small cell lung carcinoma. J Thorac Dis 4(5):456–458
Budd GT (2009) Let me do more than count the ways: what circulating tumor cells can tell us about the biology of cancer. Mol Pharm 6(5):1307–1310
Chin CD, Linder V, Sia SK (2007) Lab-on-a-chip devices for global health: past studies and future opportunities. Lab Chip 7(1):41–57
Cohen SJ, Punt CJ, Iannotti N et al (2008) Relationship of circulating tumor cells to tumor response, progression-free survival, and overall survival in patients with metastatic colorectal cancer. J Clin Oncol 26(19):3213–3221
Cristofanilli M, Budd GT, Ellis MJ et al (2004a) Circulating tumor cells, disease progression, and survival in metastatic breast cancer. N Engl J Med 351(8):781–791
Cristofanilli M, Budd GT, Ellis MJ et al (2004b) Circulating tumor cells, disease progression, and survival in metastatic breast cancer. N Engl J Med 351(8):781–791
Cristofanilli M, Hayes DF, Budd GT et al (2005) Circulating tumor cells: a novel prognostic factor for newly diagnosed metastatic breast cancer. J Clin Oncol 23(7):1420–1430
Dey SS, Kester L, Spanjaard B et al (2015) Integrated genome and transcriptome sequencing of the same cell. Nat Biotechnol 33(3):285–289
Dong Y, Skelley AM, Merdek KD et al (2013) Microfluidics and circulating tumor cells. J Mol Diagn 15(2):149–157
Eteshola E, Balberg M (2004) Microfluidic ELISA: on-chip fluorescence imaging. Biomed Microdevices 6(1):7–9
Ettinger DS, Wood DE, Akerley W et al (2015) Non-small cell lung cancer, version 6.2015. J Natl Compr Cancer Netw 13(5):515–524
Fan T, Zhao Q, Chen JJ et al (2009) Clinical significance of circulating tumor cells detected by an invasion assay in peripheral blood of patients with ovarian cancer. Gynecol Oncol 112 (1):185–191
Garnett MJ, Edelman EJ, Heidorn SJ et al (2012) Systematic identification of genomic markers of drug sensitivity in cancer cells. Nature 483(7391):570–575
Gazdar AF (2009) Activating and resistance mutations of EGFR in non-small-cell lung cancer: role in clinical response to EGFR tyrosine kinase inhibitors. Oncogene 28(Suppl 1):S24–S31
Hou HW, Warkiani ME, Khoo BL et al (2013) Isolation and retrieval of circulating tumor cells using centrifugal forces. Sci Report 3:1259
Hussain SA, Palmer DH, Stevens A et al (2005) Role of chemotherapy in breast cancer. Expert Rev Anticancer Ther 5(6):1095–1110
Hyun K-A, Jung H-I (2014) Advances and critical concerns with the microfluidic enrichments of circulating tumor cells. Lab Chip 14(1):45–56
Karabacak NM, Spuhler PS, Fachin F et al (2014) Microfluidic, marker-free isolation of circulating tumor cells from blood samples. Nat Protoc 9(3):694–710
Kartalov EP, Quake SR (2004) Microfluidic device reads up to four consecutive base pairs in DNA sequencing-by-synthesis. Nucleic Acids Res 32(9):2873–2879
Kessler DA, Austin RH, Levine H (2014) Resistance to chemotherapy: patient variability and cellular heterogeneity. Cancer Res 74(17):4663–4670
Kling J (2012) Beyond counting tumor cells. Nat Biotechnol 30(7):578–580
Lohr JG, Adalsteinsson VA, Cibulskis K et al (2014) Whole-exome sequencing of circulating tumor cells provides a window into metastatic prostate cancer. Nat Biotech 32(5):479–484
Mach AJ, Kim JH, Arshi A et al (2011) Automated cellular sample preparation using a centrifuge-on-a-chip. Lab Chip 11(17):2827–2834
Maheswaran S, Haber DA (2010) Circulating tumor cells: a window into cancer biology and metastasis. Curr Opin Genet Dev 20(1):96–99

Mark D, Haeberle S, Roth G et al (2010) Microfluidic lab-on-a-chip platforms: requirements, characteristics and applications. Chem Soc Rev 39(3):1153–1182

Muinelo-Romay L, Vieito M, Abalo A et al (2014) Evaluation of circulating tumor cells and related events as prognostic factors and surrogate biomarkers in advanced NSCLC patients receiving first-line systemic treatment. Cancer 6(1):153

Nagrath S, Sequist LV, Maheswaran S et al (2007) Isolation of rare circulating tumour cells in cancer patients by microchip technology. Nature 450(7173):1235–1239

Nahta R, Yu D, Hung MC et al (2006) Mechanisms of disease: understanding resistance to HER2-targeted therapy in human breast cancer. Nat Clin Pract Oncol 3(5):269–280

Neves RP, Raba K, Schmidt O et al (2014) Genomic high-resolution profiling of single CKpos/CD45neg flow-sorting purified circulating tumor cells from patients with metastatic breast cancer. Clin Chem 60(10):1290–1297

Ozkumur E, Shah AM, Ciciliano JC et al (2013) Inertial focusing for tumor antigen-dependent and -independent sorting of rare circulating tumor cells. Sci Transl Med 5(179):179ra147

Paguirigan AL, Beebe DJ (2008) Microfluidics meet cell biology: bridging the gap by validation and application of microscale techniques for cell biological assays. BioEssays 30(9):811–821

Peeters DJE, De Laere B, Van den Eynden GG et al (2013) Semiautomated isolation and molecular characterisation of single or highly purified tumour cells from CellSearch enriched blood samples using dielectrophoretic cell sorting. Br J Cancer 108(6):1358–1367

Peto R, Boreham J, Clarke M et al (2000) UK and USA breast cancer deaths down 25% in year 2000 at ages 20–69 years. Lancet 355(9217):1822

Pierga JY, Bidard FC, Mathiot C et al (2008) Circulating tumor cell detection predicts early metastatic relapse after neoadjuvant chemotherapy in large operable and locally advanced breast cancer in a phase II randomized trial. Clin Cancer Res 14(21):7004–7010

Powell AA, Talasaz AH, Zhang H et al (2012) Single cell profiling of circulating tumor cells: transcriptional heterogeneity and diversity from breast cancer cell lines. PLoS One 7(5): e33788

Punnoose EA, Atwal SK, Spoerke JM et al (2010) Molecular biomarker analyses using circulating tumor cells. PLoS One 5(9):e12517

Punnoose EA, Atwal S, Liu W et al (2012) Evaluation of circulating tumor cells and circulating tumor DNA in non-small cell lung cancer: association with clinical endpoints in a phase II clinical trial of pertuzumab and erlotinib. Clin Cancer Res Off J Am Assoc Cancer Res 18 (8):2391–2401

Rask-Andersen M, Almen MS, Schioth HB (2011) Trends in the exploitation of novel drug targets. Nat Rev Drug Discov 10(8):579–590

Reategui E, Aceto N, Lim EJ et al (2015) Tunable nanostructured coating for the capture and selective release of viable circulating tumor cells. Adv Mater 27(9):1593–1599

Robert D, Pamme N, Conjeaud H et al (2011) Cell sorting by endocytotic capacity in a microfluidic magnetophoresis device. Lab Chip 11(11):1902–1910

Saunders NA, Simpson F, Thompson EW et al (2012) Role of intratumoural heterogeneity in cancer drug resistance: molecular and clinical perspectives. EMBO Mol Med 4(8):675–684

Schubert C (2011) Single-cell analysis: the deepest differences. Nature 480(7375):133–137

Spencer SL, Sorger PK (2011) Measuring and modeling apoptosis in single cells. Cell 144 (6):926–939

Stoecklein NH, Hosch SB, Bezler M et al (2008) Direct genetic analysis of single disseminated cancer cells for prediction of outcome and therapy selection in esophageal cancer. Cancer Cell 13(5):441–453

Swennenhuis JF, Reumers J, Thys K et al (2013) Efficiency of whole genome amplification of single circulating tumor cells enriched by CellSearch and sorted by FACS. Genitourin Med 5 (11):106

Swennenhuis JF, Tibbe AG, Stevens M et al (2015) Self-seeding microwell chip for the isolation and characterization of single cells. Lab Chip 15(14):3039–3046

Tan SJ, Yobas L, Lee GY et al (2009) Microdevice for the isolation and enumeration of cancer cells from blood. Biomed Microdevices 11(4):883–892

Thorsen T, Maerkl SJ, Quake SR (2002) Microfluidic large-scale integration. Science 298 (5593):580–584

Tsiatis AC, Norris-Kirby A, Rich RG et al (2010) Comparison of Sanger sequencing, pyrosequencing, and melting curve analysis for the detection of KRAS mutations: diagnostic and clinical implications. J Mol Diagn 12(4):425–432

VanDelinder V, Groisman A (2006) Separation of plasma from whole human blood in a continuous cross-flow in a molded microfluidic device. Anal Chem 78(11):3765–3771

Wang D, Bodovitz S (2010) Single cell analysis: the new frontier in 'omics'. Trends Biotechnol 28 (6):281–290

Wang J, Fan HC, Behr B et al (2012) Genome-wide single-cell analysis of recombination activity and de novo mutation rates in human sperm. Cell 150(2):402–412

White AK, VanInsberghe M, Petriv OI et al (2011) High-throughput microfluidic single-cell RT-qPCR. Proc Natl Acad Sci U S A 108(34):13999–14004

Whitesides GM (2006) The origins and the future of microfluidics. Nature 442(7101):368–373

Williams SC (2013) Circulating tumor cells. Proc Natl Acad Sci U S A 110(13):4861

Xu X, Hou Y, Yin X et al (2012) Single-cell exome sequencing reveals single-nucleotide mutation characteristics of a kidney tumor. Cell 148(5):886–895

Yang Y, Rho HS, Stevens M et al (2015) Microfluidic device for DNA amplification of single cancer cells isolated from whole blood by self-seeding microwells. Lab Chip 15 (22):4331–4337

Yeo T, Tan SJ, Lim CL et al (2016) Microfluidic enrichment for the single cell analysis of circulating tumor cells. Sci Report 6:22076

Chapter 15
Glycan Markers as Potential Immunological Targets in Circulating Tumor Cells

Denong Wang, Lisa Wu, and Xiaohe Liu

Abstract We present here an experimental approach for exploring a new class of tumor biomarkers that are overexpressed by circulating tumor cells (CTCs) and are likely targetable in immunotherapy against tumor metastasis. Using carbohydrate microarrays, anti-tumor monoclonal antibodies (mAbs) were scanned against a large panel of carbohydrate antigens to identify potential tumor glycan markers. Subsequently, flow cytometry and fiber-optic array scanning technology (FAST) were applied to determine whether the identified targets are tumor-specific cell-surface markers and are, therefore, likely suitable for targeted immunotherapy. Finally, the tumor glycan-specific antibodies identified were validated using cancer patients' blood samples for their performance in CTC-detection and immunotyping analysis. In this article, identifying breast CTC-specific glycan markers and targeting mAbs serve as examples to illustrate this tumor biomarker discovery strategy.

Keywords Glycan markers • Breast circulating tumor cells • Carbohydrate microarray • Breast cancer

15.1 Introduction

Breast cancer (BCa) is among the most prevalent cancers and accounts for the highest number of cancer-related deaths among women worldwide (Chatterjee and Zetter 2005). Identifying biomarkers of immunological significance is important in developing precision diagnostic and therapeutic strategies to advance current BCa

D. Wang (✉) • L. Wu
Tumor Glycomics Laboratory, Biosciences Division, SRI International, 333 Ravenswood Avenue, Menlo Park, CA 94025-3493, USA
e-mail: denong.wang@sri.com

X. Liu
Biosciences Division, SRI International, 333 Ravenswood Avenue, Menlo Park, CA 94025-3493, USA

M.J.M. Magbanua, J.W. Park (eds.), *Isolation and Molecular Characterization of Circulating Tumor Cells*, Advances in Experimental Medicine and Biology 994,
DOI 10.1007/978-3-319-55947-6_15

healthcare. Recognition of abnormal glycosylation in virtually every cancer type has raised great interest in exploration of the tumor glycome for biomarker discovery (Hakomori 1989, 2001; Fukuda 1996; Dube and Bertozzi 2005). Potential glycan markers of BCa identified may include, but are not limited to, mucin-1 (CA 15-3) (Persson et al. 2009), carcinoembryonic antigen (Haidopoulos et al. 2000), sialyl Lewis x (Renkonen et al. 1997; Nakagoe et al. 2002), and glycoforms of a number of serum acute phase proteins, such as α1-acid glycoprotein, α1-antichymotrypsin, and haptoglobin β-chain (Abd Hamid et al. 2008). Since carbohydrate moieties are often surface-exposed and easily accessible by antibodies, some targets have been employed for antibody therapeutics (Vassilaros et al. 2013; Apostolopoulos et al. 2006; Shibata et al. 2009; Tomlinson et al. 1995).

Exploring glycan markers of breast circulating tumor cells (bCTCs) represents a new development in tumor biomarker discovery. Although bCTCs are rare in blood, they play a key role in tumor metastasis (Jacob et al. 2007; Hayashi and Yamauchi 2012). Detection of CTCs has been explored as a non-invasive "liquid biopsy" for tumor diagnosis and prognosis (Somlo et al. 2011; Das et al. 2012; Liu et al. 2012). Glycan markers of bCTCs may have unique value in BCa healthcare, especially in the personalized therapy that targets specific immunotypes of BCa. Thus, our team has worked to establish a practical strategy to facilitate identification and characterization of potential glycan markers of bCTCs. Figure 15.1 highlights two core technologies explored in this investigation.

15.2 Carbohydrate Microarray Identifies Blood Group Precursors as the Natural Ligands of Anti-tumor Antibody HAE3

Antibody responses elicited by native tumor glycoprotein antigens may target glycan-based antigenic determinants in addition to conventional protein epitopes. MAbs established by such immunization strategies are highly valuable for tumor biomarker discovery (Wang et al. 2015a; Wang et al. 2015b; Codington et al. 1972; Gao et al. 2014; Newsom-Davis et al. 2009). In this study, an anti-tumor mAb, HAE3, served as a key reagent for probing bCTC-glycan markers. This mAb was raised against epiglycanin, the major sialomucin glycoprotein (~ 500 kDa) of murine mammary adenocarcinoma TA3 cells (Codington et al. 1972). Interestingly, HAE3 was found to strongly cross react with a number of human epithelial tumors in tissues, including lung, prostate, bladder, esophagus, and ovarian cancers (Li et al. 2004; Liang et al. 2004; Somlo et al. 2011; Yao et al. 2004). This cross-species tumor binding profile suggests the possibility that HAE3 may recognize a conserved tumor glycan marker that is co-expressed by both mouse- and human-derived epithelial cancers.

We produced, therefore, a comprehensive carbohydrate microarray to explore potential tumor glycan markers using antibody HAE3. As shown in Fig. 15.2, a

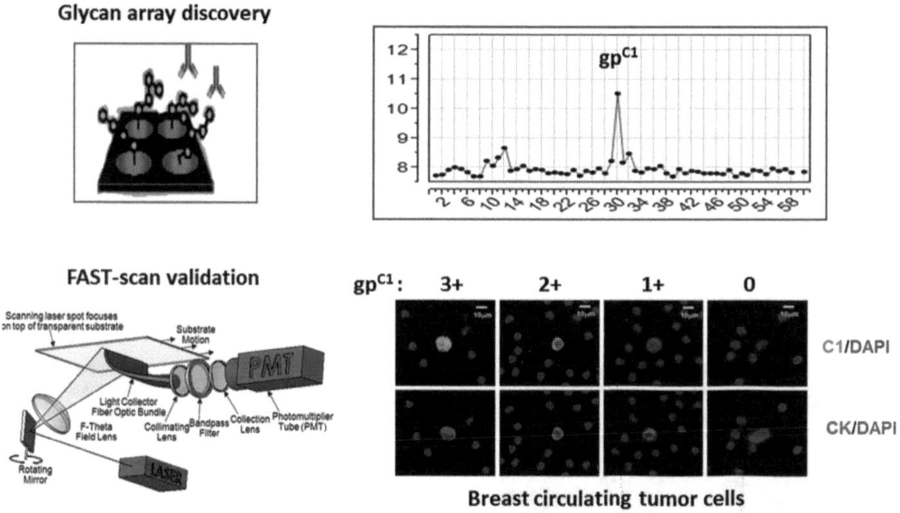

Fig. 15.1 Glycan array discovery and FAST-scan validation of a novel glycan marker gp^{C1} of bCTCs (Adapted from Wang et al. 2015a)

large collection of purified natural carbohydrate antigens was applied for carbohydrate microarray construction. Blood group substance reference reagents (Kabat 1956) used include Cyst 9 and Cyst 14, A active; Beach phenol insoluble, B active; Hog, H active; JS phenol insoluble, H and Le^b active, and N-1 20% from the second 10%, Le^a active. Importantly, a number of blood group precursor references, including OG, Tij II, Beach P1, and McDon P1 ($29^{\#}$–$32^{\#}$), were spotted in this carbohydrate microarray. These precursor substances were prepared to remove most of the α-L-fucosyl end groups that are essential for blood group A, B, H, or Lewis active side chains, but possess the internal domains or core structures of blood group substances. A large panel of other autoantigens and microbial polysaccharides were also spotted in the same microarrays to critically examine the antibody binding specificity. A preparation of HAE3-reactive human carcinoma-associated antigen (HCA) served as a positive control for this assay (Li et al. 2004).

In Fig. 15.2a, HAE3 binding signal (red column) are plotted with corresponding local background reading (blue column) as an overlay plot. Each data point represents the mean of triplicate detections; these are shown in the Fig. 15.2b microarray image with the number of positive antigens labeled. Each error bar is constructed using one standard deviation from the mean. As illustrated, HAE3 is strongly positive with HCA ($1^{\#}$ and $2^{\#}$) as expected. Importantly, this antibody selectively binds to four blood group precursor antigens, Beach P1 ($29^{\#}$), McDon P1 ($30^{\#}$), Tij II ($31^{\#}$), and OG ($32^{\#}$). By contrast, HAE3 has no detectable cross-reactivity with blood group substances A, B. O, or Lewis antigens, or the large panel of other carbohydrate antigens spotted in the same array.

Figure 15.2c is a schematic of blood group substance structure with the common blood group precursor core structure highlighted. The four branched structure in the

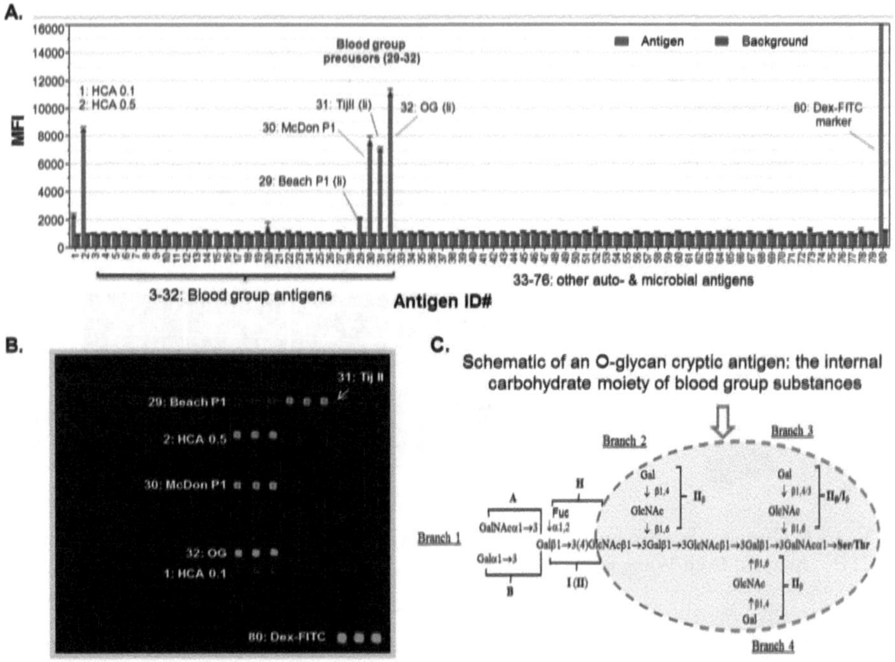

Fig. 15.2 Carbohydrate microarray analysis of anti-epiglycanin mAb HAE3. Seventy-six glycoproteins, glycoconjugates, and polysaccharides were spotted in triplicates in 1 to 2 dilutions to yield the customized microarrays for antibody screening. (**a**) Microarray detections were shown as the mean fluorescent intensities (MFIs) of each microspot with antigen-binding signal in *red* and background reading in *blue*. Each error bar is constructed using one standard deviation from the mean of triplicate detections. The labeled antigens include HCA (ID# 1 and 2), a number of blood group precursors ($29^{\#}$–$32^{\#}$), and a microarray spotting marker ($80^{\#}$). (**b**) Images of a microarray stained with HAE3 (5 μg/ml). (**c**) Schematic of a blood group substance structure with the conserved *O*-glycan core highlighted (Adapted from Wang et al. 2015b)

circle represents the internal portion of the carbohydrate moiety of blood group substances, which was proposed based on extensive immunochemical characterization of precursor OG and other P1 fractions of blood group precursors that were isolated from ovarian cancer cyst fluids (Vicari and Kabat 1970; Feizi et al. a, 1971b; Wu et al. 2007). Selective detection of these blood group precursors from a large panel of blood group substances by HAE3 illustrated that this antibody is specific for a shared cryptic glyco-epitope of these precursor substances.

15.3 Flow Cytometry Analysis to Examine Tumor Cell Surface Expression of HAE3^{+} Glyco-Epitopes

We further examined whether the HAE3^{+} glyco-epitopes were expressed as cell surface tumor markers. To ensure the observed cross-species antigenic reactivities are not owing to the unexpected presence of oligoclonal populations in the original

HAE3 hybridoma cell line, we further subcloned HAE3 and produced antibody from a single clone, HAE3-C1 (C1). Antibody C1 was verified by carbohydrate microarrays and a glycan-specific ELISA to be highly specific for a conserved O-glycan cryptic glyco-epitope gp^{C1} in human blood group precursors (Wang et al. 2015a).

In the first set of experiments, we screened a panel of four tumor cell lines by cell surface staining in flow cytometry. These include (a) a BCa line, T-47D, which was selected owing to the fact that breast cancer patients were found to produce substances in circulation that are highly effective in inhibiting AE3-binding of epiglycanin (Codington et al. 2002; Codington et al. 1997); (b) a lung cancer (LCa) line, A549, which is known to produce an HAE3-positive substance in cell culture; (c) a prostate cancer (PCa) line, PC3, which is found to express a blood group B-related F77 glyco-epitope (Gao et al. 2014; Nonaka et al. 2014); and (d) a melanoma cell line SKMEL-28, which is derived from skin but not epithelial tissue. As shown in Fig. 15.3a, melanoma SKMEL-28 and prostate cancer PC3 were negative for HAE3. The A549 lung cancer cell line was weakly positive. By contrast, the breast cancer cell line T-47D was strongly positive in HAE3-cell surface staining.

Given these results, we extended the flow cytometry analysis to a panel of seven human breast cancer cell lines, including two estrogen receptor positive (ER^+) and progesterone receptor positive (PR^+) lines (T-47D and MCF-7), one ER^+ (SK-BR-3), and four triple-negative (TN) cancers that lack the estrogen, progesterone, and Her2)/neu receptors (BT-549, Hs 578 T, MDA-MB-231, and MDA-MB-468). Fig. 15.3b shows that two ER^+PR^+ lines, T-47D and MCF-7, and two triple-negative lines, BT-549 and MDA-MB-468, are HAE3 strongly positive. SK-BR-3 is intermediately positive. By contrast, the two remaining triple-negative cell lines, Hs578T and MDA-MB-231, were HAE3 negative.

15.4 Detection of Glycan Marker-Positive bCTCs in Stage IV Breast Cancer Patients

With antibody C1 as a key probe, we investigated whether gp^{C1} is applicable for detection and immunotyping analysis of CTCs in patients with metastatic breast cancer. In a pilot clinical case study, we characterized blood samples from five Stage IV breast cancer patients using the FAST-scan technology. Figure 15.4a illustrates how CTCs captured from the Stage IV breast cancer patients were scored as 3+, 2+, 1+, and 0, left to right. Four representative bCTCs are shown in which the epithelial-derived cells were labeled by anti-cytokeratins (CK) antibodies in red, and the gp^{C1} positive cells were stained in green in the background of the DAPI-blue labeling of white blood cells. Figure 15.4b and c show that all subjects characterized had gp^{C1}-positive CTCs. Approximately 40% of CTCs captured in these patients expressed higher levels (2+ and 3+) of the gp^{C1} markers; gp^{C1}-positive and -negative CTCs were found to co-exist in four subjects. Notably, a

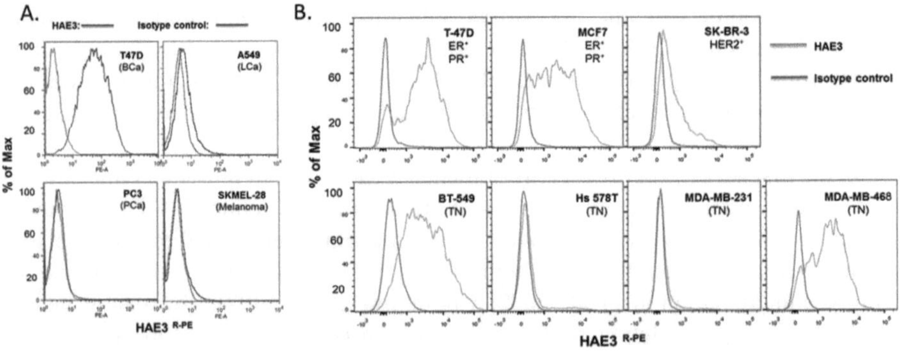

Fig. 15.3 HAE3 cell surface staining detected selective expression of the HAE3-cryptic glycan markers in human cancer cell lines. (**a**) Four tumor cell lines, T-47D, A549, PC3, and SKMEL-28, were stained with the C1 preparation of HAE3 (IgM) at 1:6 dilution or with an isotype control IgM, 9.14.7 (5.0 μg/ml). (**b**) Seven breast cancer cell lines were stained with purified mAb HAE3 (5.0 μg/ml) or 9.14.7 (5.0 μg/ml). These cell lines are T-47D, MCF-7, SK-BR-3, BT-549, Hs578T, MDA-MB-231, and MDA-MB-468. An R-PE-conjugated goat anti-mouse IgM antibody was applied to quantify the cell surface-captured IgM antibodies. *Blue line*: HAE3 stain; *Red line:* 9.14.7 IgM isotype control (Adapted from Wang et al. 2015b)

triple-negative patient (ID# 189370) produced predominantly gp^{C1}-positive CTCs (37 of 40 CTCs) with 50% scored gp^{C1} 2+/3+. In this patient, metastatic tumors were seen in multiple sites, including bone, liver, and skin.

It is noteworthy that more than 1 million global cases of BCa are diagnosed each year and approximately 15% are triple negative. Owing to the lack of an effective therapeutic target, a younger age at onset, and early metastatic spread, patients suffering triple-negative BCa often have poor prognoses and clinical outcomes (Anders and Carey 2009; Brenton et al. 2005). If gp^{C1} were confirmed to be significantly associated with the triple-negative BCa in a larger cohort validation study, this O-core cryptic glycan marker could be used for immunotype-enhanced precision diagnosis and prognosis of BCa and targeted immunotherapy against BCa metastasis.

15.5 Summary

Although tumor-associated abnormal glycosylation has been recognized for years, identifying glycan markers of CTCs remains technically challenging. We describe here a practical approach to overcome this difficulty. Conceptually, we take advantage of the fact that the immune systems of many animal species are able to recognize subtle changes in sugar moieties displayed by cells or soluble antigens and produce specific antibodies for abnormally expressed tumor glycan markers. Experimentally, we first screened anti-tumor mAbs using carbohydrate microarrays to identify those that are specific for glycan markers. Subsequently, we determined whether the selected mAbs are specific for the cell-surface glycan markers using

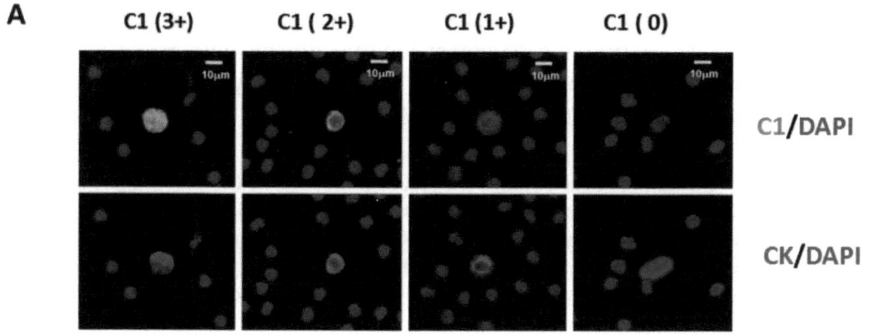

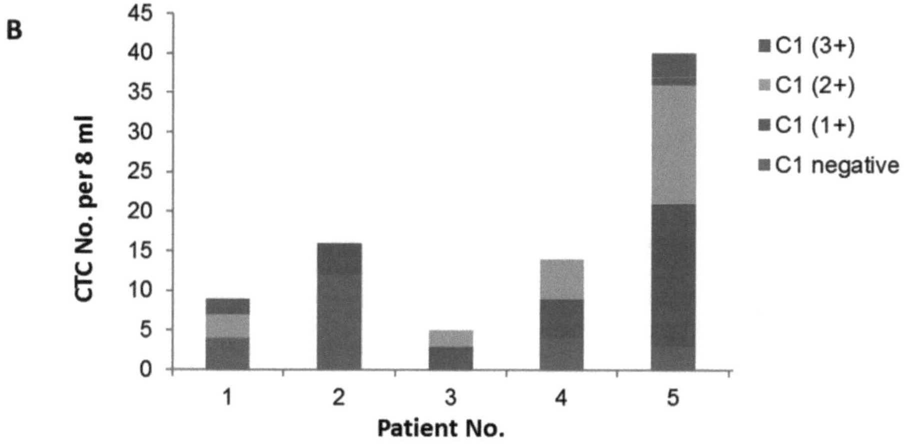

C

Demographics and clinical characteristics of Stage IV metastatic BCA patients

Patient ID	Age	ER	HER2	PR	Location of Metastases	Line of therapy	Time point	CTCs (no. per 8 ml)
194563	62	+	-	+	brain, lung	3rd line	9 month	9
211980	51	+	-	-	bone	3rd line	24 month	16
254439	54	+	-	+	bone	2nd line	9 month	5
265783	47	+	-	+	ovaries	2nd line	baseline	14
189370	68	-	-	-	bone, liver, skin	2nd line	12 month	40

Fig. 15.4 Glycan marker gp^{C1} is expressed in significant numbers of CTCs in Stage IV breast cancer patients. (**a**) FAST-scan images of bCTCs. *Upper panels*: Co-staining of C1 (*green*) and DAPI (*blue*); *Bottom panels:* co-staining of anti-CK (*red*) and DAPI (*blue*). (**b**) Distribution of gp ^{C1}–positive and -negative bCTCs in five subjects. C1-staining of bCTCs was semi-quantitatively measured by the FAST scan as antibody negative (*blue*), 1+ (*purple*), 2+ (*green*), and 3+ (*red*) as described. A patient with triple-negative BCa (ID# 189370) was measured gp^{C1}–positive in 37 of 40 CTCs with 50% scored as strong positive (2+ and 3+). (ER, estrogen receptor; PR, progesterone receptor; HER2, human epidermal growth factor2). (**c**) A summary of patients' demographics and clinical characteristics (Adapted from Wang et al. 2015a)

flow cytometry and FAST-scan technology. Finally, we used the new antibody probe to monitor CTC-expression of corresponding glycan markers in advanced breast cancer patients. This approach is likely to be generally useful for exploring potential glycan markers of CTCs of epithelial cancers.

Acknowledgments The authors acknowledge the Kabat Collection of Carbohydrate Antigens at SRI International for a number of carbohydrate antigens that were applied in this study.

This work was supported in part by NIH grants U01CA128416 (DW) and R56AI118464 (DW), and by SRI International IR&D funds (DW and XL). The content is solely the responsibility of the authors and does not necessarily represent the official views of the National Institutes of Health.

Conflict of Interest There are no conflicts of interest to declare for any of the authors involved in this work.

References

Abd Hamid UM, Royle L, Saldova R et al (2008) A strategy to reveal potential glycan markers from serum glycoproteins associated with breast cancer progression. Glycobiology 18 (12):1105–1118

Anders CK, Carey LA (2009) Biology, metastatic patterns, and treatment of patients with triple-negative breast cancer. Clin Breast Cancer 9(Suppl 2):S73–S81

Apostolopoulos V, Pietersz GA, Tsibanis A et al (2006) Pilot phase III immunotherapy study in early-stage breast cancer patients using oxidized mannan-MUC1 [ISRCTN71711835]. Breast Cancer Ress: BCR 8(3):R27

Brenton JD, Carey LA, Ahmed AA et al (2005) Molecular classification and molecular forecasting of breast cancer: ready for clinical application? J Clin Oncol Off J Am Soc Clin Oncol 23 (29):7350–7360

Chatterjee SK, Zetter BR (2005) Cancer biomarkers: knowing the present and predicting the future. Future Oncol 1(1):37–50

Codington JF, Sanford BH, Jeanloz RW (1972) Glycoprotein coat of the TA3 cell. Isolation and partial characterization of a sialic acid containing glycoprotein fraction. Biochemistry 11 (14):2559–2564

Codington JF, Mass N, Haavik S et al (1997) Antibodies to human carcinoma antigen. US Pat No 5,693,763, Dec 2, 1997

Codington JF, Haavik S, Nikrui N et al (2002) Immunologic quantitation of the carcinoma specific human carcinoma antigen in clinical samples. Cancer 94(3):803–813

Das M, Riess JW, Frankel P et al (2012) ERCC1 expression in circulating tumor cells (CTCs) using a novel detection platform correlates with progression-free survival (PFS) in patients with metastatic non-small-cell lung cancer (NSCLC) receiving platinum chemotherapy. Lung Cancer 77(2):421–426

Dube DH, Bertozzi CR (2005) Glycans in cancer and inflammation – potential for therapeutics and diagnostics. Nat Rev Drug Discov 4(6):477–488

Feizi T, Kabat EA, Vicari G et al (1971a) Immunochemical studies on blood groups. XLVII. The I antigen complex – precursors in the A, B, H, Le^a, and le^b blood group system – hemagglutination-inhibition studies. J Exp Med 133(1):39–52

Feizi T, Kabat EA, Vicari G et al (1971b) Immunochemical studies on blood groups.XLIX. The I antigen complex: specificity differences among anti-I sera revealed by quantitative precipitin studies; partial structure of the I determinant specific for one anti-I serum. J Immunol 106 (6):1578–1592

Fukuda M (1996) Possible roles of tumor-associated carbohydrate antigens. Cancer Res 56 (10):2237–2244

Gao C, Liu Y, Zhang H et al (2014) Carbohydrate sequence of the prostate cancer-associated antigen F77 assigned by a mucin O-glycome designer Array. J Biol Chem 289 (23):16462–16477

Haidopoulos D, Konstadoulakis MM, Antonakis PT et al (2000) Circulating anti-CEA antibodies in the sera of patients with breast cancer. Eur J Surg Oncol: J Eur Soc Surg Oncol Br Assoc Surg Oncol 26(8):742–746

Hakomori S (1989) Aberrant glycosylation in tumors and tumor-associated carbohydrate antigens. Adv Cancer Res 52:257–331

Hakomori S (2001) Tumor-associated carbohydrate antigens defining tumor malignancy: basis for development of anti-cancer vaccines. Adv Exp Med Biol 491:369–402

Hayashi N, Yamauchi H (2012) Role of circulating tumor cells and disseminated tumor cells in primary breast cancer. Breast Cancer 19(2):110–117

Jacob K, Sollier C, Jabado N (2007) Circulating tumor cells: detection, molecular profiling and future prospects. Expert Rev Proteomics 4(6):741–756

Kabat EA (1956) Blood group substances, their chemistry and immunochemistry. Academic, New York

Li R, Yao JL, Bourne PA et al (2004) Frequent expression of human carcinoma-associated antigen, a mucin-type glycoprotein, in cells of prostatic carcinoma. Arch Pathol Lab Med 128 (12):1412–1417

Liang S, Yao J, Bourne PA et al (2004) Overexpression of human carcinoma-associated antigen in esophageal adenocarcinoma and its precursor lesions. Am J Clin Pathol 122(5):747–751

Liu X, Hsieh HB, Campana D et al (2012) A new method for high speed, sensitive detection of minimal residual disease. Cytometry Part A J Int Soc Anal Cytol 81(2):169–175

Nakagoe T, Fukushima K, Itoyanagi N et al (2002) Expression of ABH/Lewis-related antigens as prognostic factors in patients with breast cancer. J Cancer Res Clin Oncol 128(5):257–264

Newsom-Davis TE, Wang D, Steinman L et al (2009) Enhanced immune recognition of cryptic glycan markers in human tumors. Cancer Res 69(5):2018–2025

Nonaka M, Fukuda MN, Gao C et al (2014) Determination of carbohydrate structure recognized by prostate-specific F77 monoclonal antibody through expression analysis of Glycosyltransferase genes. J Biol Chem 289(23):16478–16486

Persson J, Backstrom M, Johansson H et al (2009) Molecular evolution of specific human antibody against MUC1 mucin results in improved recognition of the antigen on tumor cells. Tumour Biol J Int Soc Oncodev Biol Med 30(4):221–231

Renkonen J, Paavonen T, Renkonen R (1997) Endothelial and epithelial expression of sialyl Lewis^{x} and sialyl Lewis^{a} in lesions of breast carcinoma. Int J Cancer 74(3):296–300

Shibata S, Raubitschek A, Leong L et al (2009) A phase I study of a combination of yttrium-90-labeled anti-carcinoembryonic antigen (CEA) antibody and gemcitabine in patients with CEA-producing advanced malignancies. Clin Cancer Res Off J Am Assoc Cancer Res 15 (8):2935–2941

Somlo G, Lau SK, Frankel P et al (2011) Multiple biomarker expression on circulating tumor cells in comparison to tumor tissues from primary and metastatic sites in patients with locally advanced/inflammatory, and stage IV breast cancer, using a novel detection technology. Breast Cancer Res Treat 128(1):155–163

Tomlinson IP, Whyman A, Barrett JA et al (1995) Tumour marker CA15-3: possible uses in the routine management of breast cancer. Eur J Cancer 31A(6):899–902

Vassilaros S, Tsibanis A, Tsikkinis A et al (2013) Up to 15-year clinical follow-up of a pilot phase III immunotherapy study in stage II breast cancer patients using oxidized mannan-MUC1. Immunotherapy 5(11):1177–1182

Vicari G, Kabat EA (1970) Structures and activities of oligosaccharides produced by alkaline degradation of a blood group substance lacking A, B, H, Le b specificities. Biochemistry 9 (17):3414–3421

Wang D, Liu X, Hsieh B et al (2015a) Exploring glycan markers for immunotyping and precision-targeting of breast circulating tumor cells. Arch Med Res 46(8):642–650

Wang D, Tang J, Liu S et al (2015b) Blood group precursor cryptic glyco-epitopes as breast cancer cell surface markers for immune recognition and targeting. J Immunol Res 9:510810

Wu AM, Khoo KH, Yu SY et al (2007) Glycomic mapping of pseudomucinous human ovarian cyst glycoproteins: identification of Lewis and sialyl Lewis glycotopes. Proteomics 7 (20):3699–3717

Yao JL, Bourne PA, Yang Q et al (2004) Overexpression of human carcinoma-associated antigen in urothelial carcinoma of the bladder. Arch Pathol Lab Med 128(7):785–787

Chapter 16
Significance of EGFR Expression in Circulating Tumor Cells

María José Serrano, María Jesús Alvarez-Cubero, Diego De Miguel Pérez, Alba Rodríguez-Martínez, Lucas Gonzalez-Herrera, Inmaculada Robles-Fernandez, José Exposito Hernandez, Jose Luis García Puche, and José Antonio Lorente

Abstract This chapter focuses on a deep description of the epidermal growth factor receptor (EGFR) expression in circulating tumor cells (CTCs) and its main role in cancer progression, genetic changes related to metastasis, and resistance to treatment. The aberrant behavior of cancer cells is caused by genetic mutations and altered patterns of gene expression. These changes can be responsible for an increase in cell motility but also an ability of CTCs to survival in different microenvironments, as well as developing therapy-resistant clones. Finally, CTCs can acquire the ability to invade distant organs, where metastatic foci can develop.

Keywords Circulating tumor cells (CTCs) • Dormancy • Epidermal growth factor receptor (EGFR) • Epithelial mesenchymal transition (EMT) • Invasion • Mutations • Migration • Resistant clones

---

M.J. Serrano (✉)
GENYO. Centre for Genomics and Oncological Research, Pfizer/University of Granada/Andalusian Regional Government, PTS Granada Av. Ilustration, 114, 18016 Granada, Spain

Integral Oncology Division, Clinical University Hospital, Av. Dr. Olóriz 16, 18012 Granada, Spain
e-mail: mjose.serrano@genyo.es

M.J. Alvarez-Cubero • I. Robles-Fernandez • J.L.G. Puche
GENYO. Centre for Genomics and Oncological Research, Pfizer/University of Granada/Andalusian Regional Government, PTS Granada Av. Ilustration, 114, 18016 Granada, Spain

D. De Miguel Pérez • A. Rodríguez-Martínez • L. Gonzalez-Herrera • J.A. Lorente
GENYO. Centre for Genomics and Oncological Research, Pfizer/University of Granada/Andalusian Regional Government, PTS Granada Av. Ilustration, 114, 18016 Granada, Spain

Faculty of Medicine, Department of Forensic Medicine, University of Granada, Av. de la Investigación, 18071 Granada, Spain

J.E. Hernandez
Integral Oncology Division, Clinical University Hospital, Av. Dr. Olóriz 16, 18012 Granada, Spain

M.J.M. Magbanua, J.W. Park (eds.), *Isolation and Molecular Characterization of Circulating Tumor Cells*, Advances in Experimental Medicine and Biology 994,
DOI 10.1007/978-3-319-55947-6_16

16.1 Introduction

The metastatic paradigm defines "metastasis" as the process that involves the release of tumor cells from a primary tumor to other target organs with no direct anatomical relationship with this primary site, where it can grow and develop a new tumor focus (Valastyan and Weinberg 2011; Gupta and Massagué 2006). For the development of this process, the circulation of tumor cells through blood or the lymph system is necessary.

Metastasis is a multiple-step process in which: cells shed from primary tumor, invade the local tissue, enter into blood or lymphatic vessels (a process known as 'intravasation'), and are passively transported to the secondary site where the cells relapse from vessels (a process known as 'extravasation') and enter into tissue (details in Fig. 16.1) (Fidler 2003; Kim et al. 2009). A fundamental step in the metastatic cascade is the dissemination tumor cell phase; where tumor cells acquire the capacity to circulate through the bloodstream and colonize different organs to develop a metastasis (Pantel and Brakenhoffn 2004). These tumor cells with the ability to circulate through the bloodstream are referred as circulating tumor cells (CTCs). Circulating tumor cells are hypothesized to be the origin of incurable metastatic disease, and are an active area of cancer research (Massard and Fizazi 2011). The first observation of tumor cells in blood was made by Thomas Ashworth in 1869 (Ashworth 1869), and as technology advanced, it became possible to detect the presence of CTCs in lower concentrations (Panteleakou et al. 2009; Sleijfer et al. 2007).

In recent years, studies have tried to analyze the complex biology of these CTCs, which involves numerous genetic and phenotypic changes (Alix-Panabières and Pantel 2014). In fact, CTCs undergo substantial changes associated with invasiveness, motility, and survival in hostile microenvironments, such as peripheral blood. Furthermore, the acquisition of these biological properties involves the activation of several genes for differentiation, activation of anti-apoptotic mechanisms, dormancy activation mechanism, or phenotypic changes such as cellular characteristics alterations from epithelial to mesenchymal cellular profiles (Epithelial-Mesenchymal-Transition) (Pantel and Speicher 2016).

The regulation of these mechanisms depends on the different signaling pathways involving cytokines or growth factors (Geho et al. 2005). Growth factors mediate diverse biological responses (regulation, differentiation, migration and cellular survival) by binding to activate cell surface receptors, named receptor tyrosine kinases (RTKs), with intrinsic protein kinase activity. The ErbB receptor family of RTKs comprises four distinct receptors: the EGFR (also known as ErbB1/HER1), ErbB2 (neu, HER2), ErbB3 (HER3) and ErbB4 (HER4). ErbB family members are often overexpressed, amplified, or mutated in many forms of cancer, making them important therapeutic targets.

In summary, the success of metastasis depends on the ability of CTCs to adapt to new microenvironments and new homing, through the activation of specific genetic

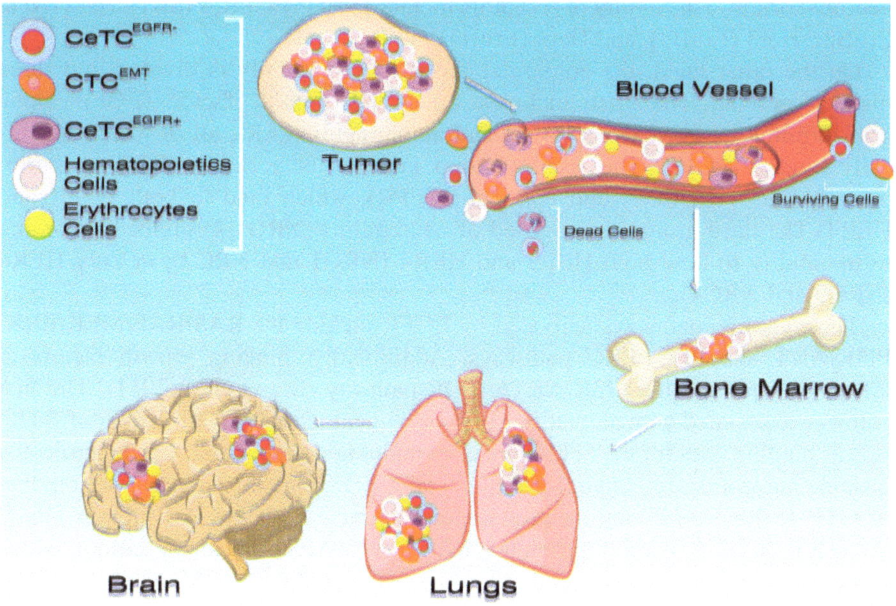

Fig. 16.1 CTC subpopulations according with the EGFR expression and acquisition of EMT phenotype. EGFR overexpression can enhance the ability of tumor cells to invade locally, the enhancement of intravasation could be due to the enhanced ability to approach the blood vessel, or to cross the blood vessel barrier

pathways. These pathways are associated with survival, competence to colonize, and proliferation in distant organs (Baccelli et al. 2013; Hodgkinson et al. 2014).

Furthermore, these biological changes adopted by CTCs, have methodological and clinical consequences. From the methodological point of view, their isolation and detection involves the use of multiple markers, since multi-CTC subpopulations can be present (Toom et al. 2016). From the clinical point of view, it implicates an increase in the probability of developing treatment failure, due to the existence of multiple subpopulations with different phenotypes, increasing the risk of disease relapse (Fig. 16.1) (Wang et al. 2016; Aparicio et al. 2015).

16.2 Methodology: EGFR and Its Role in the Dissemination Process

16.2.1 EGFR Biology

It is known that the epidermal growth factor receptor family is ubiquitously expressed in various cell types including those of epithelial, mesenchymal and neuronal origin. This family of receptors includes Her1 (EGFR, ErbB1), Her2 (Neu, ErbB2), Her3 (ErbB3), and Her4 (ErbB4).

On the other hand, the epidermal growth factor family is divided into three distinct groups. The first includes epidermal growth factor (EGF), alpha transforming growth factor (TGFα) and amphiregulin (AR), all of which specifically bind to EGFR. The second group includes betacellulin (BTC), heparin-binding EGF (HB-EGF) and epiregulin (EPR), which bind to both EGFR and HER4. The third group is composed of neuregulins (NRG1-4) divided according to the ability to bind both HER3 and HER4 (NRG1 and NRG2); or only HER4 (NRG3 and NRG4).

The signaling pathways activated by EGFR include the RAS/RAF/MEK/ERK, PI3K/AKT and PLCγ/PKC pathways. Additionally, binding growth factors to RTKs also initiates the PI3K/AKT/mTOR pathway (Brand et al. 2011). The first pathway associated with activation, and subsequent autophosphorylation, of RTKs acts as binding sites for the SH2-domain-containing protein Grb2. Grb2 recruits the guanine nucleotide exchange factor SOS via its SH3 domain, and promotes binding of GTP to Ras. GTP-binding protein Ras interacts with the Raf protein kinase (MAPK). RAF activation promotes ERK1/2 (MAPK) phosphorylation, which involves the activation of several other kinases, including MNK1, MNK2, MSK1, MSK2, and RSK. MAPK also involves the activation of several transcription factors like Elk-1, peroxisome-proliferator-activated receptor γ (PPARγ), signal transducer and activator of transcription 1 and 3 (STAT1 and STAT3), C-myc and AP-1 (Plotnikov et al. 2011). The activation of these transcription factors increases the expression of genes involved in cellular proliferation.

The second important pathway involves the activation of PI3K/AKT/mTOR pathway by growth factor binding to RTKs. The protein kinase C (PKC) pathway plays an important role in activating growth factor receptors (Brand et al. 2011; Plotnikov et al. 2011). After EGFR activation, phospholipase C (PLC) interacts with phospho-tyrosine sites on EGFR via its SH2 domain. This leads to the specific phosphorylation of PLC and dissociation from EGFR. Activated PLC in turn to interact with plasma membrane, most likely mediated by PIP_3 via a PH domain, where it cleaves PIP_2 to inositol triphosphate (IP_3) and diacyglycerol (DAG). IP_3 can diffuse into cytosol and bind IP_3 receptors on the endoplasmic reticulum (ER) to induce calcium influx into the cell from the ER. DAG remains in the membrane where it can activate PKC via conformational change that removes the pseudosubstrate region from the catalytic active site. Activated PKC (a potent serine/threonine kinase) is capable of phosphorylating a plethora of substrates leading to complex cellular processes including proliferation, apoptosis, cell survival, and cell migration.

16.2.2 Modulating Role of EGFR in Circulating Tumor Cells Migration and Invasion

Active migration of cancer cells from primary tumor via lymphatic or blood vessel routes is an indispensable prerequisite for metastasis formation. Regulation of cancer cell migration processes is dependent on many different signaling pathways, as well as, their interaction with extracellular matrix components. Cytokines and growth factors, which regulate kinases receptors and their associated receptors, play an important role in cancer cell migration (Lemmon and Schlessinger 2010). Indeed, ErbB family receptor tyrosine kinases includes EGFR, ErbB2, ErbB3, and ErbB4. Recently, EGFR/ErbB signaling has been involved in the initiation of the EMT process and cancer cell migration.

EGF was discovered in 1960, and was shown to be a polypeptide able to stimulate growth and cell differentiation (Cohen 1983). Further studies showed that EGF is able to bind with a high affinity to a specific receptor located in the cell membrane, and is able to stimulate intrinsic kinase activities (Wieduwilt and Moasser 2008).

Cancer cell migration and invasion allows tumor cells spread into peripheral blood to circulate and invade surrounding tissues. Cell migration is a highly coordinated process involving precise regulation of cell adhesion and loss of adherence to extracellular matrix (ECM). Currently, the study of CTCs as the origin of new metastases, and as an important hallmark of poor prognosis is ongoing (Friedl and Wolf 2003). In this context, EGF induces signaling that is often associated with tumor invasion (Lindsey and Langhans 2015; Lu et al. 2001). Futhermore, EGFR overexpression has been found in lung, colon, breast, prostate, brain, head and neck, thyroid, ovarian, or renal carcinoma and associated with a higher incidence of distant metastases and poor prognosis (De Luca et al. 2008; Giltnane et al. 2009).

16.2.3 Influence of EGFR in the Migration of CTCs Through the EMT Process

Metastasis is an extremely complex process which involves a series of biological events, ranging from departure of metastatic cells (detachment and migration), invasion through base membrane, intravasation into the blood vessel, survival during circulation, extravasation from the blood stream, and finally proliferation at a secondary site.

Under normal circumstances, cells will undergo apoptosis (programmed cell death) when detached from its original tissue, a phenomenon referred as anoikis. However, in the case of CTCs this process can be evaded. One of the biological cell processes involved in the acquisition of anoikis evasion is EMT, characterized mainly by the transformation of highly differentiated, polarized, and organized epithelial cells into undifferentiated, isolated and mesenchymal-like cells with migratory and invasive properties. Interestingly, EGFR signaling has also been associated to tumor cell proliferation, motility, survival and metastasis, and it is known to be overexpressed in breast cancer (BC), especially in triple negative BC types (Ueno and Zhang 2011; Serrano et al. 2014). It has been demonstrated that EGFR inhibition suppresses EMT and consequently decreases cell migration and invasion ability (Chang et al. 2012).

In fact, the EMT process means a distinct change in the expression profile, characterized by downregulation of epithelial markers and upregulation of mesenchymal markers (Vimentin) and transcription factors (Snail family) (Serrano et al. 2014). In this context, several molecular mechanisms have been identified as EMT inducers in cancer cells, and growth factors, such as EGF, have been deemed responsible for triggering signaling cascades through their related receptors.

Along the acquisition of a mesenchymal phenotype, transcriptional repression of epithelial markers such as E-cadherin can be observed, and it is accepted that the lack of E-cadherin expression is associated with the acquisition of a motile phenotype. However, C. Holz et al. observed E-cadherin expression during the EMT process in head and neck cancer cells lines (Holz et al. 2011). According to their results, the lack of E-cadherin was not necessary to acquire the motile phenotype, so they observed the E-cadherin expression in tumor cells with migratory activity induced by EGFR activation. Nevertheless, they detected an internalization of E-cadherin from cell to cell junction to perinuclear region. Therefore, the ability of migration and invasion of these tumor cells involves the disruption of cell-to-cell contacts, which is mediated by surface expression of E-cadherin. Taken together, the data suggested EGFR activation promotes cell migration and invasion by inducing EMT-like phenotypic change (Zuo et al. 2011).

In fact, EGFR overexpression is showed to affect *in vivo* invasiveness, intravasation, and metastasis without affecting primary tumor growth (Xue et al. 2006). Intravasation is usually measured as the number of CTCs in the blood or lymphatic vessel. Since EGFR overexpression can facilitate the ability of tumor cells to invade locally, increased intravasation could be due to enhanced ability of CTCs to approach blood vessels, or to cross the blood vessel barrier (Fig. 16.1). Comparison of studies on EGFR inhibitors to ErbB2 inhibitors suggests that EGFR signaling may be more important for the approach to the vessel, whereas ErbB2 signaling could be involved in the intravasation process (Kedrin et al. 2009). According to this hypothesis, EGFR is associated with the regulation of development and the maintenance of vascular architecture for sustaining cancer cell intravasation (De Luca et al. 2008). In a recent study by Minder et al. (2015), they demonstrated new mechanisms involving EGFR in cell dissemination, through the development of intravasation-sustaining vasculature within primary tumor. EGFR-mediated induction and maintenance of intratumoral angiogenic vessels allow the activation of powerful regulators of vascular permeability like IL-8, MMP-9 and VEGF to CTCs (Minder et al. 2015).

In line with the hypothesis that EGF family members play a fundamental role in the migration and survival of tumor cells, EGFR has been involved in the initial steps of EMT. Molecular mechanism of EGFR leading to EMT process activation, involves down-regulation of caveolin-1 which leads to a loss of E-cadherin, transcriptional activation of β-catenin, and enhanced invasiveness (Lu et al. 2003). Decreased E-cadherin levels involve an increase of N-cadherin, vimentin, and SNAIL or Twist expression. N-cadherin is a cell-to-cell adhesion molecule that plays a role in cancer metastasis. In this way, N-cadherin upregulation in malignant cells was shown to enhance cell motility, invasion and metastasis. N-cadherin adhesion can lead to phosphatidylinositol 3-kinase (PI3K)-mediated activation of AKT and activated AKT signaling can stimulate β-catenin signaling (Zhang et al. 2013). The mechanism of activation the P13K/Akt signaling pathway remains controversial. Some studies showed that the direct activation of PI3K/Akt signaling pathway by the RhoA signaling pathway, can also affect EGF expression and induce the intracellular localization of EGFR. This action in turn activates PI3K/Akt signaling pathway (Xu et al. 2015). AKT activation regulates Twist phosphorylation, promotes TGF-β2 transcription, and activates TGF-β receptors. The activation of the latter can induce excessive PI3K/Akt signaling pathway activity, which further provides positive feedback for EMT induction. In this line, a decrease of ERK expression has been correlated to cell motility increase dependent on EGFR, simultaneously with an elevation of EGF-induced Akt activity (Huang et al. 2003).

In conclusion, EGFR-mediated signaling causing motility in CTCs can be seen through the activation of different genetic pathways, including TGF-β, SNAIL or AKT. In addition, the roles of divergent signaling pathways in trafficking EGFR regulation may enable the development of more effective therapies.

16.2.4 Role of EGFR in the Dormancy Process

Cancer patients can develop metastatic disease years to decades after diagnosis. This process can be explained through the existence of micrometastasis composed of disseminated tumor cells (DTCs) with the ability to acquire a non-proliferative status. This non-proliferative status is similar to a dormancy phenotype (Sosa et al. 2014).

Dormancy is a stage of cancer progression in which asymptomatic residual disease is present but clinically undetectable and resistant to conventional chemotherapy (Klein 2011). Dormant tumor cells are generally considered to be growth arrested, although there are some debates about whether micrometastatic disease sites exist as a balance between proliferation and death only appearing as an arrested state.

The mechanisms involved in the dormancy process are complex and poorly understood. Among the different pathways associated with this process are specially important those associated with EGFR (Humtsoe and Kramer 2010). In this line, reduced PI3K–AKT signaling has been linked to dormancy-like phenotypes (Sosa et al. 2014). In fact, under stressful conditions, like metabolic stress, cancer cells secrete factors that inhibit PI3K pathway, resulting in quiescence and autophagy induction (Jo et al. 2008). In tumor cell spheroids, loss of adhesion and nutrient deprivation promotes short-term growth arrest. This arrest is linked to epidermal growth factor receptor (EGFR)-Y1086 autophosphorylation, which inhibits AKT activation and cyclin D1 induction (Garay et al. 2015). In the study of Shen and Kramer (2004), it was demonstrated that EGFR-mediated survival effects were primarily through activation of ERK, not AKT. EGFR can trigger PI3K mediated AKT activation. Despite activated EGFR, phospho-AKT was not detected. These results, may represent an example of context-dependent EGFR-mediated PI3K/AKT signaling. Defining the underlying cellular events involved here may provide insights on the mechanism by which EGFR modulates tumor cell survival and growth, in the adverse and dynamic microenvironment encountered during tumor progression.

Cellular tumor dormancy may result from the ability of tumor cells to attain a differentiated state. Their growth and aberrant organization is dependent on β1-integrins and EGF signaling, as inhibition of these signals leads to the re-differentiation of these tumor cells into non-proliferating state (Aguirre-Ghiso 2007). Blocking of β1-integrin signaling in these tumor cells *in vivo* ablates tumor growth, but it is not clear whether this is due to induction of a protracted state of growth arrest.

An example of switch between proliferation and growth arrest controlled by tumor cell–microenvironment crosstalk was observed in head and neck carcinomas. In this model, the metastasis-associated urokinase receptor (uPAR) drives tumor growth by interacting and activating α5β1 integrin (Aguirre-Ghiso et al. 1999). This complex in turn recruits focal adhesion kinase (FAK) and EGFR, which propagates mitogenic signals through the Ras–extra-cellular signal-regulated kinase (ERK) pathway. Blocking uPAR, β1-integrins, FAK or EGFR, singly or in combination with each other, resulted in tumor suppression *in vivo*, which is due to induction of dormancy (Aguirre-Ghiso et al. 1999). In these studies, although dormant tumor cells expressed the appropriate integrins and were surrounded by fibronectin, the downregulation of uPAR and loss of integrin function prevented these cells from transducing proliferative signals from the fibronectin-rich microenvironment (Aguirre-Ghiso et al. 2001).

The disruption of the uPAR complex activates the p38 mitogen-activated protein kinase (MAPK) signaling pathway (Koul et al. 2013). Furthermore, growing metastatic lesions show sustained ERK activity but greatly reduced p38 signaling, suggesting that proliferation in primary and secondary tumors requires a high ERK/p38 signaling ratio whereas the opposite ratio, induces cellular dormancy.

On the other hand, Ossowski et al. established a model of tumor dormancy in human squamous carcinoma (HEp3) (Aguirre-Ghiso et al. 2001). They detected that *in vivo* HEp3 remain tumorigenic (T-HEp3) and metastatic. However, the prolonged *in vitro* passaging of these cells, results in the acquisition of a dormant (D-HEp3) phenotype upon re-inoculation *in vivo*. These studies have revealed that HEp3 cells maintain a tumorigenic and metastatic phenotype by overexpressing the uPAR, which in turn signals through a complex comprising of α 5β1-integrin and

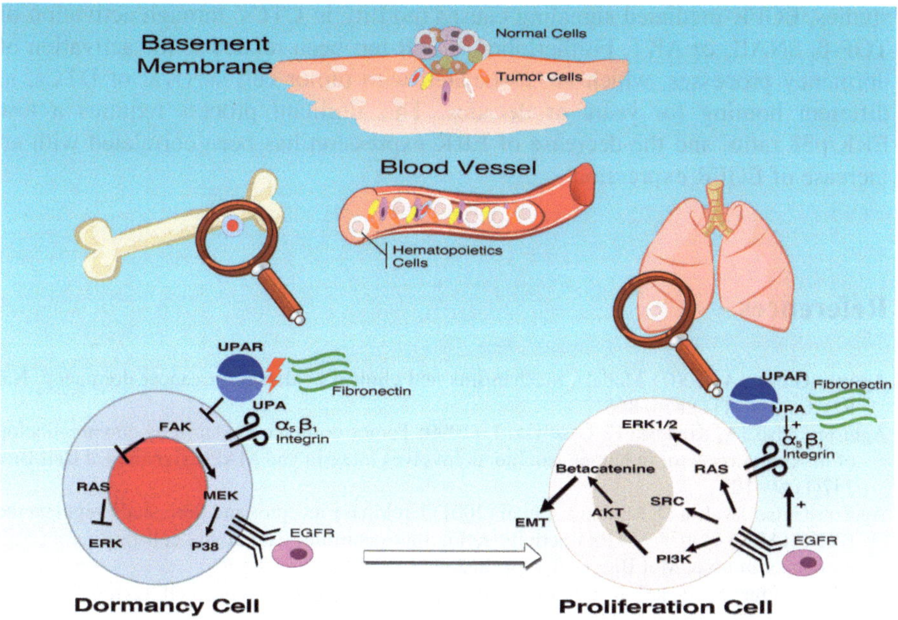

Fig. 16.2 uPAR role in the regulation of the balance between tumor cells proliferation and tumor dormancy. Downregulation or blocking of uPAR, beta1integrin, FAK or EGFR, alone or in combination causes activation of p38/MAPK pathway resulting in a cell cycle arrest and dormancy. However, if uPAR interacts and activates the fibronectin receptor alpha5b1 integrin, this receptor α5β1 Integrin causes the cell cycle arrest and dormancy. uPAR –α5β1 Integrin complex recruits focal adhesion kinase (FAK) and EGFR, and promotes mitogenic signals through the ERK pathway

EGFR. Signaling from the uPAR-integrin-EGFR complex culminates in the activation of ERK mitogenic pathway and the inhibition of p38 stress activated/growth suppressive pathway. Such cells have high ERK/p38 ratio that favors tumorigenesis. Forced or nonclonal spontaneous loss of the uPAR – α5β1- EGFR signaling complex results in p38 activation and in a low ERK/p38 ratio (Fig. 16.2) (Ranganathan et al. 2006).

16.3 Conclusion

The biological and functional framework of tumor metastasis involves a complex network of interaction between tumor cells and their microenvironment. Once the tumor cell acquires the ability to migrate, the success of the metastatic process depends on the ability of the CTC to survive in the different microenvironments they encounter. Numerous studies have shown EGFR involvement in migration and survival of CTCs, through EMT associated pathway activation. According to these studies, EGFR-mediated signaling causes motility in CTCs, through activation of TGF-β, SNAIL or AKT. Furthermore, EGFR has been related to the activation of dormancy processes, which are associated with tumor cell survival of DTCs, in different homing for years or decades. This dormant process requires a low ERK/p38 ratio, and the decrease of ERK expression has been correlated with an increase of EGFR expression.

References

Aguirre-Ghiso JA (2007) Models, mechanisms and clinical evidence for cancer dormancy. Nat Rev Cancer 7(11):834–846

Aguirre-Ghiso JA, Kovalski K, Ossowski L (1999) Tumor dormancy induced by downregulation of urokinase receptor in human carcinoma involves integrin and MAPK signaling. J Cell Biol 147(1):89–103

Aguirre-Ghiso JA, Liu D, Mignatti A et al (2001) Urokinase receptor and fibronectin regulate the ERK(MAPK) to p38(MAPK) activity ratios that determine carcinoma cell proliferation or dormancy in vivo. Mol Biol Cell 12(4):863–879

Alix-Panabières C, Pantel K (2014) Challenges in circulating tumour cell research. Nature reviews. Cancer 14(9):623–631

Aparicio LA, Blanco M, Castosa R et al (2015) Clinical implications of epithelial cell plasticity in cancer progression. Cancer Lett 366(1):1–10

Asworth T (1869) A case of cancer in which cells similar to those in the tumors were seen in the blood after death. Aust Med J 14:146–149

Baccelli I, Schneeweiss A, Riethdorf S et al (2013) Identification of a population of blood circulating tumor cells from breast cancer patients that initiates metastasis in a xenograft assay. Nat Biotechnol 31(6):539–544

Brand TM, Iida M, Wheeler DL (2011) Molecular mechanisms of resistance to the EGFR monoclonal antibody cetuximab. Cancer Biol Ther 11(9):777–792

Chang ZG, Wei JM, Qin CF et al (2012) Suppression of the epidermal growth factor receptor inhibits epithelial-mesenchymal transition in human pancreatic cancer PANC-1 cells. Dig Dis Sci 57(5):1181–1189

Cohen S (1983) The epidermal growth factor (EGF). Cancer 51:1787–1791

De Luca A, Carotenuto A, Rachiglio A et al (2008) The role of the EGFR signaling in tumor microenvironment. J Cell Physiol 214(3):559–567

Fidler IJ (2003) The pathogenesis of cancer metastasis: the "seed and soil" hypothesis revisited. Nat Rev Cancer 3(6):453–458

Friedl P, Wolf K (2003) Tumour-cell invasion and migration: diversity and escape mechanisms. Nature reviews. Cancer 3(5):362–374

Garay C, Judge G, Lucarelli S et al (2015) Epidermal growth factor-stimulated Akt phosphorylation requires clathrin or ErbB2 but not receptor endocytosis. Mol Biol Cell 26(19):3504–3519

Geho DH, Bandle RW, Clair T et al (2005) Physiological mechanisms of tumor-cell invasion and migration. Physiology (Bethesda, Md.) 20:194–200

Giltnane JM, Moeder CB, Camp RL et al (2009) Quantitative multiplexed analysis of ErbB family coexpression for primary breast cancer prognosis in a large retrospective cohort. Cancer 115(11):2400–2409

Gupta GP, Massagué J (2006) Cancer metastasis: building a framework. Cell 127(4):679–695

Hodgkinson CL, Morrow CJ, Li Y et al (2014) Tumorigenicity and genetic profiling of circulating tumor cells in small-cell lung cancer. Nat Med 20(8):897–903

Holz C, Niehr F, Boyko M et al (2011) Epithelial-mesenchymal-transition induced by EGFR activation interferes with cell migration and response to irradiation and cetuximab in head and neck cancer cells. Radiother Oncol 101(1):158–164

Huang Y, Kim SO, Jiang J et al (2003) Growth hormone-induced phosphorylation of epidermal growth factor (EGF) receptor in 3T3-F442A cells: modulation of EGF-induced trafficking and signaling. J Biol Chem 278(21):18902–18913

Humtsoe JO, Kramer RH (2010) Differential epidermal growth factor receptor signaling regulates anchorage-independent growth by modulation of the PI3K/AKT pathway. Oncogene 29(8):1214–1226

Jo H, Jia Y, Subramanian KK et al (2008) Cancer cell-derived clusterin modulates the phosphatidylinositol 3′-kinase-Akt pathway through attenuation of insulin-like growth factor 1 during serum deprivation. Mol Cell Biol 28(13):4285–4299

Kedrin D, Wyckoff J, Boimel PJ et al (2009) ERBB1 and ERBB2 have distinct functions in tumor cell invasion and intravasation. Clin Cancer Res 15(11):3733–3739

Kim MY, Oskarsson T, Acharyya S et al (2009) Tumor self-seeding by circulating cancer cells. Cell 139(7):1315–1326

Klein CA (2011) Framework models of tumor dormancy from patient-derived observations. Curr Opin in Genet Dev 21(1):42–49

Koul HK, Pal M, Koul S (2013) Role of p38 MAP kinase signal transduction in solid tumors. Genes Cancer 4(9–10):342–359

Lemmon MA, Schlessinger J (2010) Cell signaling by receptor tyrosine kinases. Cell 141(7):1117–1134

Lindsey S, Langhans SA (2015) Epidermal growth factor signaling in transformed cells. Int Rev Cell Mol Biol 314:1–41

Lu Z, Jiang G, Blume-Jensen P et al (2001) Epidermal growth factor-induced tumor cell invasion and metastasis initiated by dephosphorylation and downregulation of focal adhesion kinase. Mol Cell Biol 21(12):4016–4031

Lu Z, Ghosh S, Wang Z et al (2003) Downregulation of caveolin-1 function by EGF leads to the loss of E-cadherin, increased transcriptional activity of B-catenin, and enhanced tumor cell invasion. Cancer Cell 4(6):499–515

Massard C, Fizazi K (2011) Targeting continued androgen receptor signaling in prostate cancer. Clin Cancer Res 17(12):3876–3883

Minder P, Zajac E, Quigley JP (2015) EGFR regulates the development and microarchitecture of intratumoral angiogenic vasculature capable of sustaining cancer cell intravasation. Neoplasia 17(8):634–649

Pantel K, Brakenhoffn RH (2004) Dissecting the metastatic cascade. Nat Rev Cancer 4(6):448–456

Pantel K, Speicher MR (2016) The biology of circulating tumor cells. Oncogene 35(10):1216–1224

Panteleakou Z, Lembessis P, Sourla A et al (2009) Detection of circulating tumor cells in prostate cancer patients: methodological pitfalls and clinical relevance. Mol Med 15:101–114

Plotnikov A, Zehorai E, Procaccia S et al (2011) The MAPK cascades: signaling components, nuclear roles and mechanisms of nuclear translocation. Biochim Biophys Acta, Mol Cell Res 1813(9):1619–1633

Ranganathan AC, Adam AP, Zhang L et al (2006) Tumor cell dormancy induced by p38SAPK and ER-stress signaling: an adaptive advantage for metastatic cells? Cancer Biol Ther 5(7):729–735

Serrano MJ, Ortega FG, Alvarez-Cubero MJ et al (2014) EMT and EGFR in CTCs cytokeratin negative non-metastatic breast cancer. Oncotarget 5(17):7486–7497

Shen X, Kramer RH (2004) Adhesion-mediated squamous cell carcinoma survival through ligand-independent activation of epidermal growth factor receptor. Am J Pathol 165(4):1315–1329

Sleijfer S, Gratama JW, Sieuwerts AM et al (2007) Circulating tumour cell detection on its way to routine diagnostic implementation? Eur J Cancer 43(18):2645–2650

Sosa MS, Bragado P, Aguirre-Ghiso JA (2014) Mechanisms of disseminated cancer cell dormancy: an awakening field. Nat Rev Cancer 14(9):611–622

Ueno NT, Zhang D (2011) Targeting EGFR in triple negative breast cancer. J Cancer 2(1):324–328

Valastyan S, Weinberg RA (2011) Tumor metastasis: molecular insights and evolving paradigms. Cell 147(2):275–292

van der Toom EE, Verdone JE, Gorin MA et al (2016) Technical challenges in the isolation and analysis of circulating tumor cells. Oncotarget 7(38):62754–62766

Wang H, Stoecklein NH, Lin PP et al (2016) Circulating and disseminated tumor cells: diagnostic tools and therapeutic targets in motion. Oncotarget. doi:10.18632/oncotarget.12242

Wieduwilt MJ, Moasser MM (2008) The epidermal growth factor receptor family: biology driving targeted therapeutics. Cell Mol Life Sci 65(10):1566–1584

Xu W, Yang Z, Lu N (2015) A new role for the PI3K/Akt signaling pathway in the epithelial-mesenchymal transition. Cell Adhes Migr 9(4):317–324

Xue C, Wyckoff J, Liang F et al (2006) Epidermal growth factor receptor overexpression results in increased tumor cell motility in vivo coordinately with enhanced intravasation and metastasis. Cancer Res 66(1):192–197

Zhang J, Wyckoff J, Liang F et al (2013) AKT activation by N-cadherin regulates beta-catenin signaling and neuronal differentiation during cortical development. Neural Dev 8(1):7

Zuo JH, Zhu W, Li MY et al (2011) Activation of EGFR promotes squamous carcinoma SCC10A cell migration and invasion via inducing EMT-like phenotype change and MMP-9-mediated degradation of E-cadherin. J Cell Biochem 112(9):2508–2517

Index

M.J.M. Magbanua, J.W. Park (eds.), *Isolation and Molecular Characterization of Circulating Tumor Cells*, Advances in Experimental Medicine and Biology 994,
DOI 10.1007/978-3-319-55947-6